POINTERS
TO THE
COMMON REMEDIES

POINTERS
TO THE
COMMON REMEDIES

DR. M. L. TYLER
(M.D., Brux.; L.R.C.P., L.R.C.S., Edin.; L.R.F.P.S., Glas.)

B. Jain Publishers Pvt. Ltd.

Export Edition

Price : Rs. 55.00

Reprint Edition 1995

Publish by :
B. Jain Publishers Pvt. LTD.
7, Wazir Pur Printing Press Complex,
Ring Road, Delhi-110 052 (INDIA)

Printed in India by :
J.J. Offset Printers
7, Wazirpur, Delhi-110 052

ISBN 81–7021–036–4

BOOK CODE B-2527

CONTENTS

ON PRESCRIBING

MANY drugs have produced the symptoms of, and can therefore cure the common cold : but alas ! only the one that has evoked the exact conditions of the individual patient will CURE that patient : i.e. not merely palliate while he recovers, but CURE.

Why ? Because there is Law behind cure ; and if we desire to evoke Power, we must conform to its conditions. The only known Law of Healing is Hahnemann's *similia similibus curentur*. In acute work, if you can get exact correspondence between the symptoms of the patient and the symptoms evoked in healthy persons by some drug, it is a mathematical certainty that you will cure—*because of the Law of Similars*. If you do not get the correspondence it is equally certain that you will NOT cure—*because of the Law of Similars*. Law does not fail. It is we who fail in our attempts to put it in action. We may do bad work and call it Homœopathy, discrediting it in the patient's eyes and in our own : only it did not happen to *be* Homœopathy ! When an aeroplane crashes no one says, " The laws of gravitation—motion—physics—have failed in *this* case ! " —the fault is sought in faulty adaptation. Law is inexorable.

At times the question of an epidemic has to be reckoned with, Hahnemann says that by taking the symptoms of a number of cases you can select a drug that covers the lot, and cure, practically, every case of THAT epidemic. We have all found that the medicine that was so widely curative one year, was useless the next. One has often heard, " This is a *Bryonia* year ! " " *Mercurius* is curing all the colds just now. . . ." Then, wind and weather change, and another set of remedies *for another set of patients* crops up.

If the blighting influence that bowled over people of a certain temperament was a cold, *dry*, East wind, such drugs as *Aconite, Bryonia, Hepar, Nux* will suggest themselves. Whereas a sudden cold *wet* spell would play havoc with the people who cannot stand *cold wet* conditions, and here *Dulcamara, Natrum sulph.*, or *Rhus* would come up for consideration. Why is it that good prescribers will find that they are suddenly getting quite a number of *Lycopodium* cases ? It is not that they are framing their questions to lead up to that drug, but because conditions—perhaps social—economic—or even meteoric are putting a severe strain on persons of the *Lycopodium* make-up.

Among the remedies of the Common Cold, then, some suit the illness brought on by dry cold, some by damp cold, some even by warm wet. The affected mucous membranes may be dry—or they may pour. Relief may come in cold, open air, or there may be utter intolerance of cold air, of open air, of draughts, of uncovering, and so on. Without precision, results are poor.

COMMON REMEDIES OF THE COMMON COLD*

Camphor — A person who has been chilled, and cannot get warm. For the cold stage, before catarrhal symptoms have ultimated, to prevent.

A couple of drops of *Camphor* (strong tincture) on a lump of sugar, repeat till warm.

BUT " as *Camphor* antidotes most of our drugs, the *Camphor* bottle should be put away in the other end of the house." *Kent.*

Aconite .. Sudden onset from exposure to COLD ; TO COLD DRY WINDS.

NOSE. Coryza dry, with headache, roaring in ears, fever, thirst, sleeplessness.

Checked coryza, better open air, worse talking.

Fluent coryza, frequent sneezing ; dropping of a clear hot water : fluent mornings.

THROAT. Acute inflammation of the throat with high fever, dark redness of the parts, burning and stinging in fauces.

Larynx sensitive to touch and inspired air, as if denuded.

Laryngitis with inflammatory fever ; also with suffocative spasms (spasm of glottis).

CROUP : child in agony, tosses about : dry short cough, not much wheezing . . .

After exposure to dry, cold winds.

CHEST. Tightness and oppression. Stitches when breathing.

Cough clear ringing and whistling, caused by burning, pricking in larynx and trachea.

Cough hoarse, dry, loud: spasmodic. Breath hot.

Cough wakes him from sleep, is dry, croupy, suffocating : *Great anxiety.*

Sputum absent—scanty : bloody or blood-streaked : bright red blood.

Early stages of pneumonia, bronchitis, croup.

Aconite is RESTLESS, ANXIOUS, FRIGHTENED : Onset sudden. Worse at night.

* *These drugs are arranged, more or less, for acuteness, and for comparison.*

Allium cepa .. Coryza, streaming eyes and nose, with headache; frequent sneezing, profuse *acrid* discharge from nose, corroding lip and nose.

Lachrymation also profuse, but *bland* (reverse of *Euphrasia*).

Hot and thirsty: worse evenings: indoors: warm room. Better open air.

Violent catarrhal laryngitis. Tickling in larynx.

Cough seems to split and tear larynx: grasps larynx, feels as if cough will tear it.

Cough from inhaling cold air.

Belladonna .. Suppressed catarrh with maddening headache.

Throat raw and sore: very red and shining

Hoarseness with painful dryness of larynx.

As if larynx inflamed and swollen, with snoring breathing and danger of suffocation.

Acute catarrhal laryngitis.

Cough with red, injected throat.

Dry, tearing cough, which scrapes throat.

Belladonna is red, and hot, and dry.

Bryonia .. Often begins in the nose, sneezing, coryza, running at nose, lachrymation, aching eyes, nose and head the first day. then trouble goes down to posterior nares, throat, larynx, with hoarseness, and a bronchitis comes on: may end in pleurisy and pneumonia.

Trouble travels down from the beginning of respiratory tract. (Reverse of *Lyc.*)

Dry, spasmodic cough, worse at night; after eating and drinking; on entering a warm room; on taking a deep inspiration.

Cough with *stitches in chest,* with headache as if the *head would fly to pieces.*

Cough shaking the whole body.

Stitches in chest and pleura: worse breathing and coughing.

Cough dry, hard, racking, expectoration scanty

Bryonia is irritable: thirsty for long drinks: wants to lie still and be let alone. Dryness of mucous membranes. (*Bell.*)

Lips parched and dry.

Worse cold, dry weather.

Euphrasia .. Nasal catarrh bland, with lachrymation which is excoriating (exact opposite of *Allium cepa*).

Severe fluent coryza, apt to extend down to larynx with hard cough.

Coryza worse at night; lying down: cough worse by day, and better lying down.

Hepar .. From cold, dry weather (*Acon.*, *Nux*). Catarrh of nose, ears, throat, larynx and chest.

Cold in nose, with much discharge: with *sneezing every time he goes into a cold wind*.

Sneezing and running from nose, first watery; then thick, yellow, *offensive*.

Every time he goes into *dry*, *cold wind*, gets hoarse, and coughs: worse inspiring cold air: or putting hand or foot out of bed.

Sweating all night without relief (*Merc.*).

Hypersensitive, to touch, pain, draughts, cold air. Wants to hit anybody who makes a draught in room.

Better moist, wet weather (reverse of *Gels.*).

(Farrington (only) says, *Hepar* is not indicated in the early stages of a cold; apt to stop it in the nose, while it goes down to chest: " here *Phos.* follows and cures ".)

Nux .. Colds from DRY COLD WEATHER (*Acon.*) (reverse of *Dulc.*). *Acon.* is anxious; *Nux* irritable.

Nose stuffed and dry, initial stage: throat rough as if scraped; raw, sore.

Sneezing, nose stuffed up at night and in open air.

Fluent coryza in warm room and by day.

Coldness of whole body, not better by warmth of stove, or by any amount of covering.

Chills, back, limbs, or whole body, not relieved by warmth.

Can't stir from fire.

Shivering after drinking: from slightest contact with open air; *from slightest motion.*

Chill as soon as he moves the bed clothes.

Chill alternating with heat. Heat with internal chilliness.

Nux is oversensitive: irritable; touchy; sensitive to least draught. (*Hepar.*)

Dulcamara .. Colds from COLD WET WEATHER (*Rhus*) and snow.
From getting wet, or chilled when heated.
Worse sudden changes from hot to cold.
Dry coryza, sore throat, stiff neck.
Coryza worse in open air.
More fluent in house, in warmth ; less fluent in cold air—cold room. (*Nux.*)
Starts sneezing in a cold room.
Eyes become red and sore with every cold.
Nose stuffs up when there is cold rain.
Profuse discharge of water from nose and eyes, worse in the open air.
Stiff neck : sore throat, back and limbs painful.

Mercurius sol. .. *Creeping chilliness* in the beginning of a cold.
Much sneezing, fluent discharge, *corrosive.*
Acrid, offensive matter flows from nose : greenish, fetid pus.
Nose red, swollen, shining.
Catarrhal inflammation of frontal sinuses, etc.
Hoarse voice ; dry, rough, tickling cough.
Feels bad in a warm room, yet cannot bear the cold.
Taste sweet, salty, metallic, putrid.
Creeping chilliness.
Profuse offensive sweats, and worse from sweating. (Reverse of *Nat sul.*)
Swollen, flabby tongue, tooth-notched.
Offensive breath : offensive salivation.

Gelsemium .. Catarrhs of *warm, moist, relaxing weather* (*Carbo veg.*), (reverse of *Hepar.* and *Dulc.*).
Discharge excoriating : nostrils sore.
As if red-hot water passing through nostrils.
Gels. colds " develop several days after exposure : the *Acon.* cold comes on in a few hours ".
Suits the colds and fevers of mild winters.
Teasing, tickling cough, better near the fire.
Great weight and tiredness of the whole body.
Chills up and down the back.
Headache.
(One of the greatest of 'flu medicines.)

Iodium .. Loss of smell. Nose dry and stuffed up.
Dry coryza, fluent in open air.
Severe coryza, with fever, severe headache, excessive secretion and much sneezing.
Catarrh, thin, excoriating. Hot water drops out.
The *Iodine* patient is lean and hungry and can't stand heat.

Kali iod. .. Colds from every exposure—from DAMP.
Nose red, swollen, ACRID watery discharge.
Eyes smart and lachrymate.
Catarrhal headaches with inflammation of mucous membranes of FRONTAL SINUSES, eyes, throat and chest.
Forehead heavy ; dull and stupid.
Violent sneezing, eyes bloated, profuse lachrymation. Violent acrid coryza.
Nose tender, face red. Uneasy. Tongue white.
Nasal voice ; violent thirst.
Catarrhal inflammation of frontal sinuses, antra and fauces.
Hot and dry, then, alternately drenched with sweat. Alternate heat and chill.
Heat with intermittent shuddering.

Arsenicum *Thin watery discharge from nose which excoriates upper lip : while nose is stuffed up all the time.*
" Sneezing no joke ! "—and affords no relief.
Sneezing from irritation in one spot (like a tickling feather), after sneeze, irritation as before.
Always taking colds in the nose, and sneezes from *every change of weather*.
Colds begin in the nose and go down to the chest.
Always chilly, suffers from draughts (*Hep*.).
Always freezing : hovers round fire : can't get enough clothes to keep warm. (*Nux*.)
Ars. is chilly : with *burnings, relieved by heat* :
Is restless : anxious : morbidly fastidious.
During rigors and chills feels as if blood flowing through vessels were ice-cold water : a rushing through body of ice-cold waves.
With fever, intensely hot, with feeling of boiling water going through blood vessels.

Natrum mur. .. Catarrhs watery, or thick whitish, like white of egg " raw or cooked ".
Catarrhs with abnormal quantity of secretion.
Paroxysms of sneezing.
Fluent alternating with dry catarrh.
Worse exposure to fresh air.
Watery vesicles about lips and wings of nose.
Cough with bursting headache (*Bry.*).
Hoarseness.
Urine spurts when coughing (*Caust., Scilla.*).
Nat mur. loves salt : hates fuss : weepy, but no one to see. Depressed.

Pulsatilla " One of our sheet anchors in old catarrhs with loss of smell, thick yellow discharge, and amelioration in the open air (in the nervous, timid, yielding). Discharge NOT excoriating.
Stuffing up of the nose at night and copious flow in the morning."
Fluent in open air : stopped up in house. (Reverse of *Nux.*)
Well in open air, but violent catarrh as soon as he enters a room, and in the evening.
Lips chapped and peel.
Stuffed coryza, with blowing of blood from nose.
A weepy patient : craves sympathy. Craves air : cool air ; better motion.

Rhus tox. .. From COLD DAMP weather : exposure to cold damp when perspiring. (*Dulc.*)
Violent coryza : redness and oedema of throat.
Nose stopped up with every cold.
Worse cold : better warmth.
Thick yellow offensive mucus.
Fear and restlessness at night.
Hoarseness, rawness, roughness : worse first beginning to sing or to talk : wears off after singing a few notes or talking a little while.
Thirst for cold drinks especially at night : but cold drinks bring on chilliness and cough.
Worse uncovering.
Bones ache : sneezing and coughing : worse evening and night : tickling behind upper part of sternum.

Ipecacuanha .. Simple common colds : settle in nose : blowing of blood from nose with excessive sneezing.
Bronchitis of infancy : to break it up. (Later stages *Ant. tart.*)
Colds begin in nose, spread very rapidly to chest.
Stopping of nose.
Violent chill : frame shakes and teeth chatter.
No thirst : overwhelming nausea.
NAUSEA is a guide to *Ipecac.* in most sicknesses.

Carbo veg. .. Worse *warm moist weather.*
Worse evening.
Aphonia every evening (*Phos.*).
Dry tickling cough.
Rawness larynx and pharynx.

Natrum c. .. Fluent catarrh, provoked by the least draught.
With a periodical aggravation *every other day.*
Entirely relieved by sweating. (Reverse of *Merc.*)

Phosphorus .. Frequent alternations of fluent and stopped coryza (*Nux. Puls.*).
Sore throat : head dull : Feverish.
Secretion dries to crusts which adhere tightly.
Hoarseness and bronchial catarrh.
Discharge from one nostril and stoppage of the other.
Sneezing causes pain in throat or head.
Blowing blood from nose.
Nose red, shiny, painful.
Chest tight.
Cough hard, tight, dry, racks the patient : worse open air.
Phos. colds generally begin in chest or larynx.

Kali bich. .. Catarrh with thick yellow or greenish, ropy, stringy mucous discharges, or tough and jelly-like.
Discharge offensive.
Adherent mucus. which can be drawn out into long strings
Plugs in nostrils.
Dryness nose with pressive pain at root of nose.

ESPECIALLY IN LATER STAGES OR TO CLEAR UP

Sulphur .. Subject to coryza : constant sneezing, stoppage of nose.
Fluent, like water trickling from nose.
Nasal discharges acrid and burning.
Cannot take a bath, cannot become overheated, cannot get into a cold place, cannot overexert without getting this cold in the nose.
The typical *Sulphur* patient likes fat : gets hungry about 11 a.m. : feels the heat.

Calcarea .. Lingering catarrhs ; thick yellow discharge.
Great crusts from nose.
Breathes part of night through nose, then it clogs up, and has to breathe through mouth.
Chilly : perspires much.
So sensitive to cold he finds it difficult to dress to protect himself.

Tuberculinum .. Persons with a family history of T.B.
Always catching cold.
Always tired.
Worse in warm room.

MINIATURE REPERTORY OF THESE REMEDIES OF THE COMMON COLD

Easily chilled	*Ars. Bry. Hep. Merc. Nat m. Nux. Phos. Puls.*
COLD. Worse cold air	*All c. Ars. Dulc. Hep. Nux. Phos.*
,, cold dry weather	*Acon. Bry. Hep. Nux. Caust.*
,, cold-wet	*Calc. Dulc. Rhus. Nat s.*
,, inhaling cold air	*All c. Hep. Phos. Rumex.*
,, draught	*Ars. Bell. Hep. Nat c. Nux. Sul. Dulc. Merc.*
WET. ,, wet	*Calc. Dulc. Kali iod. Merc. Rhus. Puls. Sul.*
,, warm wet	*Gels. Carbo v.*
Better warm wet	*Hep.*
Warm room. Worse	*Puls. Tub. All c. Merc. Nux* (more fluent).
,, ,, entering	*Bry.*
Open air. Worse	*Nux. Nat m. Phos. Bry. Hep.*
,, Better	*All c. Puls. Acon.* (See *Ars. Dulc.*)
Uncovering head. Worse	*Hep. Nat m.*
Much sneezing	*All c. Dulc. Hep. Ipec. Kali iod. Merc. Nat m. Phos. Rhus. Sul.*

Catarrh. Copious	*All c. Ars. Kali iod. Nat m.*
,, Fluent	*Acon. All c. Ars. Nat c. Hep. Nux.*
,, ,, in warmth	*Dulc. Sul.*
,, Fluent alt. dry	*Ars. Nat m. Nux. Phos. Puls. Sul.*
Dry coryza	*Bell. Bry. Nux.* (early), *Dulc.* (in cold air). *Kali bich.*
Nose stopped	*Nux. Dulc. Puls. Rhus. Ipec. Carbo v.*
With lachrymation	*All c. Bry. Euphr.* (acrid tears), *Kali iod.*
Discharge acrid	*All c. Ars. Gels. Kali iod. Merc. Nux. Sul.*
,, bland	*Euphr. Puls.*
,, ,, with acrid lachrymation	*Euphr.*
,, offensive	*Hep. Merc. Calc. Kali bich. Nat c. Puls.*
,, crusts	*Calc. Kali bich. Phos. Tub.*
,, greenish	*Kali bich. Kali iod. Merc. Puls.*
,, purulent	*Calc. Hep. Kali bich. Kali iod. Merc. Phos. Puls. Tub.*
,, blows out blood	*All c. Ars. Bell. Hep. Phos. Puls.*
With chilliness	*Nux. Ars. Gels. Merc. Rhus. Calc. Bry. Phos.*
,, chills	*Nux. Gels. Ipec.*
,, shivering	*Kali iod. Ipec. Bry. Nux. Rhus.*
Alternate heat and chill	*Kali iod.*
Sweating. Better from	*Nat c. Kali iod.*
,, Worse from, or not better	*Hep. Merc.*
With nausea	*Ipec. Ant tart.*
Cold travels down	*Bry. Ipec. Carbo v. Ars.* etc.
Hoarseness	*Bell. Phos.* etc.
Begins in chest and goes up	*Phos.*
Frontal sinuses affected	*Merc. Kali iod. Ars. Lyc. Sil.*
Larynx affected	*Acon. All c. Bell. Bry. Carbo v. Euphr. Hep. Merc. Nat m. Phos. Rhus.*
With pain in head from sneezing or coughing	*Bry. Nat m. Phos.*
With pain in abdomen, from sneezing or coughing	*Bry. Dros.*
With sore throat	*Merc. Nux. Phos.*

* * *

Drugs produce peculiar symptoms. Where these agree in drug and patient, the ailment is cancelled, and health results. (This is most strikingly seen in acute and uncomplicated sickness.)

When you give to a patient a remedy that can produce his symptoms, you must give it in the small dose to which his sensitive condition will respond without undue aggravation and suffering.

THE COMMONER INFLUENZA REMEDIES

Aconite .. Sudden onset of fever, with chilliness, throbbing pulses, and great restlessness—*from anxiety.*

A remedy of cold, dry weather, bitter winds (opp. to *Gels.*).

Gelsemium .. Heaviness and tiredness of body and limbs.

Head heavy ; eyelids heavy ; limbs heavy.

Colds and fevers of mild winters (opp. to *Acon.*).

Chills in back. "Chills and heats chase one another."

Bursting headache, from neck, over head to eyes and forehead ; relieved by copious urination.

No thirst.

Eupatorium perf. Intense aching limbs and back, as if BONES were broken.

Dare not move for pain (opp. of *Pyrogen*).

Aching in all bones, with soreness of flesh.

Bones feel broken : dislocated : as if would break.

Bursting headache : dare not move for pain.

Shivering ; chills in back. (*Gels., Pyrog.*)

Chill begins 7 to 9 a.m.

Eyeballs sore. (*Bry., Gels.*)

There may be vomiting of bile.

Like the "break-bone fever" (Dengue).

Pyrogen .. *For the fever of violent pulsations and intense restlessness.*

Pulse very rapid : ratio between pulse and temperature disturbed. High temperature with slow pulse, or the reverse.

Chilliness no fire can warm. (*Nux, Gels.*)

Creeping chills in back, with thumping heart.

Bursting headache, with intense restlessness.

Hard bed sensation : feels beaten, bruised (*Arn.*).

Better beginning to move (opp. to *Rhus*), has to keep on moving, rocking, wriggling, for momentary relief.*

Copious urination of clear water, with fever.

* *One very bad 'flu year, all the cases one came across cleared up in twenty-four to forty-eight hours with* Pyrogen 6 *six-hourly. The symptoms, besides the thumping heart and the fever, were agonizing pain in lumbar and upper thigh muscles that made it impossible to keep still one moment.*

Baptisia .. Rapid onset. Sinks rapidly into a stupid typhoid state.

Dull red face : drugged, besotted appearance.

High temperature : red : dusky : comatose.

Drops asleep while answering.

" Gastric 'flu ": sudden attacks of violent diarrhœa and vomiting. Great prostration. (In such cases *Baptisia* will ensure as sudden a recovery.)

'Flu-pneumonias with this besotted appearance.

In the worst cases, mouth and throat are foul, and discharges very offensive. (*Merc.*)

(Curious symptom) dissociation of parts : " scattered and can't get himself together ". (*Petrol.*, *Pyrogen.*)

Bryonia .. White tongue : thirst for much cold fluid. (*Phos.*)

From every movement, every noise, attacked with dry heat (rev. of *Nux*, *Gels.*, etc.).

Wants to lie quite still, and be let alone.

Especially with pleurisy, or pleuro-pneumonia.

Headaches and pain all better for pressure, and worse for movement. (*Eup. per.*)

The anxiety, dreams and delirium of *Bry.* are of business ; in delirium he " wants to go home ".

Pains in head from coughing. Irritable.

Rhus tox. .. Stiff, lame and bruised on first moving (opp. of *Pyrogen*), passes off with motion, till he becomes weak and must rest : then restlessness and uneasiness drive him to move again.

The worst sufferings when at rest and kept without motion (opp. of *Bry.*).

Illness from cold, damp weather : from cold damp when perspiring. (*Dulc.*)

Anxiety, fear : worse at night. (*Acon.*)

Restlessness : intense fever : thirst : great prostration. Weeps without knowing why. (*Puls.*)

Typhoid forms of fever. (*Bapt.*)

Severe aching in bones. (*Eup. per.*)

A mental symptom of *Rhus* is fear of poison.

Mercurius sol. Profuse, very *offensive* sweat.

Very foul mouth. (*Bapt.*)

Salivation. Offensive.

Worse from sweating ; or no relief from sweating.

Colds extend to chest.

Camphor and *Nux* in Influenza

Hahnemann discusses the effect of *Camphor* in the influenza epidemics " endemic in Siberia ", which come among us occasionally. . . " *Camphor,*" he says, " is of service, only as a palliative certainly—but an invaluable palliative, seeing that the disease is one of short duration."

" *On the other hand, Nux vomica, in a single dose, and that the smallest possible, will often remove the disease homœopathically in a few hours.*"

Read the pathogenesis of *Nux*, and see that this must be so. . . .

Nux .. " *After drinking, immediately shivering and chilliness.*

Chilliness on the slightest movement. On the slightest exposure to the open air, shivering and chilliness for an hour ; dreads to go into open air.

By the slightest draught of air he gets chilled.

He cannot get warm.

Great coldness not removed by heat of stove, or by bed coverings.

Attack, as of fever : shivering and drawing in the limbs. . . ."

No wonder that Hahnemann says, " *Serious ailments from catching cold are often removed by it.*"

After Influenza Badly Recovered from

Gelsemium .. Patients sometimes come to hospital, " cannot get well after 'flu a few weeks ago." They are found to have a temperature of somewhere about 99°. Not ill : *not well.*

If they are chilly, with heats and chills ; if they feel a weakness and *heaviness* of limbs and eyelids, *Gels.* quickly puts them right.

China .. *Continued debility, with chilliness.*

Anæmic : pallid : weak.

Sensitive to touch : to motion : to cold air.

Worse alternate days.

Weariness of limbs, with desire to stretch, move, or change position.

Kali phos. .. General weakness and gloom.

Arsenicum .. *Chilliness : restlessness : anxiety : fear : fear of death* (*Acon.*) *: prostration.*
Burnings, relieved by heat.
Oversensitive : fastidious.
Queer symptoms :—red-hot-needle pains.
Sensation of ice-water running through veins.
Or boiling water going through blood-vessels.
Thirst for sips of cold water.

Pulsatilla .. Flitting chilliness : chills in spots.
Cold creeps in back. Chilly in warm room.
Profuse morning sweat.
Heat as if hot water thrown over him.
One-sided chilliness—heat—sweat.
External warmth intolerable. Worse in a close room.
Palpitation with anxiety : must throw off clothes.
Better out of doors.
Better for slow motion (opp. *Bry.*, *Eup. per.*, etc.).
Dry cough at night, goes on sitting up : returns on lying down again (*Hyos.*).
Thirstless : no hunger. Tearful ; peevish.

Sulphur .. Partially recovers and then relapses.
Frequent flushes of heat. Uneasiness in blood.
Very sensitive to open air ; to draughts (opp. to *Puls.*) ; worse for washing and bath. Takes cold.
Oppression, burning, stitches, congestion in chest.
Heat crown of head with cold feet.
Soles burn at night, must be put out of bed.
Hungry—starving at 11 a.m.
Drowsy by day : restless nights. Starts from frightful dreams.

* * * *

" *Cyprepedium pubescens*, *Cyprepedin* and *Scutellaria lat.* have been my sheet anchors in post-influenzal neuroses." BURNETT.

ONE OF THE CASES THAT JUSTIFIES DR. BURNETT HERE

J.M., ill and away from work for a year after an attack of influenza which lasted six weeks, till he " collapsed "

Said his heart was weak. He couldn't walk. Was suicidal. " Couldn't restrain himself." He complained of depression : despondency : felt his brain would burst. *Scutellaria* 30.

A week later : " different : livelier : stronger." Went back to work—absolutely himself again.

SOME THROAT REMEDIES

Aconite .. Throat *very red* : tingling.
Uvula feels long : comes in contact with tongue.
" Acute inflammation of all that can be seen and called throat." (Kent.)
Burning, smarting, dryness, great redness.
" Sudden onset in the night after exposure to cold, raw wind.
Plethoric person, wakes at night with violent, burning, tearing sore throat.
Cannot swallow. High fever, with great thirst for cold water.
Anxiety and fever."

Gelsemium .. A *Gels*. develops several days after exposure : *Acon*. comes on in a few hours.
Gels. for colds and fevers of mild winters : *Acon*. for those of violent winters and great cold winds (*Bell*.).
Gels. catarrhs excited by *warm, moist, relaxing weather*.
Sore throat, tonsils red : difficulty in swallowing, from weakness of muscles of deglutition. (*Bell*. from spasm, not weakness.)
Shuddering, as if ice rubbed up the back.
Hot skin : high temp. with cold extremities.
Weight and tiredness of whole body.
Sore throat, comes gradually : with muscular *weakness*, so that food and drink come back through nose. (*Bell*. from spasm.)
Great remedy of diphtheritic paralysis. (*Phyt*.)

Belladona .. Inflammation of throat. Tongue *bright red* or " strawberry " : dry burning.
Fauces and tonsils inflamed and bright red. Esp. right side ; extends to left (*Lyc*.).
Rapid progress. Constriction on attempting to swallow : ejection of food and drink through nose and mouth. (*Gels*. from paresis : *Bell*. from spasm.)
Dryness of fauces. Aversion to liquids.
Typical *Bell*. has congested, red, hot face and skin : big pupils, heat and dryness marked.

Phytolacca .. Throat sore. Isthmus congested and dark red.

Dark red inflammation of fauces: tonsils swollen.

Feeling of a lump when swallowing saliva, or when turning head to left.

Dryness, roughness, burning and smarting (fauces).

"As if a ball of red-hot iron had lodged in throat."

Throat so full, as if choked: or

Pharynx dry, feels like a cavern.

Every attempt to swallow sends shooting pains through ears (*Nit. a.*).

Unable to swallow even water.

Diphtheritic inflammation and ulceration of throat.

Diphtheria, with above symptoms. Here *Phyto.* has made notable cures.

Tongue fiery-red: feels burnt: or pain at root of tongue and into ear on swallowing.

In less severe sore throats—ordinary ones!—one sees, not the smooth red swelling of *Bell.*, but a bluish-red inflammation (*Lach.*).

Nux .. Sore throat.

Colds settle in nose, throat, chest, ears.

Sensitive to *least draught:* sneezing from itching in nose, and to throat and trachea.

"Great heat: burning hot, but cannot move or uncover in the least without feeling chilly."

Nux is hypersensitive (*Hep.*) irritable.

Apis .. Burning, stinging pains in throat, better for cold, *worse for heat.*

Œdematous condition: uvula and throat looks as if water would flow if pricked.

Pains like bee-stings, with the thrust, and the burning following.

Absence of thirst (*Gels.*).

Must be cool: worse for heat: wants cool things.

Especially worse from fire and radiated heat.

Much throat trouble—even to diphtheria—with above symptoms.

.. Hoarseness and loss of voice (*Phos.*, *Dros.*).
Catches cold with every exposure to fresh air.
" Lump in throat, must be swallowed."
Stinging pains when swallowing (*Apis*).
Uvula long, and neck stiff.
Always taking cold, and it settles in throat.
Chilliness: perspires much. Worse: cold air, water, draughts: better warmth.
" Fish-bone sensation in throat " so soon as he catches, or becomes, cold. (*Hep.*, *Merc.*, *Nit. a.*, etc.)
Hawks and hems.

Hepar .. " Seldom good in incipient colds and throats—more for ripened cold."
Fish-bone or crumb sensation (*Merc.*, *Alum.*, *Nit. a.*, *Arg. nit.*).
Worse any exposure: *worse cold dry wind.*
Intensely sensitive, mind and body.
Easily angry, abusive.
Throat extremely sensitive to touch (*Lach.*). Pain as if full of splinters: (*Nit. a.*) pain on swallowing.
The whole pharynx in a catarrhal state with copious discharge.
Larynx painful: painful as a bolus of food goes down behind the larynx.
Putting hand out of bed will increase the pain in larynx and cough. Croup after exposure to cold, dry wind (*Acon.*).

Dulcamara .. Sore throat from *damp, cold weather.*
Tendency to ulceration, which eats and spreads.
Catarrhal angina after catching cold.
Sore throat; fills with mucus: with yellow slime.
The tonsils inflamed, even quinsy (*Baryt. c.*).

Phosphorus .. Larynx raw, sore, furry. " Cotton " in throat.
Tonsils and uvula much swollen: uvula elongated: with dry, burning sensation.
Worse passing from warm to cold air.
Worse talking and coughing.
Hoarseness and aphonia, worse evening.

Arum triph. .. *Sore throats of speakers and singers.*
"Clergyman's sore throat" from straining voice, or a cold.
Arum triph. has a marked effect on larynx.
Hoarseness: lack of control over vocal cords.
If raises voice, it goes up with a squeak.
Graph. also for "uncertainty of voice: cannot control vocal cords: voice cracks".
And *Carbo veg.* has "deep voice, fails when he attempts to raise it".
But *Phyto.* also with real bad sore throats.
Corners of mouth and tongue cracked.
Excoriating saliva.
Tingling and pricking, lips, tongue, throat, nose: "in spite of soreness they pinch and scratch, and *pick and bore into sore parts*".
Stinging pain in throat, which is ulcerated, raw and bleeding.

Alumina .. Like "Clergyman's sore throat" (*Arum triph.*).
Throat dry on waking, with husky weak voice.
It is dark red: uvula long.
Better hot drinks.
Splinter sensation, swallowing (*Hep.*, *Nit. a.*, etc.).

Ignatia .. "A plug in throat", worse when not swallowing.
Tonsils studded with small, superficial ulcers.
Constriction about throat, with nervousness and insomnia. (Aphthous sore throat.)
Constriction also of larynx: "a feather there".
The more he coughs the worse the tickling.

Capsicum .. Throat feels "constricted, spasmodically closed".
Worse when not swallowing (*Ign.*).
The pain is smarting, *as from cayenne pepper.*
Chill or shuddering after every drink.
Odour from mouth like carrion.
"*Caps.* is loose, flabby, red, fat and cold."
"Throat looks as if it would bleed, so red. It is puffed, discoloured, purple, mottled."
Throat remains sore a long time after a cold, or sore throat. (*Sulph.*) Does not get very bad, but gets no better.
Nose and cheeks red, and cold.

Aesculus .. Useful in coryza and sore throat.
Coryza, thin, watery, burning: with *rawness.*
Sensitive to inhaled cold air. (*Phos., Rumex.*)
Violent burning in throat, with raw feeling.
Fauces dark, congested.
"After the sore throat, engorged veins left."
HOT, DRY, STIFF, ROUGH. Full feeling internally, throat and anus.
Chronic sore throat with hæmorrhoids.

Pulsatilla .. Catarrh of throat. Veins distended: throat bluish-red.
Redness and varicose condition of tonsils.
Stinging pains (*Apis*) worse swallowing saliva.
Better cold, fresh, open air (opp. to *Phos.*).
Worse warm air, room; worse getting feet wet.
(A *Puls.* patient: weepy: wants fuss and help.)

Sulphur .. Sore throat with great burning and dryness.
Chronic sore throat. Tonsil enlarged, with purplish aspect lasting for weeks and months; a sore and painfully sensitive throat.
Inflammation purplish, venous. . . .
In a sulphur patient: "the ragged philosopher": argumentative and speculative. Intolerant of heat. Loves fat. Intolerant of clothing: kicks covers off, and thrusts feet out.

Baryta mur. .. "Less greasy than *Merc.*" Warm, damp skin.
Saliva sticking round tonsils.
Tonsils very large, look like big plums.
"A lump in throat" pain.
Pains shoot to neck (*Phyt.* to ears).

Baryta carb. .. Every little exposure to *damp or cold* awakens anew inflammation of tonsils—throat—fauces (*Dulc.*).
Granulations, throat: worse every cold spell.
A very sore throat that comes slowly after days of exposure.
Children with big tonsils; intellectually and physically dwarfish: slow to develop.
Even the sore throat is of very slow development.

Sepia .. Left side inflamed: much swelling but little redness.
Sensation of lump in throat (*Ign.*).
Waked with sensation as if had swallowed something which has stuck in throat.
Contraction of throat when swallowing.
Sepia is chilly: indifferent; intolerant alike of cold and of close places.

Cinnabaris. .. Throat swollen: tonsils enlarged and red.
" Sensation of something pressing on nose, like a heavy pair of spectacles."
Throat very dry, awakening from sleep.

Natrum ars. .. Throat dark-red, swollen, covered with yellow, gelatinous mucus which gags the patient when he attempts to hawk it out.
Sneezing from draught, or breathing cold air.

Mercurius .. Smarting, raw, sore throat.
Sore throat with every cold.
Tongue: thick, yellow, moist covering.
Profuse sweating without relief.
Thirst with salivation.
Bad smell from mouth.
Discharge (nose) yellow-green, thick, muco-purulent.
Worse at night: worse in bed.
(" Rarely give *Merc.* if tongue is dry.")

Nitric acid .. One of the " fish-bone in throat " remedies.
Ulcers in throat, irregular in outline.
" A morsel stuck in pharynx ", " as if pharynx constricted ".
Swallowing difficult: distorts face and draws head down.
Swallowing even a teaspoonful of fluid causes violent pain extending to ear (*Phyto.*).
Suddenly appearing, or slowly creeping ulcers on fauces and soft palate.
Large deep ulcers, with bluish margins.
Nit. a. is chilly: loves salt and fat: is depressed and anxious. Its pains are splinter-like, as if sticking in the part, worse for touch.

Aurum .. Tonsils red and swollen; parotid gland on affected side feels sore (*Phyto.*).

Ulceration of palate and throat (*Nit. a.*) and especially after *Mercury* and Syphilis.

Aurum especially where the patient is depressed to the verge of suicide. Loathing of life.

Kali bich. .. Ulcers, throat, which tend to perforate.

Tonsils swollen and inflamed: ulcerated: deep ulcers: dropsical, shiny, red, puffy.

Discharges ropy and stringy.

Nose, throat, bronchi, bladder, all partake of this catarrhal condition, with discharges thick, yellow, ropy and stick like glue; tough, jelly-like: form hard masses.

Exudate in throat looks like fine ashes sprinkled on the part.

Cantharis .. Inflammation of throat with severe *burning* and rawness. Vesication.

Great constriction of throat and larynx, with suffocation on any attempt to swallow water. (*Bell., Merc. cor., Ars., Arum triph., Caps.*)

Mercurius cor. Symptoms "almost identical with *Canth.* But *Merc. cor.* has more swelling, throat and tongue, and deep ulcers, rather than the extensive vesication of *Canth.*"

Intense burning in throat (*Ars., Ars. iod., Caps.*).

Uvula swollen, elongated, dark-red.

Throat symptoms very violent.

"Any attempt to swallow=violent spasms of throat (*Bell.*) with ejection of the solid or liquid; but distinguished from *Bell.* by its intense *destructive* inflammation of throat."

Mercurius cy. .. Throat feels raw and sore.

Looks raw in spots, as if denuded.

Broken-down appearance of mucous membrane, bordering on suppuration.

One of our most frequently-useful remedies in follicular tonsillitis: in diphtheria also, for which it has a great reputation.

In poisonings *Merc. cy.* has produced membrane in throat, mistaken for diphtheria.

Lycopodium ..	Has peculiar hours of aggravation: 4-8 p.m. Affects right side (in throats, quinsy, diphtheria): but may extend across to left side. Also extends from above downwards, as when diphtheria begins in upper part of pharynx, or in nose, and spreads downwards. Generally better from swallowing warm fluids: or better from holding cold water in mouth. (*Lach.* is better for cold, and has spasms of throat from attempting to drink warm drinks.) " The throat is extremely painful, it has all the violence of the worst cases of diphtheria."
Lachesis ..	Left throat especially affected: left tonsil: tends to pass from left to right (opp. to *Lyc.* which goes from right to left). *Lac. can.* (in throats also, and in diphtheria) goes *from side to side and then back again.* Throat bluish-red (*Phyt., Nat ars., Lach.*). Sense of constriction: " Throat suddenly closing up " or " lump in throat that he must constantly swallow." Rawness and burning. External throat is *excessively sensitive to touch* (*Hep.*). Can swallow solids better than liquids: worse empty swallowing. Even relief from swallowing solids. *Nothing must touch larynx or throat.* All worse after sleep: sleeps into an aggravation: or wakes smothering. One of our great diphtheria remedies—left side, or left to right; with above symptoms; but without the filthy mouth and tongue of the *Mercs*.
Merc. iod. flav.	Throat right side, then left (*Lyc.*). Left to right (*Lach., Merc. iod. rub.*). Tongue yellow at base. Better cold drinks.

Lac caninum .. " Throat closing : will choke ! "

Very sensitive to external touch (*Lach.*).

Swallowing almost impossible.

Pain in throat pushes towards left ear. (*Phyto.*, shoots to ears.)

Pain, membrane, goes from side to side and back.

Throat dry, husky, as if scalded.

Sore throat before menses since diphtheria, with patches of exudation on tonsil. Glazed, shiny red throat. A grey, fuzzy, coating. Better cold, or warm drink : Worse empty swallowing.

Has cured tonsillitis, diphtheria : has been used as prophylactic against diphtheria.

Lac can. is intensely sensitive and obsessed : sees faces :—sees spiders, snakes, vermin.

Cannot bear to be alone.

Thinks she has a loathsome disease : that everything she says is a lie.

Baptisia .. Pain and soreness of fauces.

Fauces dark-red ; dark putrid ulcers : tonsils and parotids swollen.

Unusual abscence of pain, in an extremely bad throat, is a characteristic of *Baptisia.*

Œsophagus feels constricted : can only swallow water.

But all this with the *Baptisia* " typhoid condition " :—drowsy, dull red : as if drugged ; lapses into a comatose condition. *Rapid onset of very severe symptoms, and rapidly curative in the Baptisia case.*

Pyrogen .. Septic throats, with extreme fetor.

Taste as if mouth full of pus. Carrion-like odour. Offensive sweats.

Tongue, red glazed ; then dark red, intensely dry, or flabby : yellow-brown streak down centre.

Pulse very high : or out of proportion to temp.

Diphtheria with extreme fetor.

Quinsy with rapid suppuration.

A symptom of *Pyrog.* extreme restlessness.

SOME COUGH MEDICINES

Aconite .. Constant short *dry* cough, with feeling of suffocation, which increases with every respiration.

Cough hoarse, dry, loud; spasmodic: dry, hard ringing.

Cough wakes him from sleep, dry, croupy, suffocating.

Anxiety and fear. Restlessness. Worse at night.

Comes down suddenly *after exposure to cold, dry winds.*

Dry cough. Sensation of dryness whole chest. "No expectoration except a little watery mucus and blood. Otherwise dry."

Belladonna .. *Dry* cough, from *dryness* larynx.

Cough with red injected throat.

Violent scraping in larynx exciting dry cough.

Tickling and burning in larynx with violent paroxysms of cough. As if head will burst. (*Phos.*, *Nux.*, *Bry.*, etc.)

Child begins to cry immediately before cough comes on.

Attacks of cough end with sneezing.

The typical *Belladonna* patient is red, and burning hot, with dilated pupils.

Cough begins with peculiar clutching in larynx as if a speck of something had got into larynx.

Dry cough: spasmodic barking, short.

Kent. The *Bell.* cough is peculiar. As soon as its great violence and effort have raised a little mucus, he gets peace, and stops coughing. *Then air passages grow drier, and drier, and begin to tickle, then comes the spasm,* as if all air passages were taking part in it, and the whoop, the gagging and (?) vomiting. (A great whooping-cough medicine with spasms larynx, causing whoop and difficulty of breathing.)

Bryonia .. Hard, *dry* cough, with soreness in chest.
Dry spasmodic cough: worse night, after eating and drinking, when entering a warm room, after taking a deep breath.
Cough with stitches in chest: with headache, as if head would fly to pieces. (*Bell., Phos.,* etc.)
When coughing must press hand to sternum.
Cough compels to spring up in bed.
Cough shakes whole body.
Wants to sigh: to breathe deeply, which hurts.
Bry. is one of the worse cold, dry medicines: worse East wind (*Hep., Nux, Spong.,* etc.).
Bry. is always worse from movement: better for pressure.
Irritable: wants to be let alone: thirsty.

Nux .. .. Dry, teasing cough with great soreness of chest.
Coryza travels down to chest.
Feverishness, when patient *cannot move or uncover without feeling chilly.*
Spasmodic cough with retching (*Dros., Rumex*).
Worse cold, dry, windy weather.
Cough causes headache as if skull would burst: *Bell., Phos.,* etc.—or bruised pain about umbilicus, as if shattered and torn.
Tickling and pain in larynx with cough.
Acute catarrhal laryngitis: asthma—whooping cough
"Something torn loose in chest."
Nux is hypersensitive, mentally and physically. Angry, easily offended.

Hepar .. .. *Worse for cold, dry weather.*
Better in warm, moist weather.
Cough when any part of the body becomes uncovered (*Rhus, Rumex*).
Worse breathing cold air (*Rumex*): worse putting a hand out of bed.
Suffocative coughing spells.
Croup from cold, dry wind, or cold air.
In croup, after *Acon.* and *Spongia.*

Phosphorus .. Dry, tickling cough : irritation in larynx and below sternum.

Hard, dry, tight cough, which racks the patient and is very exhausting.

Racking cough. Violent cough.

Dry cough, with pain in head as if it would burst. (*Bell.*, *Nux*, etc.)

Violent pain in chest with coughing, obliged to hold chest with hand. (*Bry.*)

Cough with pain chest and abdomen, obliged to hold abdomen with hand. (*Dros.*)

There may be involuntary stool when coughing.

Oppression and constriction, as if a great weight lying on chest.

Tightness across chest, better external pressure.

Violent, shaking cough. Trembles with cough.

Cough worse laughing, talking, reading aloud eating, lying on left side.

Sputum saltish, yellow, sour, purulent, bloody, rusty.

Cold sputum, tasting sour, salt or sweet.

Worse open air. Going from warm to cold room (*Rumex*) *or vice versa.*

The typical *Phos.* patient is chilly, with thirst for cold drinks. Thirst for ice-cold water.

Craves salt.

Sensitive to thunder.

Nervous alone—in the dark.

Suspicious. Anxious. Indifferent.

Causticum .. Dryness : rawness : hoarseness : aphonia.

Cough hard, and racks the whole chest.

Chest seems full of mucus, " Feels if he could only cough a little deeper he could get it up. Struggles and coughs till exhausted or till he finds that a drink of cold water will relieve : ice-cold."

With each cough escape of urine.

Obliged to swallow the sputum raised.

Inability to expectorate.

Part of the *Causticum* local paralyses.

Greasy (*Puls.*) tasting expectoration.

Spongia .. Chest dry. No wheezing or rattling, with respiration or cough.

Croupy cough: sounds like a saw driven through a board.

Wakes out of sleep with suffocation, with loud violent cough, great alarm, anxiety and difficult breathing. (*Acon.*)

Cough worse talking, reading, singing, swallowing, lying with head low.

Later tough mucus, difficult to expectorate : has to be swallowed. (*Caust.*)

Rhus tox. .. Dry, teasing cough, from tickling in bronchia ; from uncovering even a hand.

Nocturnal dry cough

Cough with taste of blood, though no blood to be seen.

Cough during sleep.

Worse cold, wet weather. Worse uncovering. Restlessness : must move.

Sepia .. .. Violent cough with retching and gagging.

Thick, tenacious, yellow expectoration.

Severe cough on rising in a.m., with much expectoration.

No expectoration in the evening.

Or expectoration at night, none by day.

The *Sepia* patient is tired, indifferent, wants to get away.

Offensive axillary sweat.

Scilla .. .. Gush of tears with coughing.

Cough causes sneezing, flow of tears, spurting of urine (*Caust., Phos., Rumex*, etc.), even involuntary stools. (*Phos.*)

Cough with expectoration in a.m. and none in evening.

Stannum .. Loose cough, with heavy, green, sweet sputum (or salty).

Sensation of great weakness in chest.

Chest feels empty.

Drosera .. Crawling in larynx which provokes coughing.
Violent tickling in larynx brings on cough, and wakes him.
Spasmodic cough till he retches and vomits.
Cough coming from deep down in chest.
Provokes pain in hypochondrium: must hold it in coughing.
Oppression of chest so that breath could not be expelled.
Cough, the impulses follow one another so violently that he can hardly get his breath.
Hoarseness. Clutching, cramping, constricting and burning in larynx.
Cough worse at night.
Coughs of phthisis: asthma. Whooping-cough.
(Here Hahnemann urges a single dose of *Dros.* 30, not to be lightly repeated.)

N.B.—*Dros.* is especially indicated when there is a history of weak resistance to T.B.

Rumex .. .. Cough on changing rooms, *from breathing cold air.* (*Phos.*)
Cough provoked by change from warm to cold.
Covers mouth up.
Every fit of coughing produces the passage of a few drops of urine. (*Caust.*, etc.)
Tough, stringy, tenacious mucus.
(Symptoms very like *Dros.*).
Much tough mucus in larynx with constant desire to hawk it but without relief. Hoarseness.
Dry spasmodic cough like early stage of whooping-cough (*Dros.*).
Dry at first. In paroxysms, preceded by tickling in throat pit with congestion and slight pain in head and wrenching pains right chest. The most violent paroxysms were a few minutes after lying down at night (11 p.m.), after which slept all night. Paroxysms also on waking, and through day. Later, expectoration of adhesive mucus in small quantities, detached with difficulty.
Breathlessness, as when passing rapidly through the air. Sensitive to open air.

Ipecacuanha .. Spasmodic or asthmatic cough. Suffocative cough.

Child becomes blue and stiff.

Respiration wheezing. Rattling.

Violent dyspnœa with wheezing and great weight and anxiety in chest.

Loss of breath with cough : with inclination to vomit without nausea.

Or, more often, *Ipecac.* has intense nausea—nausea unrelieved by vomiting : with clean tongue.

Arsenicum .. Wheezing respiration with cough and frothy expectoration.

Air passages seem constricted, cannot breathe fully.

Asthma type of cough.

Great prostration and debility.

Very sensitive to cold.

"Catarrh keeps travelling down. From nose to larynx, with hoarseness ; down trachea with burning and smarting worse from coughing. Then constriction of chest, asthmatic dyspnœa, with dry hacking cough and no expectoration. With the *Ars.* anxiety, prostration, restlessness, exhaustion, sweat.

"Then constriction, wheezing, suffocation. Expectorates great quantities of thin, watery discharge. Expectoration is excoriating. Burning in chest."

Patient is worse after midnight. 1 a.m.

Kali carb. .. Cough at 3 a.m. or worse at 3 a.m.

Cough asthmatic : must lean forward, head on knees.

Cough with cutting or stitching (*Bry.*) in chest, with respiration, or between breaths. (*Bry. with* only.)

Sputum, of small round lumps : of blood-streaked mucus : of pus.

Kali bich. .. Cough with white mucus, "tough as pitch, can be drawn out into strings ".

Membranous shreds with cough.

Pulsatilla .. Cough caused by inspiration.
Worse warm room : coming into warm room.
Cough in the evening : when lying ; prevents sleep.
Dry in the evening, loose in the morning.
Cough from tickling or scraping in larynx.
Paroxysmal. Gagging and choking.
Dry, teasing cough, wants windows and doors thrown open. (*Sulph.*)
Discharges thick, bland, yellowish-green.
The typical *Pulsatilla* is tearful : is intolerant of heat and of close places : better in cool, fresh air. Not hungry, or thirsty.

Sulphur .. Suffocated. Wants doors and windows open (*Puls.*) at night. Cough at night.
Congestion of blood to chest : to head.
Burning chest : head : face. In soles at night.
For coughs, and to clear up coughs in a *Sulph.* patient :—starving about 11 a.m.
Red lips, red lids : red orifices. Worse for bath.

Calcarea c. .. Tickling cough.
Sputum mucous, purulent, yellow, sour, offensive.
Worse cold : worse wet : worse wind.
Head and neck apt to sweat at night.
Cold damp feet (*Sepia*).

Tuberculinum .. Hard, dry cough. Craves air (*Puls.*).
Better in cold wind. Suffocation in warm room.
To clear up coughs or pneumonias that hang fire, where there is a T.B. history.
Night sweats.

SPASMODIC CROUP

There is a celebrated group of homœopathic remedies for Spasmodic Croup, sold for years as " Boeninghausen's Croup Powders ". They are five in number.

Aconite, Hepar, Spongia, Hepar, Spongia : in that order, and should so many be required.

Give at two-to four-hourly intervals, according to the urgency of the case.

THE COMMON REMEDIES OF ACUTE CHESTS:—

BRONCHITIS, BRONCHO-PNEUMONIA, PNEUMONIA, PLEURISY, PLEURO-PNEUMONIA

IN CHILDREN AND IN ADULTS

EARLY CASES

Aconite .. Sudden onset : from chill : in cold dry weather.
First stage of pneumonia, bronchitis, pleurisy.
Cough hard, dry, painful. Chest tight.
Dry, hot skin.
Full, hard pulse. Rapid, difficult breathing.
Worse at night.
Lungs engorged. Sits erect. (*Chel.*, *Lach.*)
May grasp larynx (*Ant. t.*, *Phos.*). . . .
Always, with *Acon. restlessness, anxiety*, FEAR.

Ferrum phos. .. Early inflammatory diseases : pneumonia, etc., with very few indications.
Lacks the restless anxiety of *Aconite*, the burning, and brain symptoms of *Belladonna*, and the intense thirst of *Phos.*
Breathing oppressed, short, panting.
Expectoration of clear blood.
Pains and hæmorrhages caused by hyperæmia.

Veratrum viride Sudden, violent congestion of lungs.
Bloated, livid face : faint, attempting to sit up.
Slow, heavy breathing. Must sit up (*Ant t.*).
Dry, red streak along centre of tongue.
Rapidly oscillating temperature.
Hyperpyrexia, with sweat.
Rapid, full pulse. Engorgement severe, with violent excitement of heart.

Belladonna .. Pneumonia, etc., with cerebral complications.
Great nervousness : delirium.
Sleepy, yet cannot sleep.
Dilated pupils.
Flushed face, congested eyes : skin dry, hot.
Bronchitis with paroxysms of dry, hard, spasmodic cough.
Pleurisy, esp. right side : great pain, extreme soreness. Worse if bed jarred.
Cannot lie on sore side (opp. to *Bry.*).

Ipecacuanha .. " Especially the infant's friend, commonly indicated in the bronchitis of infancy."

Bronchitis, broncho-pneumonia, pneumonia.

" Child coughs, gags, suffocates : coarse rattling often heard through the room."

Spasmodic cough, with nausea, and vomiting.

Rapid onset (*Acon.*, *Verat v. Bapt.*).

(Compare *Ant tart.* ; both have rattling cough and breathing, and vomiting. *Ipecac.* for stage of irritation, *Ant. tart.* for stage of relaxation.

Ipecac. comes on hurriedly : *Ant. tart.* at the close of a bronchitis, or broncho-pneumonia, with threatened paralysis of lungs : while chest is full of mucus, nothing can be raised.)

Chelidonium majus. Pneumonia, generally right-sided.

Pleura generally involved, and (?) diaphragm.

If stirs, pain shoots through him like a knife.

Sits up with pain that transfixes chest. Worse movement (*Bry.* ; but *Bry.* must lie still).

Tight girdle sensation. Apt to get jaundiced.

Tongue coated ; tooth-notched (*Merc.*, etc.).

Deep-seated pain in whole of right chest.

Pain lower angle right shoulder-blade : from chest to shoulder-angle. (Characteristic.)

Cough loose and rattling, but expectoration difficult (*Ant. t.*, *Ammon. carb.*, *Kali carb.*).

" *In catarrhal pneumonia of young children* very like *Ant tart.* ; chest seems full of mucus, not easily expectorated."

Gelsemium .. Influenzal pneumonia. Chills up and down back.

Paralytic weakness. Limbs heavy : eyelids heavy.

Dusky-red face (*Bapt.*). Confused, dull, dazed, thirstless, severe congestive headache.

Baptisia .. Sudden onset : rapidly goes into a typhoid state.

Influenzal pneumonias, typhoid pneumonias.

Face besotted : dusky : purple (*Lach.*) : bloated.

Tongue dry, brown down centre.

Besotted : mind confused : tries to answer or speak, but it flits away into stupor.

In delirium, dual personality : tries to get the pieces together.

Discharges pungent : fœtid.

Pyrogen .. " *Baptisia*, only more so."
General aching and soreness.
" Bed too hard." (*Arnica.*)
Intense restlessness. (" *Rhus*, only more so.")
Offensiveness. (*Bapt.*, *Kreos.*)
Fiery-red, smooth tongue.
Quickly oscillating temperature.
Pulse quick, or reverse: out of proportion to temperature.. Delirium with dual personality.

Opium .. .. Insensitive. Comatose.
Stertor: blows out cheeks in expiration.
Hot sweat.

Nitric acid .. Inhalation of *Nitric acid* fumes causes rapid congestion and inflammation of lungs.
Chest feels crowded: oppression, worse bending backwards. Sensation of a spring released :—of a big hole in *right* temple.
Shattering cough.
Sputum sticks like glue: yellow, acrid, bitter, salt: flaps during respiration.
Expectoration of black, coagulated blood.
Stitches in right chest.
Fear of death, anxious about his illness (*Acon.*).
The typical *Nit. a.* patient is brown-eyed, chilly, intolerant of fuss; loves fat and salt.

Mercurius .. Bronchitis: cough worse evening and night.
Tickling in chest: feels dry.
" As if chest would burst."
Copious sweating without relief; " The more he sweats the worse he is."
" Rarely give *Merc.* if the tongue is dry."
" Pneumonia with excessive, offensive sweat, offensive mouth and breath, offensive expectoration." (The action of *Merc.* is pretty in such cases !)
Broncho-pneumonia, infantile broncho-pneumonia, bilious pneumonia (*Chel.*).
Tongue foul: tooth-notched (*Chel.*).
Stabbing pains from base right lung to back.
Bloody, thick-green expectoration.
Suppuration of lungs: large quantities of pus.

More Advanced Cases

Bryonia .. Takes the place of *Acon.* when hepatization has begun.

Cough hard, painful. Expectoration thicker.

Anguish from oppressed breathing (*Acon.* from fever).

Lies perfectly still. (Opp. to *Rhus.*)

Every breath causes intense pain, in pneumonia or pleuro-pneumonia (*Kali carb.*).

Breath short, rapid, as deep breathing means great pain.

Lies on painful side, to keep it still. (Opp. of *Bell.*)

Stitching pains, better pressure: (*Bell.*, has throbbing pains, worse pressure.)

Lips dry. Tongue coated: dry.

Thirst for large quantities.

Constipation; dry, dark, hard stools.

Probably our most frequently-useful medicine in pneumonia.

Kali carb. .. Pneumonia, or pleuro-pneumonia with stabbing pains (chest) worse motion, worse respiration (*Bry.*) but (unlike *Bry.*) *also independently of respiration.*

Hepatization of lungs, with much rattling of mucus during cough.

Affects especially *lower, right chest* (*Phos.*, *Merc.*).

Hepatization right lung, cannot lie right side: (*Bry.* lies on affected side—or back).

Infantile pneumonia, or broncho-pneumonia, with intense dyspnœa, much mucus, raised with difficulty, though constantly coughing.

Child oppressed, can neither sleep nor drink.

Wheezing, whistling, choking cough (*Ant t.*).

Worse 2, 3 or 5 a.m.

Natrum sul. .. Pneumonia of *left lung*, and *left lower lobe.*

Pneumonia with asthma.

" Humid asthma of children."

Important *time aggravation*, 4 or 5 a.m.

Nat sul. is *worse in damp weather; from damp dwellings.*

Phosphorus	..	" Great weight on chest." Constriction. Pneumonia with anxiety, oppression. Expectoration of bright-red blood : or sputum rust-coloured ; purulent ; saltish, sweet, cold. Especially right lower lobe (*Kali carb.*, *Merc.*) but *Phos.* lies on right side, *Merc.* on left. Stitching pains in chest : in left chest, better lying on right side. (*Bry.* better lying on and steadying sore side, opp. to *Kali c.*) Pleurisy, pleuro- or broncho-pneumonia, typhoid pneumonia—*with Phos. symptoms.* To clear up hepatization (*Tub bov.*, *Sulph.*, etc.). Dryness of air passages. Hard, dry, tight cough ; racks him. Trembles with cough. Suppresses cough, it hurts so. Bronchitis with yellow, blood-streaked sputum Thirsty for cold water (*Bry.*). Better for sleep (opp. to *Lach.*). Wants company : fear alone. Typical *Phos.* is tall, slender, " artistic " type.
Ranunculus bulbosus	..	Acute, stabbing pains chest, with effusion. Anxiety, dyspnœa and distress. Sore spots left in chest after pneumonia. Sensation of sub-cutaneous ulceration. Everything sore, bruised, *very sensitive to touch.* Bright red cheeks with clean tongue. (*Ipecac.*) Short, very oppressed breathing. Dry heat : prostration from the start. Small, very rapid pulse. Cardiac and vascular excitement : nausea, even faintness, on motion (*Bry.*).
Rhus tox.	..	Pneumonia has taken a typhoid form. (*Bapt.*) Pleuro-pneumonia, with stitching pain. (*Bry.*, *Kali carb.*, etc.) Much fever : aching bones : marked prostration. Dry hot skin. Restlessness ; relieved by motion. *Pain and dyspnœa worse at rest.* (opp. *Bry.*) Bloody expectoration : or cold, green putrid-smelling sputum. Tongue, red tip : dry. (Red line, centre, *Verat v.*) ? Incontinence of stool and urine.

Lachesis .. Worse after sleep. *Sleeps into an aggravation.*
Throat sensitive to touch.
Cyanosis.
Fits of suffocation : must sit up : or worse sitting erect, must bend forward (*Kali carb.*).
Least thing near mouth produces suffocative dyspnœa.
Oppression of chest : constriction (*Phos.*) worse afternoon : worse after sleep. Worse lying on left side (*Phos.*). Worse covering mouth or nose.
Asthma *during* sleep (*Sulph.*).
Dry, hacking cough : worse touching throat : after sleep.
Tickling cough.
Cough " as if some food had gone into wrong passage ".
Hepatization, esp. of left lung.
Threatened paralysis of lungs with much dyspnœa, and long-lasting, suffocating paroxysms.
(< Pressure, *Lach* : > pressure *Bry.*)
Left side, may go over to right.
Face puffy, purple, mottled. (*Bapt.*, *Ant t.*)

Lycopodium .. Unresolved pneumonia.
Fever worse 4-8 p.m.
Frowning forehead, in chest troubles.
Fan-like motions of alæ nasi.
Short, rattling breathing.
Wakes up angry or cross.
A little food fills up.
Fulness and noisy flatulence.
Worse eating and drinking cold things.
Bronchitis, capillary bronchitis, broncho-pneumonia, pneumonia, *with above symptoms.*

Kali bich. .. Yellow, thick, lumpy, tough, stringy or sticky secretions. (*Sang.*) Sputum sticks to teeth, tongue, lips, draws out in strings—coughs up casts.
Worse 2-3 a.m.
Worse from cold.

Capsicum .. Chest too full : not enough room in it.
Cannot get air deep enough into lungs.
With every explosive cough, there escapes a volume of pungent, fœtid air. (*Sang.*)
Cough *causes distant pains*, or *raises foul air*.
Sputum dirty-brown, not rusty.
" Children of beer-drinkers : of over-stimulated men."
Fat ; flabby ; red, cold face. (Red, hot, *Bell.*)

Sanguinaria .. Cough ceases as soon as patient passes flatus.
Circumscribed redness of cheeks.
Distressing dyspnœa. Rusty sputum.
Hands and feet burning, or cold. Tongue red and burning.
Coughs, raises foul air (*Caps.*), tough bloody plugs or purulent sputum : ends with belching.
Feels very faint, with sweat and nausea.
" Sudden chill : burning in chest : Symptoms of pneumonia : Rusty sputum ; violent cough, felt as a concussion at bifurcation of trachea ; as if a knife were in the parts ; as if torn asunder ; and after cough copious, loud, empty eructations, no other remedy has this." (Kent.)

Desperate Cases

Cantharis .. Inflammation of lungs, gangrenous type, prostration, and *the lung affected burns like fire* (*Tereb.*, *Kreos.*, *Carbo v.*), or as if full of boiling water.
Esp. with frequent micturition with burning, cutting pain.

Antimonium tartaricum Sudden and alarming symptoms of suffocation ; oppression and short breathing : must sit up.
Accumulation of mucus in chest with coarse rattling : expectoration of thick white mucus after great efforts to raise it. Chest filling up : threatened paralysis of lungs.
Capillary bronchitis : Broncho-pneumonia.
Especially infants and old people.
Drowsiness. Weakness. Lacking in reaction. Must sit up.
Sickly, sunken, pale, bluish face : twitching : covered with cold sweat.

Ammonium carb. Somnolence: drowsiness (*Ant. t.*). Great debility.
Rattling of large bubbles in lungs.
Bluish or purplish lips (*Ant. t., Lach.*).
Coughs continually, but raises nothing, or with great difficulty (*Kali carb.*).
VERY LIKE ANT. TART.—but *Ammon. carb. is worse for cold, Ant. tart. is worse for heat.*
Chests of old people; typical winter coughs.

Kreosotum .. Dreadful burning in chest. (*Tereb., Canth.,* etc.) Constriction.
Bronchitis: bronchiectasis, with *fearfully offensive sputum.* Gangrene of lung.
Bloody, greenish-yellow, pus-like sputum.

(One remembers an elderly woman, dying of bronchitis, where the stench of breath and sputum was so terrible that she was screened. *Kreos.* 200, promptly cleared whole condition up, beginning with the intolerable odour; she made a good recovery.)

Arnica .. .. Says he is well, when desperately ill.

Carbo an. .. Pneumonia, suppuration of right lung.
Burning in chest, or coldness in chest.
Suffocative cough, shakes brain, which feels loose. Sputum greenish, brown, syrup-like.
Destruction of lung tissue, and decomposition of fluids expectorated.
On closing eyes, feels smothering.

Terebinth .. Capillary bronchitis, drowsy, lungs clogged up; urine scanty, dark with blood.
Typhoid pneumonia: *unbearable burning* (*Canth., Carbo v.*) and tightness across chest: great dryness: or profuse expectoration.
Hepatization of lungs.

Carbo veg. .. The homœopathic CORPSE-REVIVER.
Burning in chest, as from glowing coals.
Capillary bronchitis.
Pneumonia, third stage. Patient moribund.
Fœtid sputum.
Cold breath and sweat: wants to be fanned.
Air-hunger. Threatened paralysis of lungs.
Cold throat, mouth; tongue cold.
Face yellow-grey: greenish: hippocratic.
Patient collapsed—"almost gone"

BUT A PNEUMONIA MAY NEED

Calcarea .. Bronchial catarrh of teething children.

To clear up pneumonia, or broncho-pneumonia in fair fat children of "plus tissue minus quality."

Head sweats profusely in sleep. Cold, damp feet.

Rickety children : big head and big abdomen.

Apis .. .. Constant sensation (chest) as if he couldn't live.

Anguish of mind. Impossible to get another breath, so great the suffocative feeling.

"Pleurisy with exudation : one of the best remedies to bring about absorption. *Apis* and *Sulph.* will cure most cases."

Apis cannot stand heat. (*Puls.*, *Sulph.*)

Sulphur .. Torpid condition : *Bry.* helped but he does not rally.

Load on chest. Flushes without much fever.

Deficiency of reaction ; to help absorption.

Especially in the typical *Sul.* patient—shock headed : argumentative : not too tidy or clean : feels the heat : throws off the clothes and won't be covered : very red lips.

Psorinum .. Patients convalesce very slowly ; are chilly, offensive ; with despair of recovery.

Psor. is a chilly *Sulphur.*

Tuberculinum bovinum has promptly cleared up many a pneumonia, where it hangs fire, in persons of *tuberculous family history.* (In rare cases one of the other nosodes may be needed on such indication.)

N.B.—An important point in treating pneumonia, is not to imagine that you have cured because the temperature has dropped to almost normal, and so stop the medicine. Don't be happy till the patient has been normal or sub-normal for 48 hours.

* * *

It is only in the earlier stages of pneumonia in patients previously healthy, that the first prescription may be expected to finish the case. You may need to retake the symptoms and prescribe again.

* * *

Again.—At the end of pneumonias and broncho-pneumonias, treat afterwards, so as not to get further attacks.

SOME ASTHMATIC CONDITIONS WITH THEIR REMEDIES

(N.B.—The big-type remedies for Asthma in Children are CHAM., IPEC., NAT. S., PULS., SAMB.)

And N.B.—*Periodically* and *Special hours* are sometimes very important in selecting the remedy for asthma : but allow for summer-time : remedies take no account of this !

Arsenicum .. Worse at night : after midnight.
Worst hour 2 *a.m.* (1 to 2 a.m.).
Periodic attacks : spasmodic.
Worse cold air (rev. of *Puls.*).
Better bending forward (*Kali carb., Kali bi., Lach., Spong.*) ; $>$ rocking (*Kali carb.*).
Leaps from bed ; $<$ lying ; lying impossible (*Kali carb.*).
Worse motion.
Great debility and burning in chest.
Ars. is typically RESTLESS ; ANXIOUS ; IN FEAR.
ANGUISH. *Agonizing fear of death* (ACON.).
Worse for ices.
Better for heat applied and hot drinks.
Hippocratic face.

Kali carb. .. *Worst hours* 2 *to* 3, *and* 3 *a.m.* (*Samb.*), or 2 to 4 a.m.
Better sitting upright, sitting *forward*, head on table on knees ; $>$ rocking (*Ars.*).
Worse lying ; lying impossible (*Ars.*).
Worse drinking ; worse motion.
Sensation of no air in chest.
$<$ draughts (*Hep., Nux*).

Kali ars. .. *Worst hour* 2 *to* 3 *a.m.* (*Kali carb.*).
Worse touch : noise.
Can't get too warm, even in summer.
Worse every other day, or every third day.

Aralia rac. .. Asthma ; loud wheezing with cough.
Worse evening and night ; *after first sleep* ; after short sleep ; after a nap.
Would suffocate if did not sit up.
Expectoration warm and salty.

Sambucus .. *Attacks* 3 *a.m.* (*Kali carb.*). Must spring out of bed (*Ars.*).

Sudden attacks in the night. Child wakes; sits up; *turns blue*; *gasps for breath*; seems almost dying. Then it goes to sleep, to wake up with another attack, again and again.

Asthma with suffocative attacks; may be well when awake, but sleeps into the trouble (*Lach.*, *Aral.*).

Samb. has dry heat when asleep, profuse sweat when awake. (Profuse sweat when asleep *Con.*)

Cuprum .. Spasmodic asthma. Violent sudden attacks, last one to three hours, suddenly cease (*Samb.*).

Dreadful spasmodic breathing. Great rattling.

The more the dyspnœa the more the thumbs will be clenched and fingers cramped.

Spasmodic asthma, and violent dry spasmodic cough: "will be suffocated."

A characteristic: *strong metallic taste* (*Rhus*).

Natrum sulph. *Worst hour,* 4 *to* 5 *a.m.*

Worse wet weather: warm wet (*worse cold dry Acon., Hep., Nux*).

Great dyspnœa; violent attacks.

Profuse greenish purulent expectoration.

Dyspnœa with cough and copious expectoration. Humid asthma.

"If in a child, give it as first remedy."

From damp weather; cold damp dwellings; night air.

Worse lying on left side.

In pneumonia of left lower chest.

Loose cough with soreness and pain through left chest (*Bry.*, with *dry* cough).

Springs up in bed (*Ars.*) and holds chest.

Pain lower left chest (lower right chest, *Ars.*).

Dulcamara .. "Asthma humidum": loose cough and rattling of mucus. *Worse cold, wet weather* (*Nat sul.*).

From suppressed sweat. From going from heat into icy cold. (Its "chronic" is *Sulph.*)

Ipecacuanha .. " Violent degree of dyspnœa, with wheezing and great precordial weight and anxiety."

Asthmatic bronchitis. Suffocates and gags with cough ; spits up a little blood (*Ferr.*).

Has to sit up at night to breathe.

Gasps for air at the open window.

Worse warmth ; better open air (*Puls.*).

" Suffocative cough ; stiffens out, turns red or blue, gags or vomits." KENT.

" Hands and feet drip cold sweat."

Antimonium tart. .. Dyspnœa : must be supported in sitting position.

Great accumulation of mucus with coarse rattling (*Ipec.*, but *Ipec.* has great expulsive power), *filling up with it, with inability to raise it.* Especially in children and old people.

Suffocative shortness of breath. Chest seems full, but less and less is raised (*Zinc.*).

Increasingly weak, drowsy, sweaty and relaxed.

Great drowsiness—almost to coma.

Face pale, or cyanotic.

Nausea and loathing of food. Thirstless.

Irritable : won't be touched or disturbed.

Aconite .. *Aconite* is sudden, violent, acute.

" AGONY : sits straight up : can hardly breathe. Pulse a thread. Sweats with anxiety."

Asthma from active hyperæmia of lungs and brain.

Face red : eyes staring : after emotions.

" A great storm, sweeps over and passes away."

From exposure to cold, dry wind (*Hep.*, *Spong.*).

Fear : anxiety. " Going to die." Restlessness.

Anxious, short, difficult breathing (? with open mouth). (With protruding tongue, *Psor.*)

" Never give *Acon.* where the sickness is borne with calmness and patience."

Ailments from fright, shock, vexation, COLD, DRY WINDS

Spongia .. Cardiac dyspnœa, and the most violent forms of asthma.

Dryness of air passages ; whistling, wheezing, seldom rattling.

Must sit up and bend forward (*Ars., Kali carb.*).

At times, after dyspnœa, white, tough mucus, difficult to expectorate (? has to be swallowed).

Feels *as if breathing through a sponge.*

Worse cold, dry wind (*Acon., Hep*).

Anxiety and fear (*Acon.*).

Kali nit. .. Asthma with violent dyspnœa : rapid gasping breathing ; faintness ; nausea.

Thirsty, but can only drink in sips between breaths.

Dull stitches or burning pain in chest.

External coldness ; internal burning.

Stramonium .. *Violence. Face flushed. Staring look.*

Desire for light and company Cannot bear to be alone.

Worse in dark and solitude.

Yet worse bright light. Looking into light.

Chamomilla .. Asthma *after a fit of anger* (*Ars., Rhus, Ign.*).

Suffocative dyspnœa. "Chest not wide enough."

Windpipe as if tied together with a string (? with or from accumulation of flatus).

Better bending head backwards ; in cold air ; from drinking cold water.

Hard, dry cough ; coughs in sleep (*Arn.. Lach.*, etc.).

Coughs when angry. Impatience of suffering.

Irritable and capricious.

One cheek flushed.

Ferrum .. Asthma after midnight : must sit up.

Better walking slowly about and talking.

Suffocative fits, with warmth of neck and trunk, and limbs cold.

Oppression from orgasm of blood, expectoration of blood (*Ipec.*).

Apis .. .. "Cough impossible, lest something burst", or tear loose. All tense and stretched.
Throat feels strangled. Suffocation: *can't bear anything about throat* (*Lach.*).
Warm room unbearable. Worse warm drinks; heat of fire. *Better cold.*
"As if every breath would be his last."
Worse bending forwards or backwards (reverse of *Kali carb.*, etc.; reverse of *Cham.*).
Attacks with violence and rapidity.

Cactus .. Especially useful in acute attacks.
Chest constricted, squeezed, caged; as if normal movement prevented by an iron band.
Congestion of blood in chest—cannot lie down.
Cardiac asthma (*Aur.*, *Naja.*, *Lach.*).

Lachesis .. May occur in sleep (*Sulph.*) and not wake.
Attacks of suffocation in sleep; when falling asleep; on waking; after sleep (*Samb.*).
Better bending forward (*Ars.*, *Kali carb.*).
Worse covering mouth, nose; touching throat.
Worse motion of arms; after talking.
Wants doors and windows open (*Apis*, *Puls.*)
Useful in cardiac asthma (*Cact.*, *Aur.*, *Naja*).
Typical *Lach.* is purple, suspicious, loquacious.

Naja .. .. "*A great remedy for asthma, especially cardiac asthma*" (*Cact.*, *Aur.*, *Lach.*). "The breathing is so bad that he cannot lie down."
Nervous palpitation; can't speak for choking.
Wakes suffocating, gasping, choking (*Lach.*).
Inability to lie on left side.
"Our most useful remedy in a cardiac state with very few symptoms."

Aurum .. Suffocative fits with spasmodic constriction of chest.
Asthma from congestion of chest.
Face bluish red, cyanotic.
Palpitation: falls down unconscious.
Cardiac dyspnœa.
Deepest depression; hopeless; suicidal.
Worse warm wet (*Nat sul.*, *Lach.*, *Carbo veg.*).

Lobelia .. Extremely difficult breathing from constriction of chest (*Cact.*). Want of breath, *hysterical.*
Asthma with sensation of lump above sternum.
Worse shortest exposure to cold during paroxysm.
Deep breath relieves pressure in epigastrium.
Attack often preceded by prickling all over, even to fingers and toes.
Urine ; deep red. with much red sediment.

Ambra .. .. Difficult breathing with cardiac symptoms.
Asthmatic dyspnœa ; from any little *exertion ; from music ; from excitement.*
" Asthma of old people and children."
Violent spasmodic cough with eructations.
Distension with much flatulence ; < after eating.
Worse presence of others. Can only pass stool, or urinate (*Nat. m.*) when alone.
" Hysteria of old age."

Nux .. .. " Asthma from every disordered stomach."
" *Connected with imperfect and slow digestion.*"
" Something disagrees, and he sits up all night with asthma."
Nux is oversensitive ; to noise, light, least draught. Is *touchy.*
Craves stimulants ; something to brace him up.
" Selects his food, and digests almost none."
Worse morning : after eating ; *from cold air.*

Lycopodium .. *Asthma with great distension.*
Feels will burst : must loosen clothes.
Asthma and dyspnœa in catarrh of chest.
Forehead frowning; alae nasi flap; inability to expectorate (*Zinc.*).
Hours of aggravation (especially of fever), 4 to 8 p.m.

Carbo veg. .. Asthma with great flatulent distension.
Desperate cases of asthma ; patient appears to be dying.
Air hunger : " Fan me ! fan me ! "
Coldness and collapse : cold face, breath.
Asthma *ever since* whooping-cough, etc.

Bromium .. *Asthma of sailors as soon as they go ashore.*
Asthma of fair and fat children, " like *Puls.* but where *Puls.* fails ".
Gasping, wheezing, rattling; spasmodic closure of glottis.
" Can't breath deeply enough."
Must sit up in bed. Constriction.
" Air passages full of smoke."
Peculiar symptom: Coldness in larynx.
Worse from dust.

AMONG HAHNEMANN'S CHRONIC REMEDIES OF CONSTITUTIONS

(HIS " ANTI-PSORICS, ANTI-SYPHILITICS AND ANTI-SYCOTICS ")

that may be needed for Asthma, are

Sulphur .. The more chronic cases with dyspnœa and oppression of chest.
Chest, rattling and heat: *especially* 11 *a.m.*
Sensation of a band, or load.
" Every cold ends in asthma " (" *Dulc.* but the deep acting remedy to follow may be *Sulph.*").
Sulph. is warm; hungry; often craves fat; kicks off the bedclothes or puts feet out.
The " ragged philosopher " type.

Psorinum .. Asthma; anxious dyspnœa and palpitation.
Worse sitting up; *better lying; the wider apart he can keep his arms, the better he breathes.*
Worse in open air.
Thinks he will die; will fail in business.
" A chilly edition of *Sulphur.*"
From suppressed eruptions (*Ars.*, *Sulph.*).

Pulsctilla .. After suppression of rash (*Ars.*), of menses; in hysteria.
Worse evenings; after eating. As if throat and chest constricted; or as if fumes of sulphur had been inhaled. (Full of smoke, *Brom.*)
In the *Puls.* type: mild, weepy, craves sympathy; *intolerant of heat; craves air.* Not hungry; not thirsty; not constipated.
Changeable symptoms, mental and physical.

Silica	" Humid asthma. Coarse rattling. Chest seems filled with mucus ; seems as if he would suffocate. Asthma of old ' sycotics ', or children of such. Pale, waxy, anæmic, with prostration and thirst."—KENT. Asthma from suppressed gonorrhœa (*Thuja*). *Worse cold ; draught ; thunderstorms.* *From checked perspiration* or foot-sweat. Often fetid, or suppressed fetid foot-sweats. Head sweats profusely at night.
Zincum ..	Can't expectorate : if he can is relieved.
Kali bich.	With *ropy mucus* ; stringy, tough, lumpy. Worse cold, damp.
Tuberculinum ..	*In persons with a T.B. history or family history.* " Takes cold every time he gets a breath of fresh air." Yet craves fresh air.
Drosera ..	*Asthma with T.B. history*—or family history ; or after whooping cough. Asthma, where the cough is violent, especially with spasmodic and constricting pains in abdomen, throat, chest, etc. Worse at night.
Thuja	Short breath from mucus in trachea (*Ars.*). from fullness and constriction upper abdomen. Sensation of adhesion of lungs. Drops in sleep. Worse from onions. *Cases that follow vaccination ; or many vaccinations ; or bad vaccination.* *After gonorrhœa*, or offensive green discharges. Greenish expectoration (*Nat sul.*)—in a.m. Copious sweat ; offensive ; pungent ; sweetish. *Peculiar symptom, sweat only on uncovered parts.* Worse cold damp (*Nat sul.*) 3 a.m. (*Kali carb.*). A left side remedy. " Often the chronic of *Ars.*"

Medorrhinum " Asthma : choking from weakness or spasm of epiglottis.

Larynx stopped so that no air can enter.

Only > by lying on face and protruding tongue."

Better seaside (*Brom.*).

Where asthma is connected, even remotely, with gonorrhœa (*Thuja*).

Lueticum .. *Worse at night ; night a dreadful time.*

" In syphilitic-looking kids."

" Attacks only at night, after lying down, or during a thunderstorm."

Aggravation from sunset to sunrise.

Queer sensation, " as if sternum were being drawn to dorsal vertebrae " (as if navel drawn to spine, *Plat.*, *Plumb.*).

COMMON STOMACH AND DIGESTIVE REMEDIES WITH INDICATIONS FOR THEIR USE

Nux .. .. Putrid or bitter taste in mouth, but food and drink taste right.

Repugnance to food.

Want of appetite, and constant nausea.

Dislike to accustomed tobacco smoking and coffee.

Eructation of bitter and sour fluid.

Nausea in morning (*Sep.*)—after dinner :

Qualmish nausea after eating :—

Inclination to vomit.

Contractive, squeezing stomachache.

Contractive pain in abdomen.

Distension and tenderness over stomach.

Flatulent colic upper part of abdomen, in the evening, lying.

Flatulence rises and presses under short ribs.

After a meal, flatulent distension (*Lyc.*) :— immediately after drinking.

Cutting bellyache with inclination to vomit :— as if diarrhœa would occur.

Vomiting of sour smelling and tasting mucus.

Constipation from irregular peristalsis : frequent, ineffectual desire for stool : or passes small quantities with each attempt.

The typical *Nux* patient is :—

Very chilly and worse cold.

Very particular (*Ars.*), careful, zealous.

Gets excited, angry, even spiteful and malicious.

Easily offended.

Anxiety : sadness : scolding crossness.

Oversensitive to noise, slightest noise, strong odours, bright light, music.

Feels everything too strongly—music, singing.

May be suicidal, but afraid to die.

Sensitiveness ; nervousness ; *chilliness.*

Worse dry winds, east wind. Better warm wet weather. (*Acon.*, *Asar.*, *Bry.*, *Caust.*, *Hep.*, *K.c.*, etc.)

Spasms from disorderly peristalsis. Reversed peristalsis.

Pulsatilla .. In mouth, taste, as from putrid flesh, with inclination to vomit.

Dislike to butter—to all fats.

Bilious eructation in the evening.

Diminished taste to all food. Adipsia.

Frequent eructation; taste of what was previously eaten.

Sensation of sickness in epigastric region, especially after eating and drinking.

Inclination to vomit, with rumbling and grumbling in subcostal region.

Aching and drawing pain, stomach, in the morning.

Immediately after supper flatulent colic: flatulence rumbles about painfully, especially in upper part of abdomen.

Flatus discharged with cutting abdominal pain in the morning.

Bellyache as if diarrhœa must ensue, yet only a natural stool occurs. Bellyache after stool.

Urgings to stool—to soft stool with mucus.

Frequent mucus stools with a little blood.

Bad taste: dryness in mouth, with no thirst.

Worse for pastry, cakes, rich, fat foods.

Not hungry: not thirsty: not constipated.

The typical *Pulsatilla* patient is:—

Mild, gentle, yielding: cries easily:—can hardly give her symptoms for weeping.

Sandy hair, blue eyes: inclined to silent grief with submissiveness.

Conscientious about business. Loves steady work, hates hustle.

Changeableness in everything:—in disposition: in the pains that wander from joint to joint: in character of stools—menses, etc.

Pulsatilla feels the heat.

Worse warm room, warm applications.

Better in cool, open air: by walking slowly: but the pains of *Puls.* are accompanied by chilliness.

Loves sympathy and fuss.

" Little suited to persons who form resolutions with rapidity, and are quick in their movements." (The antithesis of *Nux.*)

Sepia .. Nausea. Morning nausea (*Nux*).
Nausea after eating, or, often relieved by eating.
Vomiting of food and bile in the morning.
Nausea and morning sickness of pregnancy. (*Ipec.*)
Peculiar faint, sinking emptiness and goneness at pit of stomach. (*Sulph.*)
Sagging of all viscera. Bearing-down in pelvic organs. (*Lil. tigr.*)
Aversion to food—meat—fat—bread (during pregnancy) to milk, which causes diarrhœa.
Nausea from the smell of food and cooking (*Colch.*, *Ars.*, etc.).

Characteristic symptoms :—
Indifference: indifference to loved ones. (*Phos.*)
Wants to get away : to be alone. (*Nat. mur.*)
Hates fuss and sympathy (*Nat. mur.*) :— talking ; talking of others. Hates noise.
Flashes of heat with perspiration, and faintness.
General relaxation, mental and physical. Faintness—kneeling and standing.
Often, yellow saddle across nose and cheeks.

Ipecacuanha .. Nausea, with empty eructations and great flow of saliva. VOMITING.
Vomiting with a clean tongue.
Persistent nausea : not relieved by vomiting.
Distress as if stomach hung down, relaxed.
Griping, as from a hand in abdomen : esp. about umbilicus.
Diarrhœic, as it were fermented, stools.
Sulky : despises everything: desires that others should not esteem or care for anything.

Phosphorus .. Excessive thirst. Thirst for cold drinks.
Regurgitation of food. Empty eructations.
Nausea. Vomiting. *Burning in stomach.* (*Ars.*)
Thirst for cold water. (Or unable to drink water, even the sight of it causes nausea and vomiting. Must close eyes when bathing.)
Water vomited as soon as warm in stomach.
Goneness, as if stomach had been removed.
Weak, empty, gone sensation whole abdomen.
Stomach pains better for cold food, ice cream.

Phosphorus continued—

Profuse diarrhœa. Blood in stools.

Sphincter relaxed: involuntary stool. Oozing of stool from unclosed sphincter. (Comp. *Apis.*)

The typical Phos. patient is :—

Tall, thin, the artistic type. Fine, dark hair.

Easy bleedings of bright blood. Small wounds bleed much. Bruises easily.

Desire for salt—for cold drinks—for ices.

Fear alone—dark—thunder; "someone-behind."

Relief from rubbing : from a short sleep. (*Sep.*)

Burnings ; stomach, intestines, up spine, between scapulae (*Lyc.*).

(N.B.—*Ars.* burnings everywhere are better for heat ; distinguishes from *Phos.*)

Answers slowly. Indifferent: to loved ones (*Sep.*).

Arsenicum .. *Burning* pain stomach, relieved by heat. (Rev. of *Phos.*).

Burning, violent pain, like red-hot coals.

Epigastrium sensitive to slightest touch.

Great anxiety about epigastric region.

Acute gastritis ; painful vomiting of grass-green solids : or fluids ; or after drinking.

Hæmatemesis, often with black stools.

Violent pains in abdomen with great anguish : rolls about on the floor and despairs of life.

Periodic colic.

Burning in intestines. Abdomen distended.

The great remedy of PTOMAINE POISONING.

The burning pains of *Ars.* are everywhere relieved by *heat.*

Diarrhœa, worse after midnight and after eating, with great prostration.

Vomiting and stool may be simultaneous.

Intense thirst :—for small quantities :—for cold drinks, which disagree.

Characteristic symptoms :—

Great anguish. Anxious impatience.

GREAT ANXIETY.

GREAT RESTLESSNESS.

GREAT PROSTRATION.

Worse at night : after midnight : 1 to 3 a.m.

Worse cold air: cold drinks: cold applications.

Chamomilla .. Putrid breath after dinner. Ptyalism.
The pains are aggravated by eructation.
After a meal distension, with heat of face.
Obstructed flatus. Vomiting of bile.
Typical characteristic symptoms :—
A spiteful, sudden, irritable incivility.
Moans, weeps and howls in sleep.
Shivers at cold air. Redness in one cheek.
Evenings, burning cheeks with transient rigor.
Extreme restlessness, anxious tossing, with tearing pain in abdomen.
Howling on account of a slight, even imaginary insult—perhaps of long ago. (*Staph.*)
Wants this or that; then refuses it, or knocks it away. (*Staph.*)
Oversensitive to pain. "*Unsuited for persons who bear pain calmly and patiently.*"

Sulphur .. Burning in stomach. (*Phos.*, *Ars.*: *Phos.* desires cold drinks, ices; *Ars.* hot drinks.)
Empty, weak sense (stomach) about 11 a.m.
Big appetite: craves food at 11 a.m.
Or, drinks little, but eats much. Worse for milk.
Desires sweets, fat, alcohol, beer and ale.
Liable to early morning diarrhœa.
In the typical *Sulph.* patient, worse for heat: intolerant of clothing and its weight.

Natrum carb. .. "Greedy persons: love sweets and nibbling."
Excessive flatulence: always belching with sour stomachs and rheumatism.
Better eating. When chilly eats, and is warm.
All-gone feeling and pain in stomach, which drives him to eat. (At about 11 a.m. *Sulph.*)
At 5 a.m. so hungry; is forced out of bed to eat something, which also ameliorates the pain.
At 11 p.m. hungry. (11 a.m. *Sulph.*)
Fatigue and weakness; mind and body. Nervous exhaustion. Confusion. Bad tempered.
Cannot digest milk: diarrhœa from milk.
Flatulence and looseness of bowels from starchy foods.
(Patients who take much carbonate of soda to neutralize acidity, with temporary relief. Where indicated acts curatively in potencies.)

Bryonia .. After eating, pressure in the stomach ; it was as if a stone lay there and made him cross.

Stomach extremely sensitive to touch and pressure.

Vomiting : of bile : of what has been eaten.

Mouth dry : tongue white : thirst for large quantities at long intervals. (Comp. *Phos.*)

Patient cannot bear a disturbance of any kind, either mental or physical.

Cannot sit up in bed, as it makes him so sick and faint.

Better lying quite still, and left alone.

Stools dry, hard, as if burnt ; dark.

Nausea on waking : from slightest motion.

Unnatural hunger : of loss of appetite.

Desires acids, sweets, oysters, etc.

Characteristic symptoms :—

Worse for motion. Dryness of mucous membranes. Pains stitching in character, provoked by motion.

Anxious ; irritable.

Dreams of quarrelling, and of business.

Antimonium crud. .. A characteristic symptom is *Thick, milky white coating on tongue.* (*Bry.*)

Deranged stomach from eating what does not agree. Easily disturbed digestion.

Gastric catarrh : nausea and vomiting.

Loathing ; for food and drink.

Desire for acids, pickles. Worse for vinegar.

The typical Ant. crud. patient is : Sentimental : peevish : dislikes to be touched or looked at.

Colocynth .. Frequent vomiting. Vomiting caused by PAIN.

Annoyance or distress may result in extreme pain in any part of body, causing vomiting.

Agonizing pain in abdomen, *only relieved by bending double and pressing hard into abdomen.*

Colics, better heat and pressure. (*Mag. phos.*)

Robinia .. A great remedy for HEARTBURN and acidity.

Everything turns to acid.

" The chief keynote of *Robinia* is acidity, especially if the time of aggravation is night."

Lycopodium .. Fullness, flatulence, distension and bloating of stomach and abdomen (*Arg. nit.*, *Chin.*).

Discomfort, pressure, tenderness, heaviness in stomach after eating a little. *Must loosen clothing*. Very sensitive to pressure there.

Sudden, easy repletion. Loses appetite after first mouthful:—*or*, eating increases appetite.

Acidity—waterbrash—heartburn.

Typical nervous dyspepsia of the brain-worker coming on in afternoon and better in evening after getting home and being at peace—often felt only on leaving office in evening.

Hunger headache.

The typical Lycopodium patient :—

Craves sweets (*Arg. nit.*), hot drinks.

Is worse for cold food, flatulent food, cabbage, onions, oysters.

Is generally better in the morning.

Worse 4-8 *p.m.* is very typical of *Lyc.* In fevers, and pneumonias, also.

Worse afternoons and evenings, better later.

Likes, and fears to be alone. "Wants to be alone with someone in the next room."

One of the "anticipation drugs". Dreads ordeals—speaking in public—singing.

In *Lycopodium* the intellectual predominates over the physical: and it is the intellectual that is apt to suffer—memory, etc.

Argentum nitricum .. Flatulent dyspepsia. (*Lyc.*, *Carbo veg.*, etc.)

Gastric derangements accompanied by belching.

"Belching after every meal, as if stomach would burst; belching difficult, finally air rushes out with great noise and violence."

Irresistible craving for sugar, and sweets.

Fluids "go right through him".

Red painful tip to tongue, papillae prominent.

Characteristic symptoms :—

Apprehension. Anticipation, even to diarrhœa (*Gels.*). Examination funk (*Aeth.*).

Queer fears: of high places: of corners: of walls closing in. Worse shut in anywhere.

Hurried feeling. Must walk fast (*Lil. tigr.*).

Carbo veg. .. Great distension of the abdomen with gas.
Constricting and cramping pains from distension.
Belching, and sour disordered stomach.
Burning in stomach : anxiety : distension.
Constant eructations, flatulence, heartburn, waterbrash.
If he eats or drinks, abdomen feels as if it would burst. (*China*, etc.)
Worse lying down.
Aversion to fats and to milk.
Longs for coffee (*Bry.*), acids, sweet and salt things (*Arg. nit.*).
" Aversion to the most digestible things and the best kinds of food." " Mince pie fiends."
RELIEF FROM BELCHING: headaches better from belching ; rheumatism and other sufferings better from belching. Always belching.
In *Carbo veg.* the face flushes to the roots of the hair after a little wine.
A chilly patient—with air-hunger. COLDNESS.
Burnings. Internal burnings with external coldness.
" Sluggish, lazy, turgid, full, distended, swollen, puffed." " Veins large, relaxed, paralysed."

Carbo animalis The rapid and magical relief of abdominal distension after abdominal operations that follows a dose of *Carbo an.* 200 must be seen to be believed.

Colchicum .. *Colchicum* has great meteoric distension of the abdomen. (*Lyc.*, *Carbo veg.*, *Carbo animalis*, *China.*)
Aversion to food : loathing the sight, and still more the smell of it (*Sep.*, *Ars.*).
The smell of fish, eggs, fat, meats and broth causes nausea even to faintness. Smell of cooking gives extreme nausea.
Great distension of abdomen with gas.
Violent burning in epigastrium.
His suffering seems intolerable to him : external impressions, light, noise, strong smells, contact disturb his temper (*Nux*).
Gouty patients Worse extremes of heat or cold.

Asafœtida .. In dyspepsia, "If you have seen a typical case of *Asaf.* you will wonder where all the air comes from : it comes up in volumes.

"Expulsion of wind like the sound of a small pop-gun going off almost every second."

Loud belching : flatus is not passed down, but all upwards.

Offensive : *Asaf.* is offensive everywhere : "horribly offensive" liquid stools of most disgusting smell.

Puffed, venous, purple faces. *Asaf.* is "fat, flabby and purple".

Hysterical spasm of œsophagus and trachea.

Graphites .. Aversion to animal food and sweet food.

Constrictive or *gnawing* pain in stomach : in empty stomach : with relief from eating.

Pain in upper abdomen. Great distension in abdomen.

The three characteristic symptoms of *Graphites* in stomach complaints are :—

Relief from eating.

Relief from hot food, and drink. (*Chel.*)

Relief from lying down.

Ornithogalum .. Dr. Robert Cooper's little proved, but valuable remedy in gastric ulcer, even malignant.

Distension of stomach and abdomen.

Belchings of mouthfuls of offensive flatus.

Must loosen clothes.

Writhing in agony. Pains worse at night, spread to heart and shoulders.

As if an iron brick were being forced through stomach and chest.

Cooper says, "*Ornithogalum*, in those sensitive to it, goes at once to the pylorus, causes painful spasmodic contraction of it, and distends the duodenum with flatus, its pains being invariably increased when food attempts to pass the pyloric outlet of the stomach." Cooper gave a single drop of the ϕ (allowed to act for several weeks.)

SOME REMEDIES OF CONSTIPATION*

Nux .. .. Constant urging for a stool which never comes; or a small stool is passed with urging, leaving sensation of more remaining behind.

Always as if evacuation were incomplete.

Ineffectual desire for stool.

Tearing and sticking and contracting pain, as from piles in rectum and anus after a meal; and especially *on exerting the mind, and studying.* (Comp. *Caust.*)

Bright blood with fæces, with constriction and contraction during stool.

Nux is the medicine of the sedentary, the studious, the hypersensitive and the *irritable.*

The key to the *Nux* constipation (and colic) is *irregular peristalsis.* Spasmodic constrictions (*Strych.*) which drive the intestinal contents at once backwards and forwards.

Strychnine .. Obstinate constipation, with griping pains (*Nux*).

Bryonia .. Chronic constipation, with severe headache.

No desire; or urging with several attempts before result.

Stool unsatisfactory, after much straining with rush of blood to head. (Nose bleed. *Coff.*)

Stools hard, dark, dry; as if burnt (*Sulph.*).

Stools too thick: too large (*Sulph.*).

Obstruction from induration of fæces.

Distended abdomen; rumbling and cutting, yet obstinate constipation. After stool long-continued burning in rectum (*Thuja*).

Bryonia is irritable (*Nux*): everywhere DRY: < motion; white tongue; great thirst.

Natrum mur. .. Constipation: obstinate retention of stool.

Irregular; hard, dry; on alternate days.

During M.P. Anus contracted, or torn.

Knows not whether flatus or stool escapes; dryness of mucous linings, with watery secretion in other parts.

Nat. mur. is irritable; weepy; hates fuss.

Craves salt. Aversion to fats; to bread.

* N.B.—"To every action there is an equal and contrary reaction," and most of the great remedies of constipation are also great remedies for diarrhœa.

Sulphur .. Stool with " something left behind " (*Nux*). Hard, as if burnt (*Bry*.). Extreme constipation.
Stool every 2, 3 or 4 days, hard and difficult.
Stools large, painful : held back from pain.
Sulphur is a warm patient ; hungry about 11 a.m. ; kicks off the clothes at night ; puts feet out ; hungry for fat, for everything.
Red orifices ; acrid excoriating discharges.

Lac deflor. .. Large painful stools (*Sulph.*). Dry (*Bry.*).
Invincible constipation with chronic headache.
Constipation *with coldness* ; cannot get warm.
Lac deflor. is supersensitive to cold : to least draught.
Complaints from putting hands into cold water.
Worse milk : aversion to milk.

Graphites .. Stool large, hard, knotty, in agglomerated masses, mixed with *tough slimy mucus.*
" Sometimes great quantities of mucus with hard stool, as much as a cupful of thick, tough, stinking mucus."
Hæmorrhoids with burning rhagades.
Itching ; smarting, sore pain at anus.
(Characteristics of *Graph.*) Obesity ; relief from eating ; from hot foods and drinks.
Skin troubles, with sticky oozing.

Collinsonia .. Obstinate constipation with hæmorrhoids.
Piles with constipation (even diarrhœa) bleeding, or blind and protruding ; feeling of sticks (*Æsc.*), gravel, or sand in rectum.
Chronic, bleeding, painful hæmorrhoids.
Very constipated, with colic.

Æsculus .. Hard, dry, difficult stools.
Rectum dry, hot : " full of small sticks."
Knife-like pains shoot up.
Severe lumbo-sacral backache.
Stool followed by fullness in rectum, and intense pain for hours (*Nit. ac., Aloe, Ign., Sul.,* etc.).
Painful, purple external piles, with burning (*Collinsonia's* bleed more).
(A queer sensation, a bug crawling from anus.)

Nitric acid .. Pain with stool as if something would be torn.
Sticking pain (rectum) and spasmodic constriction (anus), during stool, and lasting many hours after (*Æsc.*).
Fissures and hæmorrhoids. Great pain after stool (even soft stool) *lasts for hours.*
Burning in anus. Itching in rectum.
Nitric acid affects especially parts where skin and mucous membrane join.
Its pains are *splinter pains,* worse for contact.
Nitric acid patient is very like the *Sepia* patient, but loves fat and salt (unlike *Sepia*).

Arsenicum .. Constipation with tenesmus: with pain in bowels. (More characteristic, diarrhœa and purging.)
Hæmorrhoids: with stitching pain walking and sitting, *but not at stool:* pain like slow pricks of a hot needle: protrude like coals of fire.
Burning pains anus, *relieved by heat.*
Diarrhœa alt. constipation—in an *Ars.* patient, with restlessness, anxiety and prostration.

Opium .. Almost unconquerable chronic constipation.
Constipation from inaction, or paresis—for 6 or 8 weeks, with loss of appetite.
Peristaltic action entirely suspended: even reversed peristalsis with fæcal vomiting.
Fæces protrude and recede (*Sanic., Sil., Thuja*).
Or, stool invol. after a fright—from paresis.
Stools hard, round, black balls; obstruction from indurated fæces.
Opium has the most startling opposite conditions. Inveterate constipation—persistent diarrhœa. Coma, to complete insensibility—exalted sensibility, "Can hear the flies walk on the walls, and distant clocks chiming"; sleepy but cannot sleep; hears noises not generally noticed.

Stramonium .. Stool and urine suppressed.
Obstinate constipation.
Cannot bear solitude, or *darkness.*
Face red and bloated.
Painlessness with most complaints.

Plumbum .. Obstinate habitual constipation.

Paresis of intestines. Cannot strain at stool: cannot expel the fæces.

Obstruction from induration, from impaction.

Urging and terrible pain from constriction and spasm of anus ("Where *Platina* fails").

Violent colic. Abdominal wall "drawn to spine by a string" (*Plat.*).

As if abdomen retracted and drawn towards spine: retraction both objective and subjective.

Boat-shaped abdomen.

Stools like sheep's dung: balls in conglomerate masses.

Typical *Plumbum* has slowness; torpor; emaciation: must stretch for hours.

A keynote, "Paralysis with hyperæsthesia."

Alumen (*Alum*) Ineffectual urging: or several days without desire for stool. No ability to pass stool.

Long useless straining, then after many days stool is passed—an agglomeration of little hard balls.

After stool, sensation as if rectum still full (*Nux*).

Cramps and colic: sensation of abdomen drawn to navel (*Plumb.*, *Plat.*).

Hæmorrhoids ulcerate: prolonged suffering after stool (*Nit. ac.*, *Æsc.*, etc.).

Antidote to lead poisoning: and for lead constipation.

Symptoms very similar to lead.

Platina .. Difficult stool: sticks to anus and rectum like putty.

Frequent urging with inability to strain at stool (*Alum.*).

Inveterate constipation and unsuccessful urging (*Nux*).

Stool, hard, scanty, or sticky. Undigested.

Peculiar symptom of *Platina*. Feels tall: everything looks small to her.

Mentally also, pride, and looks down on others.

Another curious symptom, navel feels retracted by a string (*Plumb.*).

Alumina .. Inactivity rectum and bladder..
Great straining to pass even a soft stool.
Must strain at stool to urinate.
No desire for and no ability to pass stool with large accumulation. Great straining.
Rectum seems paralysed: has not strength to press the contents out.
Stool hard, knotty, covered with mucous, or soft, clayey, adhering to parts (*Plat.*).

Patients are asking for help in regard to a curious and very obstinate form of constipation, evidently from the use of aluminium cooking pots, because it promptly disappears when these are discarded, the bowels resuming their normal functioning. This is how these aluminium sensitives describe their constipation :

No desire whatever for stool.
No physical inconvenience from " No stool for days, even to a fortnight ! "
" Nothing seems to go down lower than the upper left abdomen " (the splenic flexure).
" Rectum seems not only inactive, but empty."

Veratrum alb. .. Digestion good; but defæcation almost impossible from inertia of rectum.
No desire for stool: which is large, hard, in round black balls. No expulsive action.
Verat. is cold: sweats much. Cold sweat on forehead.

Causticum .. Frequent ineffectual efforts to stool, with pain, anxiety and redness of face (with nose-bleed, *Coff.*).
Rectum inactive: fills with hard fæces, which pass involuntarily and unnoticed (*Aloe*).
Passes little balls unnoticed.
Stool tough and shiny: shines like grease.
Passes better standing.
Hæmorrhoids: impeding stool: swell; itch; stitch; worse walking; thinking of them; preaching or straining voice. (Comp. *Nux.*)
Causticum is intensely sympathetic with suffering.
A remedy of local paralysis. Urine involuntary when sneezing or coughing. Enuresis in children.

Phosphorus .. Inveterate constipation.

Fæces slender, long, dry, tough and hard, voided with difficulty. "May be compared to a dog's stool in appearance and manner of evacuation."

Paralysis of bowel, so that it is impossible to strain at stool (*Alum.*).

(*Phos.* has also a paralytic condition in which anus stands open (*Apis*) and stool oozes out.)

Hæmorrhage from bowel.

Typical *Phos.* is the slender, artistic type : fears dark—alone—thunder ; craves salt, ices, cold drinks : Chilly (*Apis*, warm).

Apis .. .. Constipation : sensation (abdomen), "something tight, will break if effort used." (See *Plumb.*, *Plat.*)

Bowels seem to be paralysed.

No stool for days—for a week.

Or stools occur with every motion of the body as if anus were constantly open (*Phos.*).

Anus swelled : oozing blood.

Apis feels the heat ; cannot stand heat.

Is *thirstless*. (Reverse of *Phos.*)

Its pains everywhere are STINGING and burning.

It is one of the remedies for dropsical conditions.

Conium .. Ineffectual urging ; hard stool.

Inability to strain at stool ; inability to expel contents because of the paralytic weakness of all the muscles that take part in expulsion.

Strains so much at stool that uterus protrudes.

At every stool tremulous weakness and palpitation.

Conium has dizziness ; numbness ; paralytic weakness, mental and physical.

A queer symptom : sweats copiously during sleep—on merely closing eyes.

Ruta .. .. Large stool evacuated with difficulty, as from loss of peristaltic action of rectum (*Alum.*, *Phos. ac.*).

Frequent urging to stool, but only rectum prolapses (*Ign.*). The slightest stooping, or crouching down, caused rectum to protrude.

Sepia	Ineffectual urging : or days with no urging, then the effort as if in labour. Stool not hard, but much straining. Constipation of pregnancy. " A ball in rectum " ; fullness, prolapse. Straining and sweating with stool. *Sepia* is dull and indifferent, has heaviness and sagging of all viscera ; tendency to prolapse.
Mezereum ..	Stool hard as stone : threatens to split anus : dark hard balls ; much painless straining. During stool prolapsus ani with constriction : it is difficult to replace. Before stool copious discharge of fetid flatus. " Frightened in the stomach " (*Calc.*, *Kali c.*, *Phos.*).
Cocculus ..	Paralytic condition rectum. Inability to press at stool, or to evacuate stool. Disposition to stool ; but peristalsis wanting in upper intestines. Inability to use muscles of evacuation. After stool violent tenesmus, even to fainting. Nausea at thought or smell of food (*Colch.*, ***Ars.***, *Sep.*).
Lachesis ..	Stool lies in rectum without urging. Drawing and constriction of anus (*Lyc.*). Pain extends from anus to navel. *Lach.* cannot bear touch (abdomen or throat). Foul stools. Piles, worse coughing. *Lach.* sleeps into aggravation of symptoms. *Lach.* is purplish and loquacious.
Calcarea ..	Old, lingering, stubborn constipation. Constipated stool white, like chalk. Patient generally better when constipated. (Diarrhœa, and no worse, or better, *Phos. ac.*) Hard, difficult, light-coloured stool. Undigested stool (*Chin.*). Smells like bad eggs. *Sour* eructations, vomit, stool, sweat. Head and neck sweat at night (*Sil.*, *Sanic.*). Coldness of single parts : sensation of cold damp stockings (*Sepia*).

Staphisagria .. Frequent desire for stool with scanty evacuations, hard or soft. Difficult evacuations.

Staph. is sensitive, angry, petulant. Dwells on old injuries, insults: on things done by himself or others.

Thuja .. .. Difficult evacuation after 2, 3, or 8 days; subsequent burning in anus (*Bry.*).

Moisture at anus. Anus fissured; painful; surrounded with flat warts.

Violent pains compel cessation of effort (*Sul.*).

Stool recedes (*Sil., Sanic.*).

Sensation of something alive in abdomen(*Croc.*).

Great remedy for the much vaccinated, or the "worse for vaccination".

Silica .. .. Stool of hard lumps: scanty; difficult; after urging and straining till abdominal walls sore. Stool already protruded slips back ("bashful stool") (*Thuja, Sanicula*).

Much urging, but inability to expel (*Alum.* no urging)

Straining with suffering and sweating head.

Silica is chilly; great want of self-confidence.

Head is apt to sweat in sleep (*Calc., Sanic.*).

Sanicula .. No desire for stool till a large accumulation.

Stool hard, impossible to evacuate; of greyish white balls (Comp. *Calc.*).

Stool, partly expelled, recedes (*Sil., Thuja*).

Odour of stool persists, despite bathing (*Sul.*).

Children, look old, dirty, greasy, brownish.

Head sweats profusely at night (*Sil., Calc.*).

Lycopodium .. No desire for days: yet rectum full, no urging.

Stool hard, difficult, small and incomplete.

Spasmodic constriction of anus preventing stool.

Lycopodium is always belching: distension of abdomen; has to loosen clothing.

Desire for sweets: hot drinks; < 4-8 p.m.

Magnesia mur. The keynote for *Mag. mur.* is *worse from salt:* salt food, salt baths, sea air.

Constipation at the sea side.

Stools dry: crumble at anus.

Brief Pointers in Acute Uncomplicated Diarrhœa

(*Compare Intestinal Conditions and Colic : also Cholera Infantum.*)

Camphor .. A couple of drops of tincture on sugar, repeated in a quarter-hour, if necessary, will generally cure acute diarrhœa.

N.B.—Keep Camphor away from other medicines.

Colocynth .. *Doubled up* with colic.

Pain only relieved by *bending double*, and *pressing into abdomen.*

Cuprum .. Diarrhœa associated with *cramps*. Cramps in abdomen, in fingers, calves, feet.

China .. .. *Painless* diarrhœa. Much flatulence.

Passes undigested food.

Veratrum alb. .. Coldness.

COLD SWEAT.

Profuse evacuations with *profuse, cold sweat.*

Cold sweat on forehead.

Arsenicum .. After eating ices ; or cold drinks when hot.

After *tainted meat and foods* or fruit.

Relentless vomiting and purging.

THE GREAT REMEDY FOR PTOMAINE POISONING.

Carbo veg. .. Diarrhœa from bad food (like *Ars.*) but with more distension.

Podophyllum .. Excessive evacuations, very offensive : with much flatus, and much colic.

Phos. acid .. Like *Podoph.* But not offensive, and no colic.

Aloe .. .. Stool urgent : at once after eating.

Dulcamara .. Diarrhœa from DAMP, OR DAMP COLD.

Baptisia .. Influenzal diarrhœa : very sudden onset : with prostration, drowsiness, putridity.

Pyrogen .. Rapidly curative in sudden, exhausting summer diarrhœa ; profuse, watery, painless : extreme restlessness.

SOME MEDICINES OF ACUTE INTESTINAL CONDITIONS, COLIC AND DIARRHŒA

Aconite

Abdominal conditions—*sudden* attacks—after exposure to violent cold : after being chilled.

Pressive weight in stomach—in hypochondria : swollen distended abdomen, like ascites.

Flatulent colic in hypogastrium, as if had taken a flatus-producing purgative.

Abdomen burning hot, tense, tympanitic, sensitive to least touch ; cutting pains ; fever ; anguish.

Before or after diarrhœa, nausea and perspiration.

Stools white (*Calc.*) : like chopped spinach : slimy, bloody, with tenesmus.

Catarrhal inflammatory troubles of all the viscera ; hepatitis, *but "with the Aconite restlessness, awful tortures of anxiety, fear of death ; red face, glassy eyes ; great thirst"*.

Belladonna ..

Abdominal pains, violent ; *come and disappear suddenly*. Are squeezing ; clawing ; as if griped by nails ; violent pinchings.

"Violent colic, intense cramping pain, face red as fire."

Tenderness of abdomen, *worst least jar*.

Frequent urging to stool, little or no result (*Nux*). Spasmodic contraction of sphincter ani.

Great pain in ileo-cæcal region : cannot bear slightest touch, even of bedclothes (early appendicitis. Local external applications to abort).

Typical *Bell.* has red, hot face ; big pupils : is sensitive to pressure, draughts, jar.

Dulcamara ..

Colic, such as is usually caused by *cold wet weather*.

Sudden attacks of diarrhœa in cold, wet weather.

Colic as if diarrhœa would occur.

Yellow watery discharge twice in a day, with tearing—cutting colic before every evacuation, as after taking cold.

Ætiology : *cold wet weather*.

Bryonia .. *Stitching* and bursting pains (*Kali carb.*)—as if stomach would burst—as if abdomen would burst. (*Aloe.*)

Effects of disordered stomach; taking cold; having been overheated: from cold drinks when heated. (*Ars.*)

Worse from pressure. (Everywhere else *Bry.* has relief from pressure: not in stomach or abdomen.)

Lies still, knees up to relax abdominal muscles.

Unable to move; breathing shallow; since movement increases the pain. (*Ars.* rolls about and is never still.)

Does not want to talk, or think.

Diarrhœa preceded by cutting in abdomen.

Nux .. .. Qualmishness: after eating.

Qualmish, anxious, nauseated, as after a violent purge. Cutting colic with qualmishness.

Pressure as from a stone in stomach. (*Bry.*)

Violent gastric symptoms.

Flatulent colic here and there in abdomen.

Better rest, sitting or lying.

Anxious, ineffectual desire for stool.

Frequent ineffectual desire for stool after evacuation.

Sensation after stool as if some remained behind.

Constipation: or, " The *Nux* diarrhœa consists of small, mostly mucous stools, with straining."

The *Nux* abdominal condition, pains and stools are due to *irregular peristalsis*. And here *Nux* cures.

Nux is irritable and hypersensitive. (*Cham.*)

Opium .. Violent griping in abdomen with constipation.

Cutting in abdomen.

Pain, pressive, as if intestines would be cut to pieces.

Almost unconquerable chronic constipation.

Constipation for weeks of small, hard dark-brown pieces.

No activity. Rectum fills with hard, black balls. (*Plumb.*)

Colocynth .. Violent griping, cutting, twisting, colic pains about umbilicus; frequent discharge of flatus, with relief.

Deep stitches, in right, or left flank.

Abdomen greatly distended, and painful.

Violent pain in abdomen, worst three fingers' breadth below umbilicus, *obliging him to bend over*. Pinching pain as if bowels were pressed inwards, with distortion of face and eyes: *pain is only relieved by pressing on bowels and doubling up*.

Pinching, "Bowels squeezed between stones."

Very violent colic in paroxysms, obliging him to bend forward. . . "unexpressible colic".

Frequent excessive urging to stool.

Stannum .. Pains slowly increase till their acme, then slowly decrease: leaving a sensation of a hole.

Intestinal obstruction.

Magnesia phos. Spasms of cramp in stomach, nipping, griping, pinching, with belching which does not relieve (*Coloc.* which does relieve).

Flatulent colic, forcing patient to bend double (*Coloc.*), *better from warmth* and rubbing.

Cramps in abdomen: violent cutting pains, has to scream out. Better bending double, pressing with hand (*Coloc.*), warmth.

Cannot lie on back stretched out.

Mag. phos. is worse cold air, cold water, touch: better heat, warmth, pressure, bending double (*Coloc.*).

Spasmodic conditions, > by heat and pressure.

(In relief from heat comp. *Ars. Ars.* has *burning* pains relieved by heat. *Mag. phos. cramping* (not burning) relieved by heat.)

Dioscorea .. Constant distress (umbilical and hypogastric regions), with severe cutting colic pains every few minutes in stomach and small intestines.

Griping in umbilical region: in lower bowels.

Rumbling in bowels and passing large quantities of flatulence.

Worse doubling up (op. of *Colocynth*).

Chamomilla .. Violent retching. Covered with cold sweat.

Cutting colic. Nightly diarrhœa with colic. Doubles up (*Coloc.*) and screams. *A wind colic.*

White slimy diarrhœa with colic: or painless green watery diarrhœa. Stool hot, smelling like rotten eggs. (*Cham.*)

Cham. is frantically irritable: impatient: oversensitive (*Nux*).

Uncivil irritability: snappish: admits it.

Excessive sensibility to pain.

Ailments from anger.

The colic of teething babies: want this and that, and then push it away.

China .. Flatulent colic (*Carbo veg.*, *Lyc.*, *Colch.*, etc.).

Abdomen feels packed full: not better by eructations. (Rev. of *Carbo veg.*)

Diarrhœa generally *painless*; watery with much flatus; *passes undigested food.* Very debilitating.

Cocculus .. Violent cramp in stomach.

Griping in upper abdomen; takes breath away.

Flatulent colic about midnight: wakened by incessant accumulation of flatus, which distends abdomen, giving oppressive pain here and there. Passed without much relief, while new flatus collects for hours.

Lies on first one side and then the other for relief.

Says, "Abdomen full of sharp sticks or stones." "Intestines pinched between sharp stones."

Worse for loss of sleep; night-nursing; overwork.

Worse for thought or smell of food. (*Colch.*, *Sep.*, *Ars.*)

Colchicum .. Very great distension of abdomen: tympanitic; Griping pain. (Membraneous colitis.)

A *Colch.* keynote, very sensitive to smell of food. (In diarrhœa, etc.)

Nausea from smell of food (*Ars.*, *Cocc.*, *Sep.*).

Lycopodium .. Abdomen bloated: distension in epigastrium after a meal.

Flatulence after eating: fermentation, rumbling, rattling, relieved by discharge of flatus.

Incarcerated flatus, with pressure up and down with frequent urging to urinate.

Immediately p.c., full, distended and tense.

So full cannot eat. Hungry, but first mouthful fills him up.

Cannot bear weight or pressure of clothes (*Lach.*). *Must loosen clothing at waist.*

Always belching. (*Asaf.*) Colicky pains.

"*Lyc.*, *Carbo veg.* and *China* are the most flatulent of remedies. *China* bloats whole abdomen, *Carbo v.* the upper part, and *Lyc.* the lower part."

Lyc. desires sweets and hot drinks: its bad hours are from 4-8 p.m. Suffers from anticipation.

Pulsatilla .. Eructations: of gas: tasting of food: of bitter fluid in the evening: like bad meat, or rancid tallow. With qualmishness.

Qualmish nausea, especially after eating and drinking.

Vomiting of food eaten long before.

Extremely disordered stomach.

Sensation of having eaten too much.

Food rises into mouth (*Phos.*) as if would vomit.

Pain, gnawing, scraping in stomach.

Colic, rumbling and gurgling in abdomen.

Flatus moves about in abdomen, rumbling and griping: worse in bed. Colic at night.

Cutting in abdomen: a stone sensation.

Diarrhœa green as bile at night, with movements in intestines before every stool.

Watery diarrhœa at night: discharge of green mucus.

Frequent evacuations of only mucus.

Typical *Pulsatilla* is tearful: must have air: is worse for heat—hot rooms.

(A curious symptom: one-sided sweat, of face or body.)

Carbo veg. .. Great accumulation of flatus in stomach.
Distension. All food turns to "wind".
Colic. Cramps in bowels and stomach.
Relief from belching. (Opp. *Lyc.* and *China.*)
Even headaches and rheumatic pains relieved by belching.

Argentum nit. .. Craves sugar: yet cannot digest it: it acts like physic and brings on diarrhœa.
Excessive flatulency.
Vomiting and purging at the same time: "gushing out both ways with great exhaustion." (*Ars.* also has this.)
Diarrhœa as soon as he drinks.

Kali carb. .. Severe pain in stomach. Will not tolerate the least amount of food: vomiting and fainting. Bloated.
Stomach as if cut to pieces.
Stitching in abdomen. (*Bry.*)
Violent cutting in intestines, must sit bent over pressing with both hands (*Coloc.*, *Mag. phos.*) or lean far back for relief. (*Dios.*)
Colic, cutting pains with distension, doubling him up (*Coloc.*). Tremendous flatulence.
Great coldness with pains. (*Verat.*)
(For cases when *Coloc.* only relieves temporarily: in colics with periodicity: that recur.)
Kali carb.'s time aggravation is 3 a.m.

Plumbum .. Nausea. Constant vomiting.
Extremely violent pains, umbilical region; shoot to other parts of abdomen. Partly relieved by pressure.
At times so violent, patient almost wild, tosses about bed: presses fists into abdomen, says must go to stool.
Abdominal muscles forcibly retracted, till navel seems to press against spine (*Plat.*). Boat-shaped abdomen.
Violent colic: screams and assumes the strangest postures for relief.
Excessive pain in abdomen, radiates to all parts of body. Hyperæsthesia.
Stools hard and scanty: like balls. (*Opium.*)

Arsenicum .. Violent pains in abdomen. Rolls about on the floor and despairs of life.

Excessive pain in abdomen, causing *great anguish and despair of life.*

Burning in intestines. Burning lancinations. Burning in intestines as from coals of fire.

Better from the application of hot things: (the *Ars.* burnings are relieved by heat).

Vomiting of everything taken: *heat relieves:* temporary relief from hot drinks.

In the abdomen all the symptoms of peritonitis. Great distension—a tympanitic state. Cannot be handled or touched, yet cannot keep still. Great exhaustion.

Ptomaine poisonings.

Excessive vomiting and purging: often simultaneous. Tongue dry—even black.

Stools bloody—watery—or black and horribly offensive.

Veratrum alb. .. One of Hahnemann's three cholera medicines. Here the indications are: *Excessive vomiting and purging, excessive cold sweat, with exhaustion.*

Gastric catarrh, great weakness, cold, sinking feeling.

Cold feeling in abdomen, or burning, as from hot coals. (*Ars.*)

Coldness of discharges: coldness of body: coldness as if blood were ice-water. Internal chill runs from head to toes.

Profuse watery discharges.

Cold sweat: especially cold sweat on forehead.

Abdomen distended: "intestines twisted into a knot."

"Flatulent colic: attacks bowels here and there, and the whole abdomen. The longer the flatus is retained, the more difficult its expulsion."

During profuse, watery stools chilliness and shivering, and extraordinary exhaustion.

"Forehead covered with cold sweat, coldness in spots over body: extremities cold as death. Full of cramps. Looks as if he would die."

Violent evacuations upwards and downwards.

Mercurius cor.	Peculiar bruised sensation about cæcum and along transverse colon. Tender to pressure. Appendicitis. (*Bell.*) Painful bloody discharges (from rectum) with vomiting. Tenesmus, persistent, incessant, with insupportable cutting, colicky pains. Diarrhœa—dysentery—*with terrible straining before, with, and after stool.* *Merc. cor. is almost specific for dysentery.* Very distressing tenesmus, getting worse and worse: nothing passed but mucus tinged with blood.
Cuprum ..	Violent intermittent colic. Violent diarrhœa. Violent pressure at stomach. Spasmodic motions of abdominal muscles. Abdomen tense, hot and tender to touch. Cramps—start fingers and toes. One of Hahnemann's *Cholera* medicines. (i.e. *Camphor, Cuprum, Verat. alb.*)
Camphor ..	Everything vomited. Tongue blue and cold: breath cold. (*Carbo veg.*) Yet there may be internal burning—or cold sensation in stomach and abdomen. Violent pain in stomach with anguished face (*Ars.*): feels he must die (*Ars.*). *In cold stage wants to uncover: in hot phase to be kept warm.*
Baptisia ..	Gastric and abdominal 'flu, with drowsiness. Fullness in abdomen with rumbling and diarrhœa. Sudden onset: rapid "typhoid" conditions. Drowsy and stupid. *Putrid conditions and discharges: fetid, exhausting diarrhœa,* causing excoriation.
Lachesis ..	Painful distension of abdomen. *Can bear no pressure,* the surface nerves are so sensitive. Worse everywhere from pressure or constriction, throat, neck, chest, abdomen. Lies on back with clothes lifted from abdomen. *Lach. sleeps into an aggravation.*

Sulphur ..	Inflation of abdomen with wind. Grumbling and gurgling in bowels. Painless diarrhœa driving out of bed about 5 a.m. Morning diarrhœa : must go immediately. Anus red. Stool acrid. Typical *Sulph.* patient, is starving about 11 a.m. Hungry an hour before usual meal. Burning soles at night, puts them out (*Cham.*, *Med.*, *Puls.*). Loves fat and sweet things. Worse after sleeping—eating—bathing. *Sulph.* " a chronic remedy " is speedily curative in acute conditions in a *Sulphur* patient.
Aloe	Has to hurry to stool immediately after eating and drinking. (*Arg. nit.*) Colicky pain in bowels from eating and drinking. Diarrhœa from drinking beer. Fullness : distension as if abdomen would burst. Loud rumbling, heard all over the room. Gurgling and spluttering stools. Early morning diarrhœa (*Sulph.*). [A queer symptom, peculiar to *Aloe* :—may strain in vain, and presently a large formed stool slips out unnoticed. Or, fæces involuntary after stool.] " Jelly-fish stools." " Lumpy, watery stools."
Croton tig. ..	Flatulence followed by urgent desire for stool. *Evacuations sudden : shot out of rectum :* of a dirty green colour and offensive. Worse least food or drink. Swashing in intestines as from water.
Raphanus ..	Post-operative intestinal stasis. Bits of intestine blown up here and there. Paralytic ileus. (*Thuja.*) Accumulation and retention of flatus, no relief up or downwards.
Thuja	Protrusion here and there as from a child's arm. " Something alive in abdomen." (*Crocus.*)

EPIDEMIC DIARRHŒA OF CHILDREN : CHOLERA INFANTUM.

Here Homœopathy, so rapidly curative in acute disease, gives splendid results. But, of course, the remedy must be, not only a "homœopathic remedy", but *homœopathic*. It must be a remedy not only of diarrhœa (every drug that can cause diarrhœa is that), but it must fit the peculiarities of *this* case of diarrhœa; otherwise there is nothing doing. One diarrhœa remedy will not do for another. A medicine, to cure, must be able to produce just the condition we seek to cure : outside that, no contact is made. Some people might express it, that the vibrations of disease and remedy must be identical—we seem to be approaching that idea. But, however that may be, and whether it is expressed in terms of electricity, or vibration, or Homœopathy, so urgent are these cases that one needs their remedies at one's finger-tips, or in portable form for easy reference.

But outside the giving of the remedy, the child should be kept warm, and, in desperate cases, when seen first at almost the last gasp, we must remember that the infant may have lost more fluid than it can afford to lose and live. Here fluid cannot be retained *per rectum*, and many a small life may be saved by slow absorption of warm saline, subcutaneously.

It is Hahnemann's teaching that not only do different cases of the same disease demand, by their peculiar symptoms, different remedies, but also that different epidemics of the same disease ask for different remedies. And here, in epidemic work, by carefully collecting the symptoms of several individual cases, the *genus epidemicus* may disclose itself in its entirety, and may be fitted with a medicine which will be found to cure the majority of the cases, even where they do not all display the complete disease picture. But it is also found that in such epidemics the cases not covered by the epidemic remedy are often very difficult to match.

One remembers an epidemic when a number of children came to Out-patients with a diarrhœa that was painless, while the stools contained much indigested food. Here *China* quickly put matters right. *Colocynth*, with its agonies of abdominal pain, that double the victim up, again and again, and demand pressure, would have been useless. To discover the epidemic remedy, whatever it may be, makes prescribing easy and most satisfactory, until—which is possible !—the type changes—perhaps with the weather, when a fresh remedy has to be sought.

Mercurius cor.	Dysenteric, scanty stools with blood, and *incessant straining, not relieved by stool.*
Cuprum ..	Diarrhœa with *intense cramps.*
Ipecacuanha ..	Violent simultaneous vomiting and purging (*Ars.*). *Great nausea* with pale face and clean tongue. Stools like a mass of fermented yeast.
Podophyllum ..	Diarrhœa, *stools profuse, offensive,* gushing, seem to drain the infant dry. Painless. Stools larger than expected from food taken. Desire for much water, none for food. Marked gurgling. Retching ; vomits green froth or food. Diarrhœa worse in the morning : in teething babies. Head sweats much during sleep. Rectum may prolapse with soft stool.
China ..	Painless and undigested stools: copious: putrid.
Mercurius ..	Slimy, even bloody diarrhœa : with straining : followed by chilliness. Profuse perspiration which does not relieve. Mouth offensive. Salivation with intense thirst. Tongue large, flabby, tooth-notched. Worse at night : from warmth of bed. Thighs and legs cold and clammy, esp. at night.
Phosphorus ..	Characteristic of *Phos.* thin stool oozes from open anus. Increased urine with diarrhœa. Or stools large and forcible. In the tall *Phos.* child : with fear alone—in the dark : thirst for cold water.
Pulsatilla ..	Colic and diarrhœa worse at night. No two stools alike. Relief from fresh air. Mild, weepy children.
Phosphoric acid	Long-continued diarrhœa, with cramps (*Cup.*). Stools white (*Calc.*), watery, painless, profuse. Pallid, weary, weedy children.
Sulphur ..	Intolerant of heat: kicks off the clothes : hungry : craves for fat. Great hurry. Stool acrid. Leaves anus red.

Baptisia .. Taken *suddenly* and frightfully ill. Sudden attack of diarrhœa and vomiting, with a rapidly typhoid condition.
Fœtid, exhausting diarrhœa, with excoriation.
Odour of stool putrid, penetrating.
Tongue swollen : dark : dry : yellow or brown centre : cracked : ulcerated. (Comp. *Ars.*)
Drowsy, as if drugged, or intoxicated.
If roused, begins to speak, then fades back into stupor.
Dark, red, besotted countenance. Hot—flushed —dusky. Influenzal cases.

Veratrum .. *Diarrhœa with violent vomiting: vomit—stools—sweat very profuse.*
Thirst for much cold water, for acid drinks.
Exhaustion after each spell.
Cold sweat on forehead from least movement.

Carbo veg. .. Putrid, or bloody, offensive stools. Acrid.
Face pale, or greenish.
Abdomen distended : in lumps.
Emission of large quantities of flatus.
Skin damp, cold : tongue and breath cold.
(The homœopathic veritable corpse-reviver.)

* * *

Aconite .. From *low temperature* in room.
From chill or fright.
Green, watery, frequent stools.
Dry heat of body : dry tongue, restlessness and fear. Fear of death.

Bryonia .. Diarrhœa *from hot weather,* and the return of hot weather.
Vomits food immediately.
Colic, with thirst for big drinks, and lumpy diarrhœa.
Dry, parched lips.

Dulcamara .. Every *change of weather to cool,* brings diarrhœa.
(Rev. of *Bry.*) Exposure to cold, or damp.
Changeable stools.
Nausea with desire for stool.
Colic before and during stool. Prostration.

Croton tig. .. Yellow, watery stools, *come out like a shot,* while nursing, or immediately after.
Any food or drink starts this sudden stool.
A hand pressing on umbilicus produced protrusion of rectum.

Aloe .. .. Hurry to stool after eating or drinking.
Inability to retain—or to evacuate—stool.
(Straining may fail to produce stool, which presently slips out unnoticed.)

Ignatia .. Colic and diarrhœa in breast-fed infants, whose mothers are suffering from grief.

Kreosote .. Cholera infantum in teething infants, with *very painful dentition* : gums painful, spongy.
Severe cases, with incessant vomiting, and stools cadaveric-smelling.
Intensely irritable (*Cham.*).
(See HOMŒOPATHY, June, 1934, pp. 178-9.)

Chamomilla .. Watery, greenish stools : excoriating : smell like rotten eggs.
Very cross (*Kreos.*). Must be carried.
Especially in teething babies.

Cactus .. .. Bilious diarrhœa, preceded by great pain.
Great weight in anus ; desire to pass a quantity, but nothing comes.

Belladonna .. Drowsiness (*Baptisia*) with dry, burning heat.
Pupils dilated.
Stools green, small, frequent.
Colic before stool : straining.
Child starts with every noise : twitches.

Colocynth .. Paroxysms of severe colicky pain precede stools. Immediately after eating.
Relief from doubling up and pressure.
Frothy stools. Stools watery, then bilious, then bloody; excoriating; frequent; not profuse.

Magnesia phos. Very like *Colocynth*, but urgently *demands heat as well as pressure.*

(A case in Hospital : *Colocynth* had helped the diarrhœa, but the Resident thought the child would die. The only relief was from a warm hand pressed on abdomen. *Mag. phos.* saved the child.)

SEVERE URGENT CASES, WITH COLLAPSE.

Aethusa .. Intolerance of milk.
Face expresses anxiety and pain.
Linea nasalis—pearly whiteness on upper lip bounded by a distinct line to angles of mouth
Violent vomiting: of milk: after milk.
Stool undigested: thin: green: bilious.
Violent straining before and after stool.
Collapse—almost as bad as Ars. *only not restless.*
A remedy of violence—violent vomiting—violent convulsions—violent pains—violent diarrhœa.

Arsenicum .. Worse at night, 1 to 3 a.m.
Rapid emaciation; *exhaustion and collapse.*
Intense restlessness. (*Pyrog.*) (opp. of *Aeth.*)
Painless, offensive, watery stools.
There may be simultaneous vomiting and diarrhœa. (*Ipec.*)
After cold drinks; when heated; in older persons after ices.
Thirst for cold water, immediately vomited.
Coldness of extremities.
Pale cadaverous face.
Skin dry, wrinkled, toneless.

Camphor .. *Skin cold as marble* (*Carbo veg.*), *but child will not remain covered.*
Great prostration and diarrhœa.*

Pyrogen .. Extreme restlessness: has to keep on moving.
Only momentary relief from moving, but has to move for that relief. (Comp. *Rhus.*)
Diarrhœa with frightfully offensive stools (*Bapt.*).
Profuse, watery, painless stools, with (?) vomiting.

(One has seen *Pyrogen* almost magic for sudden, very exhausting attacks of summer diarrhœa.)

* *Give a drop of the strong tincture on sugar. Repeat in 5 to 15 minutes if case urgent. Keep Camphor away from Homœopathic medicines.*

SOME REMEDIES OF ACUTE DYSENTERY

Mercurius cor. Persistent straining before, during, and after stool (rev. of *Nux*).
Scanty stools of bloody or shreddy slime.
Stools excoriate, burn. Burning in rectum.
" Never-get-done " sensation.
Straining to pass hot urine, drop by drop.
Merc. cor. IS ALMOST A SPECIFIC FOR DYSENTERY.
Tongue large, flabby, tooth-notched.
Mouth foul. Salivation.

Mercurius .. Bloody, slimy stools with much straining: never-get-done feeling (*Merc. cor.*); but *Merc. cor.* has a more violent attack.
Stools followed by chilliness.
Rarely indicated where there is no slime.
Rarely indicated where the tongue is dry.
" Your first prescription should cure in epidemic dysentery, and if you work cautiously you will cure every case."—KENT.

Aloe .. .. " Violent tenesmus, heat in rectum, prostration to fainting and profuse clammy sweats."
Bloody mucus passes after urging and straining. Rumbling, gurgling, sudden urge to stool.
Urine and fæces pass at the same time: cannot pass one without the other (*Mur. a.*).
Curious symptom. Stools, even solid, pass unnoticed. Sense of insecurity at anus.
Another curious verified symptom. On laying head on pillow, as if a fine globe broke at base of brain, fragments could be heard tinkling as they fell.

Nux .. . Stools of slimy mucus and blood, but small and unsatisfactory: *with relief, pro tem., after every stool* (rev. of *Merc.* and *Merc. cor.*).
Irregular peristalsis.
Griping pains, now here, now there, in abdomen. COLIC.
Nux is irritable, hypersensitive, offended.
Is chilly, with great aversion to uncovering.

Colocynth ..	With much colic, only *relieved by bending double*, and *pressing hard into abdomen*.
Sulphur ..	Stools bloody with constant straining: with the *Merc.* " never-get-done " sensation. Dysenteric stools, esp. at night, with colic and violent tenesmus. " Follows *Nux*, esp. when worse at night: discharge of blood, slime, pus, with fever." Pain so violent as to cause nausea and drenching perspiration. Stools acrid: excoriate. Characteristic symptom, *redness about anus*.
Phosphorus ..	Dysenteric stools oozing from an open anus. Patient craves COLD DRINKS and food; ices.
Apis ..	Stools with every motion of body as if anus constantly open (*Phos.*); oozes blood. " Tomato-sauce " stools—blood, mucus, food. Thirstless: can't bear heat—warm room.
Ipecacuanha ..	Dysentery with *constant nausea*. Sits almost constantly on stool and passes a little slime, or a little *bright-red blood*. Tenesmus awful: pain so great that nausea comes on and he vomits bile. *Tongue clean with nausea*.
Colchicum autumnale	Dysentery in the fall of the year, when days are warm and nights cold (*Dulc.*). Stools: shreddy and bloody like scrapings: thin, watery, but they cool to form a jelly. Great meteoric distension (*Carbo veg.*). Bloody discharges from bowels with deathly nausea. The smell of food causes nausea to faintness.
Gelsemium ..	Epidemic dysentery, malarial or catarrhal. Acute catarrhal enteritis, mucous diarrhœa. Discharges almost involuntary: intense spasmodic colic and tenesmus. *Fright, emotion, anticipation* will produce diarrhœa (*Arg. nit.*). *Gels.* has chills up and down back: trembling; and heaviness of limbs and eyelids.

Arsenicum .. RESTLESSNESS, ANGUISH, FEARFUL ANXIETY.
Worse after midnight.
Burning thirst for sips of cold water.
Internal, violent burning pain, with cold extremities. *Better heat, hot drinks.* (Rev. of *Phos.*)
Great collapse and prostration.
Tongue dry, to brown, or black.
Putrid stools: involuntary: with prostration: blood and straining.
THE GREAT REMEDY IN PTOMAINE POISONING.
(N.B.—" Don't give *Ars.* in dysentery unless there is the *Ars.* restlessness, anxiety, and thirst for frequent small drinks.")

Rhus .. .. Cases with *extreme restlessness* (*Ars.*).
Worse *damp weather: damp cold weather.*
Dry, dark-coated tongue: or triangular red tip.
Herpetic eruptions about mouth.
Copious, watery, bloody stools; drive him out of bed (*Sulph.*) as early as 4 a.m.
" Diarrhœa with tearing pains running down back of leg with every stool. Painful tenesmus with every stool."

Aconite .. Stools of pure blood, with a little slime.
With anguish, cramp, terrible urging.
Or black, very fetid stools.
Sensation, warm fluid escaping from anus.

Cuprum .. Frightful colic; > pressure.
Spouting stool of bloody, greenish water.
Cramps—abdomen, calves, soles, fingers, toes.
Strong metallic taste.

Podophyllum .. " Abdomen becomes tumultuous."
Gurgling: then sudden, profuse, putrid stools: generally painless: with perhaps prolapsus recti.

Psorinum .. Stools dark, gushing, horridly putrid.
Worse at night. Patient greasy, offensive.
Cases which do not respond to apparently indicated remedy (*Tub.*).

Capsicum .. Small frequent stools of blood and mucus.
After stool tenesmus and thirst : but drinking causes shuddering. *Thirst after every dysenteric stool :* sudden craving for ice-cold water, which causes chilliness.
Violent tenesmus in rectum and bladder at the same time (*Canth.*)
Smarting and *burning* in anus and rectum.
(*Caps.* burnings are like cayenne pepper.)
Typical *Caps.* is plump, flabby, sensitive to cold : red, cold face : nose red and cold.

Cantharis .. Stools like scrapings of intestines.
Great burning : burning at anus.
Tenesmus in rectum *and bladder* (*Caps.*).
" It is a singular fact that if there be frequent micturition with burning cutting pain attending the flow, *Cantharis* is almost always the remedy for whatever other sufferings there may be."

Carbo veg. .. " No matter what the trouble is, in *Carbo veg.* there is always burning."
Diarrhœa, dysentery, cholera, with bloody watery stool. Watery mucus mixed with blood.
Stools horribly putrid, with putrid flatulence.
The more thin, dark, bloody mucus there is, the better the remedy is indicated.
Anus red (*Sulph.*), raw, bleeding, itching.
Cold breath, cold sweat, cold nose.
Internal burning with external coldness.
Coldness and collapse, with air hunger.

Veratrum alb. .. Colic : burning, twisting, constricting, cutting. Distension, tenderness.
Stools frequent ; watery, greenish ; blackish ; bloody. Involuntary when passing flatus : from least movement of body.
May be simultaneous stool and vomiting (*Ars.*).
Sunken, hippocratic face. Characteristic symptom, *cold sweat on forehead.* (One of Hahnemann's great cholera medicines.)
The straining is not marked in *Verat.*

SOME CHOLERA REMEDIES

HOMŒOPATHY won its first great world-wide laurels in the cholera epidemics some 100 years ago, reversing everywhere the mortality: i.e. where ordinary medicine lost three-quarters of its cholera patients, Homœopathy saved three-quarters—even in some localities and under certain doctors it lost *none*.

Hahnemann never having seen the disease, but knowing its headlong rush and symptoms, laid down the remedies that would be curative: and his disciples everywhere were absolutely masters of the situation.

His three great remedies were: *Camphor*, *Cuprum* and *Veratrum album.*

Camphor .. For early stage. Promptly curative.

Dose Give a drop of the strong tincture every five minutes on sugar, till warmth and rest are restored.

(*The strong tincture is a saturated solution of camphor in rectified spirits of wine.*)

(*A lump of camphor in a small bottle of whisky, etc., will make a saturated solution. The spirit dissolves only as much as it can.*)

(*N.B.—Give Camphor on sugar. In water it nauseates and burns. Keep Camphor away from medicines.*)

Cuprum .. In the later stage of excessive vomiting and purging, and especially where CRAMPS are the feature of the case . . .

(Copper poisoning and camphor poisoning are difficult to distinguish. Copper, a plate worn on the skin, is said to protect against cholera.)

"Workers in copper mines do not get cholera."

Veratrum alb. .. For the cases with *very profuse evacuations, profuse vomiting and purging*, and *profuse, cold sweat.*

Repeat every hour or half-hour till warmth and rest are restored.

There has been the idea that *Camphor* (perhaps because of the need for frequent repetition) was not homœopathic to cholera; but that it was only proposed by Hahnemann for the treatment of cholera because of its destructiveness to the micro-organisms—which he sensed.

No greater mistake could be made. *Camphor* is *absolutely* homœopathic to cholera in its first stage—for which Hahnemann alone prescribed it. Later on, if the patient survived, *with the same organism, but changed symptoms*, camphor was no longer indicated. *Cuprum* or *Veratrum alb.*, according to symptoms, would now be homœopathic, and therefore curative.

Let us contrast the symptoms of cholera in its first stage with those of camphor poisonings, and we shall see the absolute homœopathicity of the drug.

CHOLERA SYMPTOMS— *First stage.*	CAMPHOR POISONING SYMPTOMS.
Giddy faint powerlessness.	Vertigo as if drunk. His senses leave him; he slides and falls to the ground.
Icy coldness of the body.	Icy coldness of body.
Strength suddenly sinks.	Great prostration and weakness. Could hardly be held upright. Attempted to stand, but lay down again.
Expression altered.	Face pale, distorted, sunken.
Eyes sunk in.	Eyes staring, distorted, sunken, hollow.
Face bluish and icy cold.	Face and hands deathly pale—cold—blue.
Closure of jaws, trismus.	Closure of jaws, trismus.
Whole body cold.	Body quite cold. Skin cold. Extremities icy cold.
Hopeless discouragement and anxiety.	Great anxiety.
Dread of suffocation.	Suffocative dyspnœa.
Burning in stomach and gullet.	Burning in throat and stomach.
Cramps in calves and other muscles.	Violent cramps.
On touching precordial region, he cries out.	Precordial anxiety. When spoken to loudly complained of indefinable distress in precordial region.

No thirst, no sickness, no vomiting or purging (as in the later stage).

And here, observe! Homœopathy can not only cure—abort—prevent—give instant relief in acute sickness, even before it is possible to make a diagnosis—but it can also lay down the remedy or remedies that will be curative in an unknown disease, never seen, but whose symptoms are known.

CONCERNING HOMŒOPATHY FOR CHILDREN

CHILDREN respond splendidly to the homœopathic remedy. And children's work is most fascinating: usually less complicated: the indications for the remedy are generally more clear; and the results more rapid of attainment.

Children are in the acute stage of life, rapidly growing and developing. The cell-life that clothes and binds them to earth is in a marvellous state of activity. They are hypersensitive to influences that normally exercise less power later on. They are subject to diseases that seldom attack adults. Besides which, with them, labelled diseases do not always run the same course as with their elders. For instance, what we call rheumatism—acute rheumatism—is a very different proposition, with widely different symptoms and outcome, in children and in "grown-ups".

The condition of high fever—profuse, sour sweating—tender, inflamed, painful joint or joints has very little in common with the, often trivial, "*growing pains*"—the *scarcely elevated temperature*, probably unnoticed till a thermometer is put into the mouth—the *no sweat* of the child;—where the heart is the subject of grave attack, and where extreme care and most skilful prescribing are essential if the condition is not to go on to a life-sentence of disability and suffering—to a dreary vista of cardiac break-downs, each one more damaging than the last.

Well, first—as elsewhere—one has to settle whether the ailment is acute or chronic; and, if the former, whether it occurs in a healthy or a diseased child. For a healthy child may be sick unto death, whereas a diseased child may be a museum of pathology and yet not "ill". In the latter case, treatment may have to be modified, or rather supplemented, in order to cover the whole case. A pneumonia in a child with T.B. glands or a T.B. family history, will probably not clear up till you give a dose of *Tub. bov.* And it is pathetic to find how often one has to come to *Lueticum* to make headway with the acutely sick hospital children.

In Homœopathy the essentials,—i.e. the symptoms so easy to get in the child, and so all-important, if marked, for a successful prescription, are, briefly,

(1) DISPOSITION; or, more important still, change of disposition due to illness.

(2) FEARS: habitual, or, more important, new to the child.

(3) SENSITIVENESS. One remembers a wee boy in our Children's Ward wandering about, just the right height to use the brass shields at the foot of endowed cots as a mirror (his head and

face were covered thickly with an eruption). He used to wail, "The children make such a *noise*!"—and the rattle of spoons on plates was, to him, torture. Such a symptom, in a child of his age, would be important, and must be considered when piecing together his disease-picture to be matched with the drug-disease-picture of a remedy.

(4) Food Cravings and Loathings.

(5) The Grosser Pathological Symptoms, when qualified by something that makes them rare and peculiar, and therefore diagnostic as regards the choice of the remedy.

Disposition. There is a broad distinction between the "child you want to spank" and the child you instinctively comfort and caress: and here one is at once shifted onto one or other of a totally different class of remedies. *Natrum mur.* and *Sepia* children are not amenable to sympathy. *Pulsatilla* children are weepy, but engaging little mites that claim attention and love. Then there is the heavy, lethargic, rather dull *Calcarea* type: the restless, suspicious, anxious *Arsenicum* type: the defiant, obstinate, passionate, sensitive, irritable *Nux* type: while *Chamomilla* demands a thing only to hurl it away, and cannot be placated . . . and so on. Whatever the disease, these things must be taken into consideration, if the prescription is to be successful.

Then *fears.* One little child will wander alone in the dusk through extensive school buildings where her parents are caretakers: another, put to play in the garden, hugs the window, and wants to be assured that his mother is on the other side of the glass, within call. Fears of the dark—of wind—of thunder—of strangers—of falling—of a bath.

The third useful point in determining a remedy for a child, is appetite:—*cravings and aversions.* One child craves fat, and will gnaw raw suet: another hates and is nauseated by the least morsel of fat, which has to be carefully cut off its meat (*Sulph.* has both of these). You must put the salt on a high shelf, out of reach of some children (*Nat. mur.*, *Phos.*, etc.) while the next will steal sugar, and cries for "sweeties". Some children will eat earth, chalk, and crunch slate-pencils (*Alum.*). Some cannot be made to swallow meat.

This wee girl is greedy—always hungry—"will eat anything": while her delicate little brother can hardly be induced to eat enough, so it would seem, to keep body and soul together.

There is the untruthful child; the shy child, in terror of strangers, a bit difficult for a doctor. But—children are very susceptible to flattery. Tell a child that it is opening its mouth splendidly,—" now, *just a little wider!*" and you may see its throat. The same in breathing, when you want to listen to a chest. Or you may establish relations by expressing interest or admiration for a bracelet, buttons, scraps of embroidery : or, when nothing helps, " Ta-ta ! " will abruptly suspend the sobs.

" With children, lunatics, and liars you have to observe for yourself " :—and you have to " keep your eyes skinned " where children are concerned. There is the child that always kicks the clothes off ; that never will be covered at night (*Sulph.*) : that is found with its feet on the pillow and the bedclothes on the floor. There is the infant of only a few weeks that will wriggle over to lie on its face, till the mother is in terror lest it suffocate. But it may be kept right side up by a dose of *Medorrh.*—one has seen that.

The " dirty-nosed child ", with nostrils always running, and red, and sore, is easy to prescribe for (*Sulph.*, *Kali iod.*). The puny boys that won't grow or thrive (often *Sanic.*).

Then the diseased,—or the children with heritage of poor resistance to tubercle—they are some of the joys of prescribing : children of eight years, who have never, in all their lives, been without bandages about their necks ; with glands, sinuses and scars left by cuttings, and scrapings, and aspirations :—how they respond to Homœopathy ! to *Tuberculinum—Silica—Calcarea—Drosera—Sulphur*, according to their make-up and the symptoms they present. It is to Homœopathy alone that these tuberculous gland and bone cases respond so magnificently ! and it is here especially that the homœopathic physician tastes triumph.

* * * *

SOME REMEDIES OF DENTITION

Calcarea

Fat, fair, flabby, perspiring.
Fontanelles remain open (*Sil.*, *Calc. ph.*). Deformed extremities.
Deficient, or irregular bone development.
Profuse perspiration : soaks the pillow (*Sil.*).
Sour sweat : sour diarrhœa : sour vomit.
Flabby ; FAT : lax muscles ; bones that bend.
Can't learn to walk : won't put feet to ground.
Milk crust and eruptions in the *Calcarea* child.
Teething cough or diarrhœa : in the *Calcarea* child.

Calcarea phos. Slow dentition with emaciation (reverse of *Calc.*).
Fontanelles remain open.
Soft thin skull, crackles when pressed upon.
Can't hold head up : it must be supported.
Flabby, emaciated : doesn't learn to walk.
" Great desire to nurse all the time."
Cough with rattling chest.
The *Calc. phos.* child is more wiry ; less fair ; without the sweating head of *Calc.*
Diarrhœa, stools green and spluttering.
Child shrunken and anæmic (*Sil.*).

Chamomilla .. Painful dentition.
Oversensitive to pain, which maddens.
Very irritable : snaps and snarls (*Cina*).
Excessive uneasiness, anxiety, tossing, (*Acon.*).
Only to be quieted by being carried about.
Drowsiness with sleeplessness.
Sweats with the pain.
One cheek red and hot, the other pale and cold.
Wants this or that, only to push it away.
Turmoil in temper. *Chamomilla* is frantic : " cannot bear it ! "
Dentition diarrhœa (*Calc., Kreos.*). Stools green : odour like rotten eggs : colicky pain.
Draws the legs up. Abdomen bloated.

Kreosotum .. " Child suffering from *very* painful dentition : won't sleep at night unless caressed and fondled all the time." (*Cham.*, unless carried up and down the room.)
Gums painful, dark-red or blue : teeth decay as soon as they come.
May have constipation, or diarrhœa.
Cholera infantum during teething : very severe : vomiting incessant, with cadaveric-smelling stools.

Aconite .. Feverish. Fever. Dry hot skin (*Bell.*). Child gnaws its fists ; frets and cries.
Sleepless ; excited ; tosses ; heat ; startings and twitchings (*Bell.*) of single muscles.
Convulsions of teething children (*Bell.*).
Costive, or dark, watery stools.

Coffea .. Wakeful: constantly on the move.
Not distressed: happy: but sleepless.
Remarkable wakefulness.
Over excitement of brain.

Belladonna .. Red, hot face. Dry skin. Dilated pupils.
Starts and wakes when just falling asleep.
Twitchings and jerkings.
Quickness of sensations and emotions. Sudden pains, suddenly gone.
Convulsions.
The delirium of *Bell.* bites, strikes, wants to escape.
Acute attacks in *Calcarea* children.

Zincum .. " Brain troubles during dentition.
Child cries out in sleep, rolls head from side to side: face alternately red and pale."
Incessant, fidgety feet, must move them constantly.

Podophyllum *Pod.* has a great desire to press the gums together during dentition.
Cholera infantum, stools profuse and gushing: larger than could be expected from amount of food taken: offensive.

Sulphur .. The *Sulphur* baby will not remain covered.
Rough skin and hair: red lips and eyelids.
Redness around anus, hot palms and soles.
Acrid stools (*Calc.*) that irritate and inflame wherever they touch the skin. (The *urine* of *Lyc.* irritates the parts.)

Then the nosodes must not be forgotten in delayed dentition. Burnett proved the value of *Tuberculinum* in tardy development of all kinds, where there was a family history of deficiency of reaction to tubercle. One has seen a case of delayed dentition in a girl well on in her teens, where, after a dose of *Tub. bov.*, she erupted eight teeth in a couple of weeks.

And one would think of *Luet.* where the days are happy, but the nights a terror (*Lyc.*): or *Medorrhinum,* where the infant rolls over to sleep on its stomach (*Cina*), or a child can only sleep in the knee-elbow position: or the mother has had an evil discharge.

RICKETS

The same remedies, largely, apply to both difficult dentition and rickets, yet it may be well to more or less repeat, otherwise the picture will be incomplete.

Calcarea carb. For the fat, fair, lethargic type of child, with profusely sweating head, especially in sleep (*Sil.*, *Sanic.*): with soft, fat, flabby, inadequate limbs that bend under its weight: with big abdomen.

The child of plus tissue of minus quality.

Calcarea phos. Like *Calc.* head large, fontanelles long open; but less sweating. Bones of skull thin.

Thin—even emaciated.

Sunken, flabby abdomen (reverse of *Calc.*).

Spine too weak to support body: thin neck, too weak to support head.

Child pale and cold. Seems stupid.

" Even cretinism may be developed by the continued use of *Calc. phos.*" (i.e. think of *Calc. phos.* in cretinism).

Silica .. Pale, waxen, earthy face.

Head large (the *Calcs.*, *Sulph.*), fontanelles open.

Body small and emaciated, except the plump abdomen.

Bones and muscles poorly developed: i.e. slow in learning to walk.

Worse from milk: infant unable to take any kind of milk. (*Aeth.*)

Diarrhœa from milk.

Offensive sweat, head, neck, face, feet.

Sanicula .. *Sanicula aqua* contains *Calcarea*, *Silica*, etc. and combines many of the symptoms of these remedies. Invaluable remedy for un-flourishing, ill-developing children.

Defective nutrition.

Thin and old-looking. Dirty brownish skin.

Stubborn and touchy.

Cold, clammy hands and feet.

Profuse sweat, occiput and neck.

Sulphur .. Large head (like the *Calcareas*).
Tendency to rickets. (*Calc. c.*)
Voracious appetite, defective assimilation.
Hungry yet emaciated. (*Iod.*)
Shrivelled and dried up, like a little old man.
Skin hangs in folds, yellowish, wrinkled, and flabby. (See Dentition—*Sulph.*)

Chamomilla .. Intensely sensitive. Intensely irritable.
Changeable: never satisfied.
Wants to be carried: can't keep still.
"The *Chamomilla* child can't be touched."
Painful gums, painful teething: will hold cold glass against its gums.
Pain—colic: doubles up and screams. Kicks.
Diarrhœa. Grass green stool.
One cheek red, the other pale.
Coughing or ailments from anger.
Sleepy but can't sleep.

Arnica .. Tender to touch.
Does not want to be disturbed, or irritated, or handled.
Worse from heat.
Especially if there has been any injury at birth or otherwise.

Scurvy Rickets

Manganum .. General aching, soreness, tenderness (*Arn.*).
Bones ache, especially tibiae.
Sickly face, anæmic.
Constantly whining; fretful.
Everything better lying down.
Worse cold, damp weather.

Arnica .. (See above.) *A great remedy here.*

Phosphorus .. Bruising: extraversation. Gums bleed.
Especially in nervous, slender children.

Kreosotum .. Gums bleed and ulcerate.
Offensive odours, mouth, etc.
The *Cham.* temperament (see above) but *offensive and bleeds.*

THE COMMONER REMEDIES OF MAL-NUTRITION, WASTING, MARASMUS

WITH DIAGNOSTIC SYMPTOMS

Calcarea .. COLDNESS.

Profuse sweats, head (*Sil.*) at night (*Sil.*).

Cold, damp feet : cold legs with night-sweats.

Milk disagrees. (*Calc. ph., Nat. carb., Mag. carb., Aeth., Sil., Lac. c.*)

Big head, with large, hard abdomen. (*Sil.*)

Stomach swollen, distended even with the rest of body emaciated.

" A big-bellied child, with emaciated limbs and neck." (*Sil.*) (Opp. of *Calc. ph.*)

Malnutrition, glands, bones, and skin.

Faulty bony development : late teething : rickets.

Fat, flabby, deficient bones, deficient teeth.

" Bones stop growing, and child goes into marasmus."

" Enlarged glands, emaciation of neck and limbs, while the fat and the glands of the belly increase."

Flabby : feeble : tired.

Sourness of sweat, of sweating head. Sour stool. Sour vomit.

White stools : constipation with white stools.

" Wormy babies ", pass and vomit worms.

Chew and swallow, or grit teeth in sleep (*Cina*).

Cross and fretful : easily frightened.

Calc. phos. .. Vomits milk. (*Calc., Nat. carb., Mag. carb.*)

Stools green, slimy, lienteric, with foetid flatus.

Face pale. White ; sallow.

Neck cannot support head.

Marasmus : shrunken, emaciated, and very anæmic.

Tall scrawny, children with dirty, brownish skins.

Peevish, restless, fretful.

Flabby, sunken abdomen (opp. of *Calc. carb.*).

Phosphorus .. Tall, slender, delicate : grow too rapidly.

"Children emaciating : rapidly : going into marasmus. Tendency to consumption."

Delicate : waxy : anæmic. Hectic blush.

Bleed easily : bruise easily. Sensitive to cold.

Love to be touched : rubbed.

Fear that something will happen : of thunder : of the dark : of being alone.

Indifferent.

"The sickly, sunken, earthy face of consumption, or of those going into consumption."

Desire for cold water : ices : salt : savouries.

May complain of a hot spine.

Chilly patient, yet stomach and head better for cold : chest and limbs better for heat.

Better for sleep—for short sleep. (*Sep.*)

One of the great vertigo medicines. (*Con.*)

Tuberculinum .. "Deep-acting : long-acting : affects constitutions more deeply than most remedies (*Sulph., Sil., Dros.* etc.)."

"*Tubercular taint* : debilitated and anæmic : here give *Tub.* on a paucity of symptoms."

Hopelessness : desire to travel : to go somewhere.

"Closely related to *Calc.*, to *Sil.* All go deep into life : interchangeable, i.e. one may be indicated for a while, then the other" (KENT).

Sensitive : dissatisfied. Fear of dogs.

Aversion to meat : craves cold milk.

"Gradual emaciation—increasing weakness—fatigue."

Excessive sweat in chronic diarrhœa.

Driven out of bed with diarrhœa.

Air-hunger : suffocated in a warm room.

Better riding in a cold wind. Worse damp cold.

"When at every coming back of the case, it needs a new remedy."

Old dingy look.

Very red lips (*Sulph.*) and very blue sclerotics suggest *Tub.*

Sulphur .. Farrington says, of marasmus of children, "*Ravenous, especially at* 11 *a.m. Heat vertex: with cold feet. With these three symptoms Sulphur will never fail you.*"

Wakes screaming.

Great voracity: puts everything into its mouth.

Or, "drinks much and eats little"

Thirsty, wants much water.

Craves fat: will eat raw suet.

"Slow, lazy, hungry, and always tired."

Red lips, nostrils, eyelids, anus.

Stool offensive, excoriating.

Frequent, slimy diarrhœa, or obstinate constipation. Screams before large stool.

"*Sulphur* children have the most astonishing tendency to be filthy."

Fear of bath: hates bath: worse from bath.

Limbs emaciate, with distended abdomen.

Muscles wither, even abdominal, with much distension of abdomen itself.

Emaciates with good appetite. (*Iod.*, etc.)

Eruptions: itching: worse at night. Boils.

Psorinum .. Pale, sickly, delicate children. Look unwashed (*Sulph.*).

Have a filthy smell, even after a bath.

Dread the bath (*Sulph.*).

Kent says, "*Offensive to sight and smell.*"

Very chilly: worse open air: also worse warm bed.

Stools fluid, fetid.

Works miracles in these amazingly offensive (perhaps consumptive) children. One has seen it!

Sepia .. "No ability to feel natural love." *Indifference.*

Absence of joy. "Never happy unless he is annoying someone."

Comprehension difficult.

Progressive emaciation. Skin wrinkled.

Child looks like a shrivelled, dried-up old man.

Freckled, esp. across nose and cheeks, "the *Sepia* saddle".

Child wets the bed *in its first sleep*.

Damp cold legs and feet: (*Calc.*)

Silica .. Child weak, puny, from defective assimilation.
Big abdomen from (?) mesenteric disease.
"Large head, body small, emaciated, except abdomen which is round and plump.
Face pale, waxy, earthy or yellowish.
Pinched and old-looking. Limbs shrunken.
Bones and muscles poorly developed, for that reason late walking.
Coldness : chilliness.
Head sweats profusely : in sleep (*Calc.*).
Offensive sweat head and face.
Feet sweat: offensive foot sweat (*Bar. c.*, *Petr.*).
Little injuries fester : poor healing (*Hep.*).
Boils and pustules, and sepsis.
Want of self-confidence.

Natrum mur. .. Nutrition impaired. Eats and emaciates all the time (*Iod.*), neck particularly. (*Sars.*)
Emaciation, weakness, nervous prostration, nervous irritability.
Skin shiny, pale, waxy, as if greased; or,
Skin dry, withered, shrunken.
An infant looks like a little old man (*Iod.*, *Abrot.*, *Arg. nit.*, *Sanic.*, *Sars.*, *Op.*, *Ars.*).
Collar-bones become prominent and neck scrawny : but hips and lower limbs remain plump and round. (Opp. of *Abrot.* *Lyc.* also emaciates downwards.)
Children with *voracious appetite, yet emaciate.* (*Iod*, *Sulph.*, etc.)
One of the few "mapped-tongue" remedies.
Gets herpes about lips.
Terrible headaches.
Craving for salt. Hates bread and fat.
Weeps easily : but not amenable to sympathy.

Abrotanum .. Emaciation mostly of legs. Ascending (rev. of *Nat. mur.*, *Lyc.*, etc.).
Bloated abdomen.
Cross irritable children.
Pale, hollow-eyed, old face (*Iod.*, *Nat. mur.*, *Sulph.*, etc.). Wrinkled.
Appetite very great : *ravenous while emaciating.* (*Iod.*, etc.)
In marasmus : skin flabby ; and hangs loose.

Iodine .. *General emaciation: wants to eat all the time.*
While the body withers, the glands enlarge.
"Withering throughout the body, muscles shrink, skin wrinkles, and face of child like a little old person, *but glands under arms, in groins, and belly, enlarged and hard.* (*Arg. nit., Abrot., Nat. mur.*)
Always hungry: eats between meals, and yet is hungry.
Better eating. Emaciates with an enormous appetite.
Excitement: anxiety: impulses. Worse trying to keep still.
Worse heat: better cold. (*Lyc.*) (opp. to *Sil.* etc.)
Always too hot.

Sanicula .. Child looks old (*Arg. nit.*, etc.), dirty, greasy, and brownish.
Progressive emaciation.
Kicks off clothing in coldest weather. (*Sulph.*)
Sweats on falling asleep, mostly neck. Wets clothing through. (*Calc., Sil.*)
Cold clammy sweat occiput and neck.
Child craves meat, fat bacon, *salt.* (*Nat. mur., Arg. nit., Nit. ac.*)
Child wants to nurse all the time, yet loses flesh.
After intense straining the stool, nearly evacuated, recedes (*Sil.*).
Body smells like old cheese.
Foul footsweat, chafes toes (*Sil.*).

Sarsaparilla .. Neck emaciates (*Nat. mur.*): skin lies in folds (*Abrot.*).
Weakness of mind and tissues.
Marasmus of children from heredity.
Emaciation about the neck. (*Nat. mur.*)
Dry, purple copper-like eruptions.
No assimilation.
Children emaciated: face looks old. (*Nat. m., Arg. nit.*, etc.)
Big belly: dry, flabby skin.
Screams when about to urinate. Or, *at close of urination gives an unearthly yell.*

Lycopodium ..	Emaciates from above downwards (*Sanic.*, *Nat. mur.*). Lower limbs fairly nourished. Flatulent: distended like a drum (*Arg. nit.*), can hardly breathe. So full, he cannot eat. Wakes " ugly ". Worse 4-8 p.m. No self-confidence (*Sil.*): miseries of anticipation (*Arg. nit.*, *Ars.*, *Sil.*). Cries when thanked: when receiving a gift. Withered lads with dry cough; headache. Better from cold. Worse warm room (*Iod.*). Red sand in urine: " red pepper deposit." Craves sweets (*Arg. nit.*): hot drinks. One foot hot, one cold (characteristic). Sickly wrinkled face with contracted eyebrows.
Argentum nit. ..	Child looks dried up, like a mummy (*Op.*, *Ars.*). Old-looking, pale, bluish face. Progressive emaciation. Craves sweets (*Lyc.*) which disagree. Craves salt (*Phos.*, *Nat. mur.*). Wants cold air (*Lyc.*) cold drinks (opp. of *Lyc.*). A most flatulent remedy (*Lyc.*) distended to bursting (*Lyc.*). Emotional diarrhœa: from anticipation (*Gels.*). Examination funk. Fear of high places.
Opium ..	" Shrivelled little dried up old man." Painlessness: inactivity: torpor:— Or, sleeplessness: inquietude, nervous excitability. Lack of reaction to well-selected remedy. (*Sul.*) Fear and fright. Constipation from painless paresis of bowels.
Arsenicum ..	Atrophy of infants. Marasmus. " Dried-up mummy " child. Face pale, anxious, distorted. Skin harsh, dry, tawny. Rapid emaciation: sinking of strength. Least effort exhausting. Chilliness. Diarrhœa as soon as begins to eat or drink. Stools undigested: offensive. Restlessness: constant distress. " *Ars.* has *anxiety, restlessness, prostration, burning and cadaveric odours.*"

Hepar

Sour smell (*Calc.*): white (*Calc.*) fœtid evacuations: undigested stools.
Seems better after feeding. (*Nat. mur.*)
" Does not play: does not laugh."
Chilly: oversensitive: to cold: to dry cold; to draughts (*Nux.*, *Sulph.*); to touch.
Mind also oversensitive: every little thing makes him angry, abusive, impulsive (*Nux*).
Quarrelsome (*Nux*).
Little injuries fester (*Sil.*) are fearfully sensitive. Ears discharge: threatening mastoid.
Lax, chilly, sweats all night.
Worse cold: better warm: wrapped up (*Sil.*).

Nux ..

" Oversensitive: irritable: touchy: never satisfied. Violent temper: uncontrollable."
" Jerks things about: tears them up."
Very chilly: cannot uncover (rev. of *Sulph.*).
" Always selecting his food, and digesting almost none."
Yellow, sallow, bloated face.
Constipation: alt. diarrhœa and constipation.
Irregular peristalsis: i.e. contents of intestine driven both ways: i.e. fitful or fruitless urging to stool.

Natrum carb. ..

Nervous withered infants: cannot stand milk: diarrhœa from milk. Aversion to milk.
" A nervous, cold baby, easily startled."
Better for eating: eats to keep warm.
All-gone feeling and pain in stomach, which drives him to eat; constantly " picking ".
Abdomen hard and bloated: much flatus: loud rumbling.
Worse and esp. hungry at 11 p.m. and 5 a.m.
Headache from any mental exertion.
Ankles " turn "—weak.

Magnesia carb.

Puny and sickly from defective nutrition.
Milk refused: causes pain. Passed undigested.
Griping colic. Limbs drawn up for relief.
Stools sour, green, like frog-spawn on pond: or with lumps like tallow. (*Coloc.*, but has not the green, slimy stool.)

Petroleum .. Emaciation, with *diarrhœa by day only.*
Hunger immediately after stool.
Aversion to fat, meat and open air.
"Coldness (*Calc.*) and sweating in single parts."
Offensive feet and axillæ (*Sil.*).
Dirty, hard, rough and thickened skin.
Skin fragile, cracks deeply (*Graph.*).
Eruptions worse in winter, better summer.
Hands crack and bleed : worse in winter.
Chilblains, sea and train sickness.
"Constant hunger with diarrhœa, but can't eat without pain : emaciation : eruptions : unhealthy ragged fingers that never look clean : can't wash them, as this chaps them."
"Hands and feet burn : wants palms and soles (*Sulph.*, *Cham.*, *Puls.*, *Med.*) out of bed."
("Don't be too sure of *Sulph.* because soles burn, or too sure of *Sil.* because feet sweat." —KENT.)

***Baryta** carb.* .. "Dwarfishness : mind and body. Mental dwarfishness, and dwarfishness of organs."
"Suspends development that makes child into man or woman." (*Baryta mur.*)
"Emaciation in those who have been well nourished." (*Iod.*, etc.)
"Enlarged glands : enlarged abdomen : emaciation of tissues, emaciated limbs and dwarfishness of mind. You have there the whole of *Baryta carb.* marasmus."
Shy, bashful. Easily frightened.

Other disease products may have to be considered, in cases that make no progress, such as

Lueticum .. Dwarfish (*Bar. carb.*). Marasmic.
Worse at night.
Impulse to wash hands.
Where Syphilitic taint is the bar to progress.

Medorrhinum Sycotic taint blocks progress. Poor reaction.
Lies on abdomen : sleeps in knee-elbow position.
Fiery-red, moist, itching anus (*Sulph.*).
Worse by day (opp. of *Luet.*).

TUBERCULOUS DISEASE, GLANDS AND BONES

THE homœopathic treatment of "T.B." glands and bones in children is pure joy. One has seen children of 6 or 8 years of age, "eaten up" with tubercle, who from babyhood have been "never without a bandage" and subject to repeated operations, where homœopathic treatment has not only promptly stopped further progress of the disease but has closed the wounds; while long-suffering and feeble existence are replaced by new energy and health.

One remembers a dusky child, riddled with tubercle. She had lost the phalange of one finger, was crowded with hideous scars all round her neck, on chest also—and arm—and leg. Here a couple of years' treatment not only closed wounds and sinuses, but arrested the disease.

Many of our remedies are of great service in T.B. gland and bone, but in our experience, DROSERA EXCELS THEM ALL.

Drosera .. *Drosera* has been proved *to break down resistance to tubercle in animals said to be immune; therefore, homœopathically it should, and does, raise resistance to tubercle.* Tubercular manifestations, or a strong family history of tuberculosis, put up a strong plea for the consideration of *Drosera* in any disease. Under the influence of *Drosera* glands of neck, if they have to "break", produce only very small openings; old suppurating glands soon diminish in size, and close. Old cicatricial tissue yields and softens; deep, tied-down scars relax, and come up, so that deformity is greatly lessened. While the improvement in health, in appearance, in nutrition, where *Drosera* comes into play, is rapid and striking.

Drosera has also great use in the diseases of joints and bone (in persons with a T.B. history), even when these are not tuberculous: quickly taking away pain, and improving health and well-being.

Hahnemann urged that *Dros.* should be given in infrequent doses, and the 30th potency. This, "*one of the most powerful medicinal herbs in our zone*" still (as he then said) "needs further proving"

Silica .. Hardened glands, especially about the neck: "Scrofulous glands."

A deep remedy for eradicating the tuberculous tendency when symptoms agree.

Worse in wet, cold weather, better in dry, cold weather, but very chilly.

Tendency to swelling of glands, which suppurate.

The *Silica* child is timid, lacks confidence, "grit".

Head sweats in sleep (*Calc.*).

For nearly all disease of bone.

Fistulous openings: discharges offensive: swollen; pouting round them hard, swollen, bluish-red.

Sweat of feet, often offensive feet.

Symphytum .. A case of necrosis of lower jaw, after an accident. *Sil.* and *Tub.* failed to effect improvement. Then *Symph.* was given, with the expulsion of a sequestrum, whereupon it healed. But *Symph.* has its "schmertz-punct" in that situation—left lower jaw, and is an outstanding remedy for BONE. (*Dros.*, *Phos.*)

Sepia .. A case of T.B. bone, with a sinus on each side of the right middle finger, one above and one below the first joint. Also other T.B. manifestations; in a woman who had nursed her husband dying of phthisis *Sil.* and *Tub.* failed to help, even with three weeks at a Convalescent Home. At long last, she was given *Sepia*, BECAUSE HER INDIVIDUAL SYMPTOMS DEMANDED SEPIA; whereupon the finger got well in spite of the fact that it was all day long in dirty water, scrubbing and cleaning in the public-house in which she worked. It is sometimes difficult to remember that *it is the remedy called for by the individual symptoms of the patient, that will stimulate him to put his house in order, and get well.* One is too apt to stress the disease and treat that!

The typical *Sepia* patient is indifferent: overburdened: dull. Has axillary sweats, offensive (*Sil.*), hates noise and smells: only "wants to get away alone and be quiet"

Sulphur .. "Prince of remedies in scrofula—in caries in early childhood.

"Voracious appetite: greedily clutches at all that is offered, edible or not, as if starved.

"Shrivelled and dried up like a little old man."

Tuberculinum .. Patients with a T.B. family history, or with T.B. manifestations, glands, etc.

A deep-acting, long-acting remedy.

Closely related to *Calc.*: one may be indicated for a while, then the other. (*Sil.*, *Dros.*)

Always wanting to go somewhere—to travel.

Feeble vitality: tired: debilitated: losing flesh.

Emaciation, with hunger (*Iod.*).

Worse in a close room, in damp weather; better cold wind, open air.

Desire for alcohol, bacon, fat ham, smoked meat, cold milk, refreshing things, sweets.

Calcarea .. Affects the glands of neck and all the glands.

Glands of abdomen become hard, sore, inflamed.

Useful in T.B. formations, calcareous degenerations.

But in the *Calc. child*: i.e. the child of plus quantity, minus quality: with large, sweating head, especially at night. Phlegmatic; the "lump of chalk" child, fair, pale, fat.

Necrosis of bone in such children.

Very useful in T.B. abdomen—when symptoms agree: which they generally do. (*Psor.*, when odour of child is very offensive.)

Phosphorus .. Like *Dros.* appears to break down resistance to tubercle, since workers in match factories have been esp. liable to consumption, and have suffered from caries and necrosis of bone.

Phos. helps to cure not only bone troubles, but "scrofulous glands", but always in the typical slender *Phos.* children, who grow too rapidly: delicate, waxy, anæmic.

Bruise easily: easy bleeders: with

Thirst for cold water, hunger for salt: love of ices:

Are nervous alone—fear the dark, rather apathetic and indifferent.

Iodium .. Scrofulous swellings and induration of glands: large, hard, usually painless.

"Iodine is torpidity and sluggishness. The very indolence of the disease suggests *Iod.*"

Cross and *restless*. Impulses.

Anxiety: the more he keeps still, the more anxious.

Always too hot.

Eats ravenously yet emaciates.

Dark hair and complexion. (*Brom.* fair and blue eyes.)

"Enlargement of all the glands except the mammæ: these waste and atrophy."

Compelled to keep on doing something to drive away his impulses and anxiety, (*Ars.*) But *Iod.* is warmblooded, and wants cold: *Ars.* is cold and wants heat—warm room, warm clothing, etc.

Bromium .. Very useful in enlarged glands with great hardness without any tendency to suppurate.

Glands take on tuberculosis, and tissues take on tuberculosis.

Glands that inflame for a while begin to take on a lower form of degeneration.

"It is very similar to those enlarged, hard, scrofulous glands that we often find in the neck . . ."

Swelling and induration of glands is a strong feature of the remedy.

Those needing *Brom.* for chronic glands, etc. will have a "grey, earthy colour of the face. Oldish appearance".

Or plethoric children, with red face, easily overheated.

Left-sided remedy.

Worse dampness.

Weak and easily over-heated, then sweaty and sensitive to draughts.

Glands in persons of light complexion, fair skin and light blue eyes (distinguishes from *Iod.*).

Tonsils deep-red, swollen, with net-work of dilated vessels.

Cistus can. .. Scrofulous swelling and suppuration of glands of throat.

Scrofulous hip disease, with fistulous openings leading to the bone, and ulcers on the surface, with night sweats.

A curious *Cistus* symptom, which has led to the cure of chronic colds and nasal catarrh, is *great desire for cheese.*

Theridion .. " Has an affinity for the tubercular diatheses."

Has been used with success in caries and necrosis of bone. " It appears to go to the root of the evil and destroys the cause " (Dr. Baruch).

Theridion is hypersensitive, especially to noise : shrill sounds penetrate the teeth.

Nausea from motion, and from closing the eyes.

Baryta carb. .. Glands swell, infiltrate, hypertrophy : sometimes suppurate.

Dwarfish children, late to develop : with dwarfish minds.

Slow, inept : mistrustful of strangers. Shy.

Affected by every cold.

Cold, foul footsweat. (*Sil.*)

Tearing and tension in long bones : boring in bones.

Mercury .. A curious, but useful symptom, " sensation of shivering in an abscess ", or in a sinus from diseased bone.

A Forgotten but Useful Tip

" Dr. . . . said *Calcarea iodata* was of great value in some cases of suppurating glands, sometimes causing them to reabsorb and disappear without discharging ; when there would be only a little thickening of tissue, like a tiny scar, left. She gave *Calc. iod.* to children who were typical *Calc. carb.* patients except that they were *hot* and *hungry.*"

SOME REMEDIES OF CONVULSIONS

Belladonna .. Convulsions in infants etc.; *associated with violent cerebral congestion.*

Skin burning. Hot, bright-red face.

Wild, staring eyes (*Cic.*, *Ign.*, *Mosch.*, *Stram.*).

Spasm of glottis: clutches at throat.

Suddenly rigid: stiffens out.

Violent convulsions with distortion of limbs and eyes. May begin in arm: then body thrown backwards and forwards.

Light (*Stram.*) motion and cold (rev. of *Op.*) will bring on a convulsion (*Caust.*).

Convulsions re-excited by least touch (*Nux.*, *Cic.*, *Strych.*) or draught (*Stram.*, *Cic.*, etc.).

Bell. has great excitement: has twitching, jerking, trembling, spasms, convulsions.

Convulsions come on suddenly: unexpectedly.

Convulsions of scarlet fever, meningitis: in nervous, brainy children with biggish heads.

"*Bell.* is sudden. It has no continuance, no periodicity."

N.B.—*Calcarea* is the chronic of *Bell.*, and its complementary remedy.

We are told that *Bell.* is often given when ACONITE would be more appropriate. Both are sudden: have dry, hot skin; startings and twitchings. Convulsions from teething.

But *Aconite* has anxiety, restlessness, *fear*: *Bell.*, excitement.

Stramonium .. Violent convulsions involving every muscle.

Opisthotonos: violent distortions.

Contractions of limbs: biting of tongue.

Convulsions from bright light (*Lyss.*), dazzling objects. *Renewal of spasms from light.* (*Stram.* is less rigid—less angular than *Bell.*, *Cic.*, *Cup.*). If a liquid touches lips spasms return with great violence. Shrieks.

Convulsions of head and arm with hiccough.

One side paralysed, the other convulsed.

Jerks head suddenly from pillow.

Very sensitive to light: fears the dark: yet convulsions, even cough, worse from light.

" An absolute stand-by in renal convulsions."

Hyoscyamus .. Infants go into convulsions.
Convulsions of children, esp. after a fright (*Op.*).
Convulsions after eating. Child becomes sick after eating, vomits and goes into convulsions. Shrieks and becomes insensible.
Convulsions from worms (*Cina, Art., Stann.*).
Sudden starting and twitchings : one arm will twitch, then the other.
Motions angular : frothing at mouth. Patient seems wild.
Convulsions during deep, heavy sleep.
Convulsions not general, but wandering.
Convulsions followed by squinting and disturbances of vision.
Hyosc. is suspicious, and jealous (*Lach.*).

Ignatia .. Convulsions from fear, fright, after punishment —which will bring on a convulsion (*Cina*).
Children are convulsed in sleep after punishment. Sensitives.
Face pale (opp. of *Bell., Stram., Op., Nux*), or flushed; usually deathly pale.
Convulsive twitchings. Twitches about eyelids and mouth, then stiffens out.
The child is cold and pale, has a fixed, staring look (stares *Cic., Stram., Mosch., Aeth.*).
Convulsions in first period of dentition.

Cina .. Child cannot stand any disturbance, cannot be punished (*Ign., Op.*), because it goes into a convulsion.
Grits teeth and clenches thumbs.
Chewing motions, even before teeth erupt.
Jerking, twitching, convulsions with worms.
Sleeps on abdomen (*Med.*).

Chamomilla .. Snappish. Complaints from contradiction.
Convulsions from anger (*Nux*), teething (*Calc.*).
Worse 9 p.m., and often 9 a.m.
Convulsions after every emotion.
Petulant and angry child.
One cheek red, one pale.
Hot sweat face and head.
Thumbs in palms of hands (*Cup.* and *Glon.*).

Nux .. .. Infantile convulsions from indigestion (*Ipec.*) or bad temper.
Convulsions with consciousness (*Cina, Stram.*).
Conscious or semi-conscious during spasm.
Convulsions of all the muscles of the body, with teeth clenched; with purple face and loss of breath.
The most violent convulsions with opisthotonos (*Cic., Op., Strych.*).
Twitchings, spasms; convulsions worse from the slightest touch, noise, jar* (*Cic.*, etc.), from slightest draught of air (*Lyss.*). After anger.
Patient is nervous and chilly. Oversensitive and irritable.

Oenanthe .. Involuntary stool during convulsions.
Violent convulsions: with eyeballs turned up: lockjaw (*Nux, Strych.*).
Fell back foaming at mouth, and black in face.
Spasms in rapid succession: choking noise in throat.
Complete unconsciousness.
Convulsions followed by deep sleep or coma.

Lyssin .. Spasms and convulsions. "Always associated with throat symptoms, i.e. always affects muscles of deglutition" (of jaw, *Nux, Oen.*).
Convulsions from reflex causes: i.e. attempts to swallow: to speak: a draught of air: sight or sound of running water: bright light (*Stram.*), or shining object: a loud noise: strong odours.
Convulsions with exalted state of sense of smell, taste and touch.
Violent epileptic attacks in quick succession.
Exquisite sensibility prevails over the whole body, esp. in organs of sense.

* *Week-ending in the country one summer, there was a luckless hen cooped up by herself. "Why?"—"Because at the slightest touch, or if another hen bumped into her, or even if the coop was shaken, she went down in a violent convulsion." Fresh from testing* Strychnine *on frog-muscle, and having no* Strych. *at hand, except as* Nux, *the latter was administered. Next Saturday the hen was found running about with the rest:* Nux *had promptly cured. . . . The consciousness of* POWER, *after prescribing the "like" medicine and seeing it act, is one of the joys of life!*

Cicuta .. .. Excessively *violent* convulsions. Patient is thrown into all sorts of odd shapes and violent contortions; but one of the most invariable is the *bending* of head, neck and spine backwards—*opisthotonos.* (*Bell.*, *Cup.*, *Hyos.*, *Nux.*, *Op.*, *Stram.*, *Strych.*, etc.)

Convulsions spread from above downwards.

Begin in head and go downwards. (Opp. of *Cup.*, where they start in fingers and toes.)

Head drawn back (*Op.*); limbs convulsed, rigid.

Great difficulty of breathing from spasm (*Bell.*).

Touch and draughts bring on convulsions (*Nux*, *Bell.*, *Lyssin*, *Stram.*, *Strych.*, etc.).

Head hot, and extremities cold.

" More *staring* than in any other remedy " (*Ign.*, *Mosch.*, *Aeth.*).

Between attacks, patient mild, gentle, placid, yielding (opp. of *Cup.* which is spiteful and violent between fits; and *Nux* and *Cham.*, which are very irritable).

Opium .. .. " Is full of convulsions."

Wants cool air; open air; to be uncovered.

Convulsions if room is too warm. (*Bell.* from cold, *Caust.*). Worse hot bath.

Opisthotonos: head drawn back nearly to heels (*Cic.*, *Op.*, *Strych.*), or legs and arms spread out. (See *Glon.*, *Plat.*)

Kicks covers off: skin red; face red, mottled.

Pupils contracted.

" Now if the mother puts that child into a hot bath to relieve the convulsions it will become unconscious and cold as death. If called to see such a case, be sure to give *Opium* " (Kent).

Convulsions from fright: " the object of the fright comes up before the eyes, before attack comes on."

" Sudden effect of emotions; punishment (*Ign.*, *Cina*), fright.

" Body stiffens, mouth and face twitch, exactly like *Ignatia*: only with *Opium* the face is dark red and bloated. Loud screams."

Wakes frightened, screams and cries till spasms.

Cuprum .. Convulsions of every degree of violence.

Earliest threateinngs are drawings *in fingers*, clenchings of thumbs, or twitching of muscles.

Thumbs first drawn into palms (*Cham.*, *Glon.*, *Aeth.*), fingers close over them with great violence.

Rigidity of muscles of jaw: bites spoon if attempt to give medicine.

Spasms followed by appearance as if patient were dead.

Between attacks, spiteful, violent, weeping, crying out and shrieking (opp. of *Cicuta*).

In epilepsy, clenching of fingers: falls with a shriek; and passes urine and fæces.

Eyes jerk, twitch, roll: rotate under closed lids.

Face and lips blue.

When eruptions fail to appear (*Zinc.*).

Zincum Convulsions during acute infective fevers (*Cup.*).

Feeble children: eruption does not come out: tendency to convulsions: suppression of urine: rolling of head from side to side.

Seems as if not strength for a violent spasm (opposite of *Cup.*).

Restless especially feet: "nervous feet."

Cerebral epilepsy: worse during rest.

Whole body jerks during sleep.

Cross before attack.

Bufo .. Pupils largely dilated and unaffected by light before attack (*Arg. nit.*).

Eyeballs rolled upwards and to left before attack.

(*Eyes rolled to left before attack*, led to curative use in fingers of *Bufo* in a recent case.)

Head drawn to one side, then back, before attack.

Eyes sunken during spasm.

Twitching of face muscles, extends to body.

Face bathed in sweat during convulsions.

Lapping motion of tongue: feels face, and rubs nose before attack.

Epilepsy following onanism.

Aethusa .. Convulsions with clenched thumbs (*Cup.*), red face (*Bell.*, *Glon.*) : staring (*Cic.*, *Ign.*, *Stram.*, etc.), dilated immovable pupils; teeth set.
"Dozing of the child after vomiting, after stool, with convulsions." Great weakness and prostration, with sleepiness.
Convulsions in cholera infantum.

Ipecacuanha .. *Nausea* and vomiting, before or during spasm.
Child spasmodically drawn in some direction.
Frightful spasms, affecting whole of left side.
Clonic and tonic spasms of children and hysterical women. Rigidity of body with flushed, red face, then spasmodic jerking of arms. Jerks arms towards each other.
From indigestible food (*Nux*, *Puls.*), or suppressed eruptions (*Cup.*, *Zinc.*).
"All the complaints in *Ipecac.* are attended more or less with *nausea.*"

Pulsatilla .. One of the effective medicines in epilepsy; but in the *Pulsatilla* patient—mild, irritable, changeable; easy weeping—and smiling: jealous; loves and craves fuss and affection.
Convulsions with violent tossings of limbs followed by relaxation; with disposition to vomit (*Ipec.*) and eructations.
(Later on, from suppressed menses.)

Silica .. .. Nocturnal convulsions, especially about the time of the new moon.
Before attack, coldness of left side, shaking and twisting of left arm. (Chronic of *Puls.*)

Sulphur .. Great medicine for epilepsy—in a *Sulphur* child.
Rough hair that will not lie down.
Hates a bath—even fears it.
Hungry: craves fat. Kicks off the clothes.
Spasms start with twitching of hands (*Cup.*), then general convulsed movements of body and limbs, with sensitiveness of abdomen.
Spasms after suppressed eruptions: often removes tendency to convulsions.
Aura in arms: like a mouse running. (*Bell.*, *Calc.*)

Calcarea ..	Teething convulsions. When after *Belladonna*, the convulsions persist. Convulsions in large-headed children whose heads sweat profusely: esp. in sleep; fat, lethargic, of "plus quantity minus quality"
Calcarea ars. ..	Epilepsies proceeding from valvular *heart* disease. Attacks begin with pain in heart, or constriction (even without organic disease). Rush of blood to head before attack. (Hering found it very useful in epilepsy.)
Viscum alb. ..	Convulsions with *heart* disturbance. With constant vertigo, even in bed. Feeling whole vault of skull would be raised up. Muscles of face in constant agitation.
Tarentula ..	Falls unconsciously without warning. Rigidity: grinds teeth: bites tongue. Eyes remain open, squinting (*Hyos.*). Dizziness before fit: then convulsions with *precordial anguish.* Great chorea medicine. Music soothes.
Glonoine ..	Convulsions. Great congestion to head and heart. *Heart* violent and irregular. Glowing redness of face (*Bell.*), but more dusky. *During attack spreads fingers and toes apart.* (Opp. to *Cup.*) Convulsions from exposure to sun (*Bell.*). Contracted pupils (*Op.*; rev. of *Bell.*).
Platinum ..	Convulsions of teething children: pale, anæmic. Jaws locked (*Nux, Oena., Strych.*). *Lies on back with flexed legs and knees widely separated.* Spasms without loss of consciousness. (*Nux.*)
Veratrum alb.	Convulsions of children with *face pale or blue, and cold sweat on forehead.* Cough before or after the attack.

Actea (*Cimicifuga*) .. Children wake, frightened and trembling. Periodic convulsions. Hysteric spasms. During the menses, epileptic spasms. Sadness and gloom : comes over like a cloud.

Causticum .. Convulsions at puberty : from fright (*Bell.*, *Op.*, etc.) with screams, gnashing of teeth, violent movements of limbs, jerking.
Convulsions from being chilled (*Bell.*).
Convulsions during sleep, with disturbed eyes, and icy coldness of body.
Right-sided convulsions.
Urine flows copiously and involuntarily during convulsions. (*Bufo.*, *Hyos.*, *Oena.*, *Plumb.*, *Zinc.*).

Plumbum .. Legs heavy and numb before attack. Swollen tongue.
Consciousness returns slowly, and symptoms of paralysis remain.
Plumbum is emaciated : boat-shaped abdomen, with " string from navel to back " sensation.
Great hyperæsthesia with loss of power.

Arsenicum .. " The child lies as if dead ; pale but warm ; breathless for some time ; finally it twists its mouth, first to one side then to the other ; a violent jerk passes through body, and respiration and consciousness gradually return."

Argentum nit. Cerebral epilepsy. Pupils permanently dilated hours or days before fit (*Bufo*).
Convulsions at night.
Convulsions preceded by great restlessness. (*Cup.* has great restlessness *between* attacks.)
The *Arg. nit.* patient feels the heat : craves salt and sweets.
Has all sorts of queer fears and ideas, as closing in of walls, or ceilings, etc.

For full lists of the remedies known to cause and cure convulsions one must, of course, go to a big Repertory, and, for their full indications, to Materia Medica. But the above are probably the most generally helpful, with suggestive differentiation. And here, again, there is always the final court of appeal—Materia Medica.

CHOREA

ALTHOUGH *Chorea* is supposed to be rheumatic in origin, its remedies are very different :—must be !—because the symptoms are so different.

Of course disease-names go for nothing in homœopathic prescribing. It is the sick individual whose sickness must be neutralized by a " like " drug-sickness. It does not even help to know that the microscopic changes in the nervous system are similar to those described in acute rheumatism " ; this only proves Kent's contention that, though the post mortem room may tell us a lot about disease, it has nothing to tell us about curing disease.

Old School treatment, beyond rest from " exertion—worry—the ridicule of companions "—is not illuminating. " *Arsenic* is usually given, but there is no evidence that it is of any value." Antipyrin—aspirin, etc., are suggested as " beneficial " : while what Hahnemann calls " anti-pathy " in the shape of inhalations of chloroform, is said to give its usual results :—" the movements return as the anæsthetic effect passes off."

But homœopathy gets its favourable results whenever the actual symptoms of the individual are met by a drug capable of provoking " like " symptoms in the healthy. We have no single remedy for chorea, but we have many ;—and no one will do for the other. The angular motions of *Hyoscyamus* will not yield to the graceful, gyratory attack of *Stramonium.* The jerkings that continue in sleep will be unaffected by *Agaricus*, which whatever the contortions by day, subsides into quiet sleep at night.

It is interesting to note that spider poisons affect nerves, some causing, and therefore curing, extreme jerkings and twitchings.

* * *

Agaricus .. Clumsy : drops things : tumbles over things.
On reaching for an object it is generally missed.
Frequent jumping of muscles in different parts of the body.
Involuntary movements of children when awake : *cease during sleep.* (*Mygale—reverse of Tarent.*)
Twitching of eyes—cheeks—chest—abdomen.
Jerking, twitching and trembling.
Creeping and crawling sensations.
May sweat alternate sides.
Agaricus is very chilly, and worse from cold.

Actea — Mental unbalance; gloom comes over like a cloud.
Irregular motions of left arm; or as if bound to side.

Ignatia .. Emotional chorea, after grief—fright—excitement or threats of punishment. Sighing and sobbing.
Gait affected: stumbles and falls over small objects (*Agar.*).
Drops things (*Agar.*). Constant involuntary twitchings and throwing about of arms. Motions and contortions of extremities and head.
Cannot walk, or use hands to write.
Sitting and standing extremely difficult.
Mentally unstable.
Bright child becomes almost imbecile.

Opium .. Emotional chorea (*Ign.*, *Lauro.*, *Cham.*) from fright; anger; reproaches.
Limbs tossed at right angles to body.
Spasmodic jerking of flexors.

Chamomilla .. Twitching eyes, facial muscles: of limbs.
Aversion to touch: mustn't be spoken to.
Spiteful, sudden or uncivil irritability.
Ailments from anger.

Magnesia phosphorica — Chorea: involuntary movements and contortions of limbs. Spasm of larynx, etc.
Convulsive twitchings of corners of mouth.
Mag. phos. is worse right side.
Worse from cold—air—draught—washing.
Worse from touch. Better for warmth and heat.

Mygale .. Twitchings and contractions of facial muscles especially: eyes and mouth open and close rapidly. Head jerked to esp. right side.
Words jerked out in talking.
Twitching and jerking of one arm and leg, generally right. Hand raised to head is violently jerked backwards, or down.
Uncontrollable movements of arms and legs.
Drags legs in attempting to walk.
Limbs quiet in sleep. (*Agar.* Rev. of *Tarent.*)
"One of our best remedies in uncomplicated chorea" (Farrington).

Tarentula	..	Right arm and leg especially affected. Nocturnal chorea: the contortions not even ceasing at night. (Reverse of *Agar.*, *Mygale.*) Eating causes involuntary movements of tongue, causing food to drop from mouth. Choreic, irregular movements. Very destructive. Tears or bites bedclothes. Chorea with inclination to bite and tear. Impending imbecility. (*Ign.*) Sensitive to music: amelioration from music. Worse when observed.
Tarentula cubensis	..	" Also said to be specific for Chorea, whether in children or in adults, in acute as well as in chronic cases."
Belladonna	..	Much twitching and jerking of muscles. Remarkable quickness of sensation and motion. Eyes snap and move quickly. Pupils dilated. Spasmodic motions: generally backwards. Throws body backwards and forwards when lying, like constant change from emprosthotonos to opisthotonos. Jumping, jerking, terrifying sleep (reverse of *Agar.*, *Mygale*). Starts and talks in sleep. Staggers when walking. Excitable and sensitive. Flushed face, bright eyes, big pupils, hot skin. After mental excitement.
Hyoscyamus	..	" Is full of convulsions and contractions and trembling and quivering and jerking of muscles." Convulsive jerks of the limbs, so that all sorts of *angular* motions are made. (*Stram.* is more graceful in its spasms.) Angular motions of arms. Where every muscle in the body twitches, eyes to toes. Suspicious. Loquacious. Will not remain covered. Dull mentally, if not excited. After a fright. (*Opium*, *Hyos.*, *Stram.*)

Stramonium .. Involuntary movements : spasms.
Very violent convulsive movements.
Raises arms over head : makes graceful gyratory movements (reverse of *Hyos.*).
Facial muscles constantly in play.
Chorea from fright. (*Hyos.*, *Opium.*)
Twitching of hands—feet—tendons.
"Affects all parts of the body crosswise : *or especially upper extremities.*"
Staggers when walking.
Cannot keep on feet in a dark room : falls.
Fear in dark : fear alone.

(A case of violent jerks on attempting to move or walk, after scarlet fever, improved with *Scarlatinum* ; then rapidly cleared up with *Ignatia.*)

Cuprum .. Periodic chorea.
Irregular movements : start in fingers and toes (rev. of *Agar.*) and spread over body.
Twitchings, often one-sided.
Awkward movements, with laughter, grimacing, distortion of mouth and eyes.
Terrible contortions.
Speech difficult, or imperfect.
Cramps.
Better lying down.
From a fright (*Opium*, *Hyos.*, *Stram.*).
Where eruptions " strike in " (scarlet fever, etc.)

Cicuta .. Violent jerkings : motion is convulsive. Spasms, clonic and tonic. Actions violent.
Chorea attacks twist child into curious frightful contortions, causing it to scream.
Walks feet turned in : on outer edge of foot.
Swings feet, each step describing an arc of a circle.
Strange desires, to eat coal, etc. (*Alum.*).
After accidents : concussion : injuries to head.

Arsenicum .. " Useful in stubborn cases of chorea."
Anxious: restless: fear: especially after midnight. Fastidious.

Phosphorus .. To clear up, in tall slender, nervous child : thirst for cold water : craves salt.

POINTERS IN THE RHEUMATISM OF CHILDREN

Aconite .. Intense sudden attacks due to *cold, dry* weather. Temp. to 104°. High fever, dry skin ; thirst ; red cheeks.

Shooting, tearing pains: often numbness (*Cham.*).

When rheumatism attacks heart.

Oppression of chest: hard, bounding pulse.

Palpitation of heart with great anguish.

(But, always with the *Acon.* restlessness, anxiety, and night aggravation.)

Belladonna .. Acute inflammatory rheumatism.

Blush over affected joints, which are red, hot, sore, and burn.

Worse for motion (*Bry. Spig.*) ; for *jar.*

The pains of *Bell.* come and go suddenly.

Bell. craves lemons which ameliorate.

Is worse for wetting head, or getting hair cut,—even to pains in the limbs.

Bryonia .. Joints red, swollen, stiff, with stitching pains.

Worse from the slightest motion.

Thirst for big drinks.

Dry coated tongue.

Wants to be let alone.

Bry. especially affects serous membranes, in all parts of the body: synovial membranes.

Rhus .. .. Constant movement is the patient's only relief (*Pyrog.*).

Or, must move, though movement is painful.

All sorts of rheumatic pains and lameness, ameliorated from motion: worse when keeping still: worse when beginning to move.

From cold air: from suppressed perspiration (*Dulc.*) from *cold, wet* weather. (*Dulc.*: but *Dulc.* has not the marked relief from motion.)

Can't bear cold water. Worse from washing, or a bath.

Chamomilla ..	Pains come on at night, especially early night: so violent, cannot keep still. Must be carried: or older, gets up and walks the floor. Pains with numbness: with twitching of limbs. Sleepless and restless at night. Jerks and twitches. *Oversensitive to pain.* "Cannot bear it." *Cham.* is cross, snappish, intolerant.
Mercurius ..	Rheumatism with filthy tongue. Offensive sweat. Worse for heat and cold. Worse at night. Worse for heat of bed.
Ledum ..	Chilly patient, but rheumatic pains relieved by cold. (*Puls.*). Pains worse at night: worse heat of bed: wants them uncovered. (*Merc.*—but *Merc.* has, also, profuse sweat without relief.)
Cimicifuga "*Actea rac.*" ..	Muscular rheumatism, esp. neck. Can't turn head. Stiff neck (*Rhus*). Chilly: affected by cold, by damp cold. (*Rhus.*, *Dulc.*) Hysterical and rheumatic conditions. Mental states follow disappearance of rheumatism. A black cloud comes over her. Numbness, jerking, trembling, soreness.
Pulsatilla ..	Rheumatic pains fly from one part to another. Pain, as if sprained, in joints, with redness and swelling. Rheumatic pains in spine and limbs, worse during rest, better from slow motion. (*Ferr.*) Worse wet: getting feet wet. Worse warm room: most pains better from cold. But—in the *Puls.* patient: weepy: irritable; changeable. Never wants water. Craves things that make her sick.

Natrum phos. Schüssler's great remedy for rheumatism.
" Acid muscles, with stiffness." (*Arnica*).
Tightness of muscles and tendons.
Weakness and heaviness of limbs. (*Gels.*).
Tendons feel shortened : about knees : " calves pulled tight."
Right wrist and knees especially affected.
Heart trembling, uneasy; especially when limbs are better.
A great remedy in the rheumatism of children : one has seen acute attacks subside in a couple of days.
All sorts of rheumatic conditions affecting periosteum (Comp. *Ruta*) and fibrous tissues.

Manganum .. Soreness of periosteum, esp. of shin-bones.
Soreness to touch and jarring. (*Bell.*)
Bones very sensitive to touch. Skin sensitive.
Intolerable pains in periosteum and bones.
Rheumatism wanders from joint to joint: worse touch, motion, at night.
Cannot bear weight on heels : (some rheumatic children have to walk on their toes).
Pulse soft and weak : sometimes rapid, sometimes slow.
Worse cold, damp weather. (*Dulc.*, *Rhus.*)
Face sicking, pale, sunken. (Anaemia).
Anxiety and fear: " something going to happen."
Relief from lying down.

Naja .. .. Trembling of muscles. Rheumatic diathesis : tendency of all complaints to settle about the heart.
" Young people who grow up with valvular disease.
" School boys and girls who have no symptoms : the generic remedy for this kind of " (heart) " complaint.
" The most useful of all the remedies we have in a cardiac state with very few symptoms." (KENT.)
Aching pain between shoulders with heart complaint.
Wakes suffocating, choking (*Lach.*).

Kalmia .. Wandering pains, worse motion.

Go downwards: down arms, legs; shoulders to fingers.

Shoot and tear along nerves.

Pains shift suddenly (*Puls.*). Come and go suddenly (*Bell.*).

Rheumatism (even syphilitic) that finally attacks heart, with thickening of valves.

Violent, tumultuous, visible action of heart (*Spig.*) : or, at times, remarkably slow pulse.

" Rheumatism treated externally and cardiac symptoms ensue."

Spigelia .. Rheumatic pericarditis and endocarditis.

Irregularity of heart.

Violent beating of heart, shakes the chest—the kind of heart-action " that can be seen and heard across the room ".

Must lie on right side, with head high.

(Like *Bry.*) worse from motion.

Thrusts, in chest, like a knife.

Spigelia's pains are violent, shooting, rending : —like burning-hot needles (*Ars.*) : like hot wires. Intense pains.

Pain leaves its mark, red, inflamed, sensitive.

Worse cold, damp. Sensitive to cold.

Worse stooping, motion, noise.

(Queer symptom) fear of pointed things—pins.

" Useful for acute heart attacks, and in chronic valvular disease, with attacks of violent palpitation."

Aurum .. Rheumatism which jumps from joint to joint and finally settles on heart.

Impossible to lie down : must sit bent forward.

Visible throbbing of carotids.

Face cyanotic : gasps for breath ; can hardly speak above a whisper.

Much perspiration.

Swelling of feet and legs.

Aurum is of all drugs the most depressed and despairing.

(See also Rheumatism of Adults.)

POINTERS IN ACUTE RHEUMATISM: MORE THE ADULT TYPE

(*See also previous section.*)

Aconite .. Sudden onset after exposure to *cold dry* air.
Pains, with formication and numbness (*Cham.*).
Rheumatic inflammation of joints; pains intolerable.
Intense bright-red swelling of parts. Sensitive to contact. High fever.
Worse at night.
With the *Aconite* anxiety, fear, restlessness.

Bryonia .. A " worse *cold, dry* weather " remedy (*Acon., Nux, Hep., Caust.*).
Acute articular rheumatism; swelling; tension.
Worse slightest movement. Wants to lie still.
Irritable, wants to be let alone.
White tongue; dry, dark, hard stools.
Thirsty for large drinks.
Perspiration relieves (reverse of *Merc.*).
The characteristic pains of *Bry.* are stitching.
Affects especially synovial membranes (joints, pleura, pericardium, meninges).
Local inflammation violent, parts very hot.

Nux .. " Whole body burning hot, especially face red and hot, yet cannot move or uncover in the least without feeling chilly "
" Rheumatic fever: vertigo, chilliness alternating with heat, pains in head, back and limbs; thirst; dry skin; scanty, dark urine; delayed stool. Evening fever < towards morning."
Lumbago; pains drawing and spasmodic. Must sit up to turn over.
Attacks especially trunks of muscles and large joints; pale tensive swellings.
Worse motion (*Bry.*); dread of motion.
Worse least jar (*Bell.*), and cold.
Very chilly; cannot bear to uncover.
Better for warmth, hot things, getting warm.
Nux is irritable, sullen, surly.
Is worse in dry, better in wet weather (*Caust.*).

Causticum .. From *cold dry weather* (*Acon.*, *Bry.*, *Nux*).
Better wet weather: warm wet (*Nux*).
Burning pain in joints.
Rheumatism of articulation of jaws (*Rhus*).
Stiffness, hips, back; rises with difficulty.

Rhus .. "*Worse cold, wet*" (*Dulc.*, *Colch.*, *Verat.*).
Worse wet; bathing; washing; strain.
Drawing, tearing pain, especially fibrous tissues; joints; round joints.
Restlessness; must move, though first movement painful.
Better from dry, warm applications.

Rhododendron .. Like *Rhus*. *Worse cold, wet, stormy weather.*
Better motion. But pains shift more than those of *Rhus*. Move from above downwards.

Dulcamara .. From a chill when hot; suppressed sweat or eruptions. From *cold wet weather* (*Rhus*).
Sudden change to cold weather.
Neck stiff, back painful, loins sore and lame.
Better moving about (*Rhus*).

Arsenicum .. Indicated by its periodicity and time aggravation: after midnight, and from 1-2 a.m.
And by its intense restlessness, mental and physical: its anxiety and prostration.

A recent very acute case, rapid onset, high fever, pain in knee that kept patient turning and twisting, though every movement provoked cries and both elbows were quickly worn through with the efforts to turn. Mouth and tongue were absolutely dry on waking, and there were night-sweats. *Rhus* did not help. But *Ars.* 200 gave almost instantaneous relief, and patient woke the following day after fourteen hours deep sleep with dry skin and moist mouth, and pain practically gone. That ended the attack:—but it had to be recovered from.

Colchicum .. Arthritic pains; a jar makes patient scream.
Affects periosteum and synovial membranes.
Redness, heat, swelling of affected joints.
Worse cold, wet weather; checked sweats.
Worse autumn. Better warmth.
Patient is cold, weak, sensitive, restless.
Loathes the smell or sight *of food.* (*Ars.*, *Sep.*).

Belladonna .. Joints swollen, red, hot, shining.
Exquisitely sensitive to touch or jar.
Red streaks radiate from inflamed joint.
Recurrent fever with pains attacking nape of neck.
Especially with brain symptoms.

Salicylic acid .. Acute, inflammatory rheumatism of one or more joints, especially elbows or knees.
Great swelling and redness. High fever.
Very sensitive to least jar (*Bell.*).
Motion impossible.
In potency, where symptoms agree.

Sticta .. Acute inflammatory rheumatism, esp. of knee.
Worse from motion.
Loquacity ; must talk.
Levitation ; limb as if not resting on bed.

Chamomilla .. Numbness with the pain. (*Acon.*).
"Cannot bear it!" Beside himself with anguish.
Irritable to the last degree (*Nux*). Rude.
Stitching pains jump from place to place.
Violent rheumatic pains drive him out of bed, and compel him to walk about (Has cured Trench fever).

Lac caninum .. Inflammatory rheumatism ; wanders from joint to joint, crosses from side to side (ankle to ankle, etc.) *then comes back.*
Worse by slightest motion, by touch.
Hyperæsthesia ; hypersensitive.
(?—Peculiar delusion : "Infested by snakes.")

Ferrum phos. .. "Like an acutely developed rheumatism in a *Phos.* patient."
Acute articular rheumatism ; attacking one joint after another : joints puffy, but little red ; high fever. Or red, swollen, and very sensitive. Worse from slightest movement.

Kali bichrom. .. Wanders from joint to joint (*Mang.*, *Puls.*, *Lac can.*).
Alternates with digestive troubles.

Pulsatilla .. *Changeable*, every way.
Pains shift rapidly from part to part.
Now intensely severe ; now mild.
Also with redness and swelling of joints.
From wet weather ; wet feet (*Sil.*).
Chilliness increases with the pains : yet *worse from heat*—at night—in bed.
Better uncovering ; cold drink ; cool open air.
Sensitive to jar, touch, pressure.
Can hardly give symptoms for weeping.
Changeable moods ; irritable—then tearful—then smiling.
Dry mouth but thirstless (*Merc.* moist mouth with intense thirst).
" Drawing, tearing pains in limbs, better motion and after motion ; worse warm room ; better cold applications." (Compare *Kali sulph.*)

Ledum .. Like *Puls.*, worse from heat ; better from cold.
" *Pulsatilla*, but even more so ! "
The patient that has been found " kicking ice about in a tub to relieve pains in feet "
Worse warm in bed.
Always chilly, yet pains worse heat, and better cold.
Worse moving, especially joints (*Puls.* is better slow motion).
Starts in feet and travels up (reverse of *Kalm.*).
Affected joints worse the least jar.
" *Ledum* is bloated and purple."

Phytolacca .. Acute rheumatism which is prolonged ; worse at night.
Worse from warmth of bed, and warm applications.
Restlessness ; pain unbearable (*Cham.*).
Gonorrhœal rheumatism (*Med., Thuj.*).

Medorrhinum Acute gonorrhœal rheumatism with intense pain and tenderness in affected joints.

Veratrum alb. Pains very severe, driving the patient to delirium. *Worse wet weather*.
Keynote : cold sweat, face, esp. forehead.

Eupatorium .. Feels bruised—broken—dislocated.
Bones as if broken.
Rheumatism with perspiration and soreness of bones.
Chills and high fever. Much shivering.
Joints especially affected, hip, shoulder, inside knee, foot, great toe, elbow.
Sharp pains in hip, ankle and shoulder.
Pains worse 10 a.m. to 4 p.m.
Wants to keep still, but must move.

Arnica .. Soreness, numbness, swelling of affected joint.
Dreads touch.
" Bed too hard " (*Pyrog.*). Worse moving the part.
Intercostal rheumatism, simulates pleurisy. (Here acts like a charm.)
Worse damp cold weather (*Rhus, Dulc.*).
Heart affected, with dilatation and dyspnœa.

Gelsemium .. Rheumatic pains with heaviness and loss of power in limbs. With trembling.
Fever with chills up and down the back.
Illness begins in warm weather.

Mercurius .. Profuse and persistent sweating without relief.
Worse for sweat.
Drenched in offensive sweat ; offensive mouth.
Worse night ; from heat of bed (reverse of *Nux*).
Creepy chills ; *creepy chills in affected parts.*

Hepar .. Sweats day and night without relief.
Sweats from slightest motion.
Dread of, and extreme sensitiveness to contact (*Arn.*) out of proportion to actual pain.
< Cold : *Draught.*

Actea rac. (*Cimicifuga*) Rheumatic pains in joints, with heat and swelling.
Affects the bellies of muscles ; cramping, stitching pains.
Extreme muscular soreness.
" A heavy black cloud has settled all over her."

Kalmia .. Migratory rheumatism, with the heart affected.
Pains extend downwards, and shift suddenly.
Often remarkable slowness of pulse.

Cactus .. Inflammatory rheumatism with heart trouble.
Constriction, everywhere.
Constriction of the heart, as if an iron band prevented its normal movement; or as if caged.

Anacardium .. Rheumatic affections of pericardium.
Sharp stitches through cardiac region. (*Sulph.*, *Spig.*).
Stitches being "double", i.e. one stitch quickly followed by another; then a long interval.

China .. Has cured acute inflammatory rheumatism with every-other-day aggravation of symptoms.

Drosera .. "A case of acute rheumatism, following whooping-cough, cleared up rapidly after *Drosera*."
Gnawing and shooting in the shafts of the long bones, arms, thighs and legs: with severe stitches in the joints.
Ankle bones are specially affected.
Pains as if dislocated: great stiffness.
"Bed too hard" sensation (*Arn.*, *Pyrogen.*).
Shivering when at rest: when moving, no shivering (reverse of *Nux*).
Febrile rigor all over body, with heat in face, but cold hands: without thirst.
Sweats. Night-sweats.

(But the disease-product remedies must not be forgotten.)

Medorrhinum Several joints affected—later one.
Extensive redness, swelling, pain and tenderness.
Pain very severe, < slightest movement.
Wrists and ankles especially affected—knees.
Burning palms and soles: wants feet uncovered.
Acute (and chronic) gonorrhœal rheumatism. (*Thuja. Nit. acid.*)

Thuja ..	Here the knee-joint is most affected. *Very offensive sweat* (*Merc.*)—oily: stains yellow. Night-sweats, even soaking bed : end at 2-3 a.m. A queer symptom "Sweat only on uncovered parts."
Tuberculinum *Bacillinum* ..	With a T.B. family history, or history of some previous T.B. manifestation. We have recently seen, in Hospital, two cases of protracted acute rheumatism, that only began promptly to clear up when one of these T.B. nosodes was given.

It may be helpful to roughly epitomize. Rheumatism—

Worse warmth ..	Bry., Led., Phos., Phyt., Puls., Thuja.
Better cool ..	Led., Puls.
Better warmth ..	Ars., Caust., Colch., Coloc., Lyc., Merc., Nux, Rhus., Sulph.
Worse cold wet ..	Arn., Colch., Dulc., Rhus, Verat.
Worse cold dry ..	Acon., Bry., Caust., Hep., Nux.
Better wet, or worse dry ..	Asar., Bry., CAUST., HEP, K.c., NUX, Sep., Spong.
Better warm wet ..	Caust., Hep., Nux.
Worse motion ..	BRY., Ferr. phos., Lac can., Led., Salicyl. acid, Sticta.
Better motion ..	Cham., Dulc., Rhod., RHUS, PULS.
Worse wet ..	Puls., Verat. (see "cold wet").
Shifts rapidly ..	Kalm., LAC CAN., PULS., Kali bich.
Numbness with pain	Acon., Cham., Puls.
Worse jar ..	Arn., BELL., BRY., Hep., Led., Nux, Rhus.
Worse touch ..	Arn., BELL., Bry., Cham., COLCH., HEP., Led., Med., NUX, Puls., Rhod., Rhus.
Unaffected by change of weather excludes	Dulc., Nux m., Phos., Ran. b., Rhodo., Rhus, Sil., Tub.
Not affected by wet, excludes ..	Calc., Merc., Nat. s., Ruta.

THE MORE COMMON HEART REMEDIES

WITH INDICATIONS

Arnica .. Pain in region of heart, as if it were squeezed together (*Cact.*, *Lil. tigr.*), or had got a shock, or blow. (*Angina Pectoris.*)

Heart first rapid, then extremely slow.

Stitches in cardiac region : stitches left to right.

Pulse feeble—hurried—irregular.

Horror of instant death with cardiac distress in the night.

Imagines he has heart disease.

One of our greatest remedies for tired heart : dilated after strain or exertion.

" Arnica is the most remarkable heart remedy we possess." Also " our biggest pick-me-up."

Tired out from physical or mental strain.

Feels bruised, beaten, sore : bruises easily.

Restless because bed feels too hard.

Does not wish to be touched : fears approach.

Aconite .. Great distress in heart and chest.

Dreadful oppression of the precordial region.

Inward pressing in the region of the heart.

Palpitation with great anxiety and difficulty of breathing. Anguish with dyspnœa.

Sensation of something rushing into head, with confusion and flying heat in face.

Sudden attacks of pain in heart, with dyspnœa.

Aconite is ANXIOUS ; restless ; with fears : fear of death.

Sudden acute conditions from chill, shock, fright.

All ailments and fears worse at night.

(Under *Aconite* Kent writes : " Sits up straight and can hardly breathe. *Aconite* has such a violent cardiac irritation, pulse fluttering, weak, full and bounding : sits up in bed, grasps the throat, wants everything thrown off ; before midnight a hot skin, great thirst, great fear—everything is associated together. . . . Sudden attacks of pain in the heart with dyspnœa . . . breaks into a profuse sweat . . awful anxiety.")

Spigelia .. VIOLENT beating of heart, so that he frequently could hear the pulsation, or so that the beats could be seen through the clothes.
Palpitation aggravated by sitting down and bending forward (rev. of *Kali carb.*)
Heart seemed to be in tremulous motion.
Worse for deep inspiration, or holding breath.
" Heart sounds may be audible several inches away." (Nash.)
Must lie on right side, or with head very high.
Spigelia's pains are *stitching*. Sharp neuralgic pains (chest, head, heart, eyes, etc.).
Worse for slightest motion.

Lycopus vir. .. Protusion of eyes, with tumultuous action of heart. (*Spig.*)
Eyes feel full and heavy ; pressing outwards.
Cardiac irritability. Pulse frequent, small, compressible : or quick hard, wiry, not compressible.
Trembling hands.
(*Lycopus* is useful in exophthalmic goitre.)

Kali carb. .. Stitching pains—chest—heart, extort cries.
Stitches about heart and through to scapula.
Heart's action intermittent, irregular, tumultuous, weak. Mitral insufficiency.
Leans forward resting on arms to take weight off chest (rev. *Spig.*).

(One has seen *Kali carb.* following a few doses of *Carbo veg.*, bring back to life a dying child, an old mitral case, with pericarditis with effusion, and pneumonia with pleural effusion. A visiting doctor said (she was lying forward, cold, almost pulseless, just giving last jerking gasps), " I'll eat my hat if that child pulls round," and she did !—to come into Hospital again a couple of years later for a less severe breakdown.)

Kali carb. has *stitching pains* (like *Bry.*), but also independently of motion and respiration (unlike *Bry.*).
Its worst hours are 2-4 a.m.
Has profuse sweat. Puffiness about the eyes.
Complementary to *Carbo veg.* (that " corpse reviver ").

Lilium tigr. .. Dull pressive pain in heart ; sharp quick pain, with fluttering.

Roused from sleep by pain as if heart were violently grasped, the grasp gradually relaxed, interrupting heartbeat and breathing.

Sensation as if heart was grasped or squeezed in a vice (*Cactus*) ; as if blood had all gone to heart: must bend double; (reverse of *Spig.*).

Heart alternately grasped and released.

Heart feels over-loaded with blood.

Violent palpitation with throbbing of carotids.

Depression of spirits. Weeps.

Characteristics: Hurried feeling, as of imperative duties and inability to perform them.

Pressure on rectum and bladder. Terrible urging to stool, to urinate, all the time.

Bearing down with heavy weight, as if whole contents of pelvis would issue through vagina, but for upward pressure of hand.

Cactus Palpitation of the heart : heart squeezed.

Sensation of constriction in the heart, as if an iron band prevented its normal movement.

Several violent, irregular beats of the heart, with sensation of pressure and heaviness.

" Irregular heart-beats, with necessity for deep inspiration. Congestion in chest.

Painful constriction lower chest; "a cord tightly bound round false ribs, obstructing breathing."

Great constriction (sternum) " compressed by iron pincers."

" It is the nature of *Cactus* to constrict."

Tightness and constriction about head—chest—diaphragm—heart—uterus :—clutchings.

Chest as if filled with hot gushes of blood.

" *Cactus* has a profound curative action upon the heart."

Fear and distress. Such violent suffering !

Screaming with the pain.

Determination of blood to an organ :—chest—heart. " Blood always in the wrong place."

Strong pulsations felt in strange places—stomach—bowels—even extremities.

" 11 o'clock remedy : 11 a.m. and 11 p.m."

Sepia .. Violent palpitation of the heart and beating of all the arteries, in bed. Stitches in heart.
Violent palpitations of heart, as if it would force its way through chest wall ; *relieved by walking a long distance, and walking very fast.*
The *Sepia* patient is indifferent : hates fuss.
Tendency to ptosis and dragging down, especially in pelvic organs. (*Lil. tigr.*)
Profuse perspirations, especially axillæ.
General relief from motion—food—sleep.

Digitalis .. Sensation as though heart stood still, with great anxiety : must hold breath.
Pulse very slow :—thready, slow, intermittent.
Heart has lost its force ; beats more frequent, and sometimes irregular.
Sensation as if heart would stop beating if she moved. (*Gels.* must move or it will stop.)
Respiration difficult : sighing : stops when she drops off to sleep.
Digitalis affects heart and liver : jaundice – white stools, *with very slow pulse.* (*Kalm.*)
Diarrhœa and nausea with heart disease.

Kalmia .. Violent palpitations of the heart with faint feelings : with oppressed breathing.
Wandering rheumatic pains in region of heart, extend down left arm. (*Lat. mact.*, *Med.*)
Heart disease, after frequent attacks of rheumatism, or alternating with it.
Hypertrophy and valvular insufficiency, or thickening after rheumatism ; paroxysms of anguish about heart, with dyspnœa and febrile excitement.
Remarkable slowness of pulse (*Dig.*). Pulse very feeble : or, heart's action very tumultuous, rapid and visible (*Spig.*)
" When rheumatism has been treated externally and cardiac symptoms ensue." (Kent.)

Naja .. A great heart medicine, only proved in low potencies, so we lack the finer indications.
Heart weak. Post-diphtheritic heart.
" For a heart damaged by acute rheumatism."

Aurum .. Frequent attacks of anguish about the heart, and tremulous fearfulness.

Violent palpitation of the heart.

Congestion of heart, notably with the *Aurum* mental symptoms.

Rheumatism that has gone to heart (*Kalm.*).

Acute rheumatism with desperate heart conditions; extreme dyspnœa; impossible to lie down.

A queer symptom—heart seems to shake, as if loose, when walking.

The *Aurum* mental state is profound despondency and melancholy.

Disgust for life. Tendency to suicide.

Great anguish increasing into self-destruction.

Absolute loss of enjoyment in everything.

Terrible melancholy after the abuse of Mercury.

Pains wander from joint to joint and finally settle in the heart.

Aurum mur. .. Is also very valuable in heart troubles.

Hering (Guiding Symptoms) says "Angina pectoris (next to *Arnica* indispensable)."

Heaviness, aching, sensation of rigidity in heart. Cardiac anguish. Sticking in heart.

Latrodectus mactans .. Violent precordial pains extending to axilla and down left arm and forearm to fingers, with numbness and apnœa.

Violent precordial pains and pain left arm, which was almost paralysed.

Pulse uncountable: quick and thready.

(A great medicine for angina pectoris.)

Spongia .. Constricting pain (*cardiac*) with anxiety.

Attacks of oppression and cardiac pain < lying with head low. Anxious sweat.

Palpitation: violent, with pain, gasping respiration: suddenly awakened after midnight with suffocation, great alarm, anxiety.

Awoke often in a fright, felt suffocating (*Lach.*). Lips blue (*Lach.*).

Angina pectoris: contracting pain in chest, heat, suffocation, faintness, anxious sweat.

(*Exophthalmic goitre.*)

Lachesis Cramp-like pain in precordial region, causing palpitation with anxiety.

" Heart feels too large for containing cavity."

Bluish lips. Cyanosis. (*Spongia.*)

Intolerance of touch or pressure on throat—larynx—stomach—abdomen.

As if something swollen in pit of throat would suffocate him.

Worse after sleep. (*Spongia.*)

" *Lachesis* is one of our most useful remedies in heart troubles, acute or chronic; the peculiar suffocation, cough, and aggravation from constriction being the guiding symptoms." (Nash.)

Arsenicum . Useful in advanced and desperate heart cases.

Palpitation, with anguish; cannot lie on back: worse going up stairs. Heartbeats irritable.

Palpitation and tremulous weakness after stool.

Angina pectoris; sudden tightness above the heart; agonizing precordial pain; pains extend into neck and occiput; (*Latrodect.* and *Kalm.* to left arm and hand); breathing difficult; fainting spells. Least motion makes him lose his breath, sits bent forward, or with head thrown back. Worse at night, especially 1-5 a.m.

Rheumatism affecting heart, with great prostration, cold, sticky sweat; great anxiety and oppression; burning about the heart.

Pulse small, rapid, feeble: intermittent.

Valvular disease, with dyspnœa, anasarca.

Hydropericardium with great irritability, anguish and restlessness.

N.B.—The cardinal symptoms of *Ars.* are generally present: *extreme restlessness*, driving out of bed, or from bed to bed. Thirst for small quantities, often. Aggravation from cold: relief from heat. (Reverse of *Apis.*) But one has seen *Ars.* rapidly curative in a desperate case of hydropericardium, where these were absent.

Apis .. " The lancinating, darting pains, palpitation, orthopnœa, have rendered *Apis* invaluable in cardiac inflammations and dropsy."

Sudden œdema, dyspnœa, and sudden lancinating or STINGING pains, restlessness and anxiety.

Think of *Apis* for burning and *stinging* pains—anywhere.

Apis is generally thirstless.

Is worse after sleep: from warm room, and heat: better cold air, cold room, cold applications. (Reverse of *Ars.*)

" Skin alternately dry and hot, or perspiring."

Sulphur Anxious palpitation. Violent palpitation.

Rush of blood to heart. " Too much blood in heart." (*Cact.*) Heart feels enlarged.

Great orgasm of blood, with burning hands.

Stitches heart and chest; worse deep breathing.

Sulphur is hungry—untidy—argumentative.

Worse heat: intolerant of clothing: fond of fat.

Complaints relapse. Suppressed eruptions.

Pulsatilla .. Rheumatic irritation of heart, where pains shift rapidly about the body.

Heart symptoms reflex from indigestion.

Heaviness, pressure, fullness (heart). Violent palpitation with anguish: sight obscured.

Patient nervous, weepy, intolerant of heat: craves air, and fuss.

Phosphorus .. Palpitation: violent: on slightest motion.

Violent, lying on left side.

Precordial anguish from emotion.

Heaviness, chest, as if a weight lying on it.

Constriction: pressing sensation about heart.

Burning pain between scapulae. (*Lyc.*)

The *Phos.* type: tall, fine: fear alone, **dark**, thunder. Thirst for cold drinks.

In cases that do not respond normally to treatment one must not forget the Nosodes. One of Hahnemann's "chronic parasitic diseases" may be the bar to progress in acute sickness also—and that not only with tubercle, syphilis and gonorrhoea, but also in regard to scarlet fever, diphtheria, small-pox, measles and all the rest. Therefore, one should remember :—

Tuberculinum Bacillinum .. Heart cases where there is a family, or past history of tubercular manifestations.
Palpitation : heaviness : pressure over heart.
Irritable : irritable on waking : nothing pleases : nothing satisfies.
" Wants to travel : cosmopolitan condition of mind." Suffocates in a warm room. (*Puls.*)

Medorrhinum .. Heart felt very hot : beat fast : with bursting sensation : or feeling of a cavity where heart ought to be.
Sharp pain at apex, worse motion.
Great pain, heart, extending to left arm (*Latro. mact.*) and throat.
Intense pain, heart, radiates to all parts of left chest : worse least movement.
The troubles of *Medorrh.* are worse by day—sunrise to sunset.
Those of *Luet.* by night : sunset to sunrise.
Medorrh. is rich in mental symptoms : *Everything seems unreal,* like a dream.
Time moves so slowly : things done an hour ago, as if done a week ago. (*Cann. ind.*)
Anguish : introspection : always anticipating evil happenings. "Someone behind her."
Cannot concentrate : forgets what she is reading : cannot spell simple words.
News coming seems to touch her heart before she hears it.

Lueticum .. Pain and pressure behind the sternum.
Lancinating pains in heart *at night,* base to apex (*Medorrh.* is worse by day).

Diphtherinum .. Needs proving : but with history of diphtheria.
Feeble, irregular or intermittent pulse, quick or slow, with vomiting and cyanosis.

Cratægus oxy. (Hawthorn berries) An Irish doctor is said to have made a reputation by using *Cratægus* in heart disease.

"*Weak heart muscles.*"

Pulse irregular, feeble, intermittent.

"Must be used for some time to obtain good results. (Boericke.)

CHICKEN-POX

ACONITUM NAPELLUS

Early cases, with restlessness, anxiety and high fever.

ANTIMONIUM TARTARICUM

Delayed or receding, blue or pustular eruptions.
Drowsy, sweaty and relaxed; nausea.
Tardy eruption, to accelerate it.
Associated with bronchitis, especially in children. (*Ant. crud.*)

BELLADONNA

Severe headache: face flushed; hot skin.
Drowsiness with inability to sleep.

MERCURIUS

"Should vesicles suppurate."

RHUS TOXICODENDRON

Intense itching.
"Generally the only remedy required; under its action the dise soon disappears."

DIPHTHERIA

APIS

Throat bright-red, puffy, "varnished". Uvula long; œdematous. Nothing must touch throat (*Lach.*).

ARSENICUM ALBUM

Membrane looks dry, shrivelled. The *Arsenicum* anxiety, restlessness and prostration are present.

Worse at night: 1–2 a.m.

Chilliness: incessant thirst for small quantities.

BAPTISIA

Putridity: with dull red face; drowsiness; patient as if drugged.

Membrane dark: dry brown tongue.

DIPHTHERINUM

When the attack from the onset tends to malignancy.

Painless diphtheria. Symptoms almost, or entirely objective.

Patient weak, apathetic. Stupor.

Dark-red swelling of tonsils and throat.

Breath and discharges very offensive (*Merc. cy.*).

Membrane thick, dark-grey or brownish black.

Temperature low, or subnormal. Pulse weak and rapid. Vital reaction very low.

Epistaxis, or profound prostration from the onset. Collapse almost at the very beginning.

Swallows without pain, but fluids are vomited or returned through nose.

Laryngeal diphtheria; post-diphtheric paralysis. (*Caust.*, *Cocc.*, *Gels.* and *Lycopodium.*)

When the patient from the first seems doomed, and the most carefully-selected remedies fail to relieve, or permanently improve.

To remove persistent diphtheria-organisms, in "carriers".

Like all the nosodes, it is practically worthless below the 30th potency while its curative virtues increase with the higher potencies. It should not be repeated too frequently.

KALI BICHROMICUM

Nasal diphtheria: ropy discharges.
Exudation tough and firmly adherent.

LAC CANINUM

Patients nervous, imaginative, highly sensitive.
Skin hypersensitive (*Lach.*). Touch unbearable, though hard pressure gives no pain.
Membrane pearly, or silver white.
Milky coating on tongue.
Characteristic feature is *alternation of sides.*
Pain will jump back and forth from side to side.

LACHESIS MUTA

Membrane starts on left side, spreads to right.
Face and throat look cyanotic. Choking.
Cold things more easily swallowed than hot.
Great sensitiveness of neck and throat, so that patient cannot stand the touch of bedclothes, and pulls neck of night attire open.
General and local aggravation from heat, and all symptoms are worse after sleep. The longer the sleep, the worse he is on waking.
Characteristics are loquacity and suspicion.

LYCOPODIUM

Patient worse from 4 to 8 p.m.
Starts in nose (*Kali bic.*) or right side throat, spreads to left.
Warm drinks more easily swallowed: but reverse sometimes the case.
Movement of nostrils.
Diminished urine or copious sediment of urates, or fine red sand.

MERCURIUS CYANATUS

Fairly rapid onset, with prostration.
One or both sides of throat affected.
Membrane spreads rapidly over entire throat.
Colour white, yellow, or greenish.
Tongue thickly coated, moist; salivation.
Odour always putrid. Hot sweats.
Tepid liquids better swallowed than hot or cold.
Patient (generally) worse late evening and night.
Has also proved curative in Vincent's Angina.

PHYTOLACCA

Frequently indicated.

Membrane grey or white, may start on uvula.

May spread from right tonsil to left (*Lyc.*). But, unlike *Lyc.*, the pain is worse from heat.

Fauces dark-red: complains of lump in throat; or as if red-hot ball had stuck in throat.

Pain goes to ear.

ERYSIPELAS

ACONITUM NAPELLUS

Sudden violent onset after exposure to cold wind.
Intense fever, with restlessness, and *fear of death.*

APIS

May be in patches. Great tumefaction.
High degree of inflammation, with *stinging*, *burning*, and *œdema* and vesication.
Eyelids like sacs of water.
Amelioration from cold; aggravation from heat.
Fidgety, nervous, fretful: sleepless.

ARSENICUM ALBUM

"Sudden inflammatory conditions like gangrenous and erysipelatous inflammations.
A sudden inflammation that tends to produce malignancy in the part, belongs to *Arsenicum.*"
The secretions of *Arsen.* are acrid.
Characteristic, *burnings relieved by heat:* intense *anxiety*, *restlessness* and prostration.

BAPTISIA

Drowsy, dusky, comatose; face dark-red, with besotted expression. May be roused, but falls asleep answering.
Typhoid conditions, in the course of disease.
Acts very rapidly; rapid collapse, and rapid restoration. (*Crot. h.*)

BELLADONNA

Swelling, smooth, bright-red, streaked red; or deep, dark red.
Not much tendency to œdema or vesication.
Pains are throbbing; throbbing in brain.
Brain affected. Cases with delirium.
Jerking of limbs.
Belladonna is acute, *sudden*, and violent.
Belladonna is red, and intensely hot, dry.

CANTHARIS

Erysipelas of face with large blisters.

Burning in eyes: whole atmosphere looks yellow: scalding tears.

Like *Rhus*, but when very violent, *Canth.* will be indicated.

"*Rhus* has the blisters and the burning, but in *Canth.* between your two visits the erysipelas has grown black: it is a dusky rapid change that has taken place, looks as if gangrene would set in. Burning like fire from touch: as if the finger were a coal of fire. Not so in *Rhus*.

"The little blisters, if touched, burn like fire. ***Eruptions burn when touched***" (KENT).

Erysipelas of eyes, with gangrenous tendency. "Unquenchable thirst with disgust for drinks."

CROTALUS HORRIDUS

Frequently recurring erysipelas of face.

General local phlegmonous or œdematous erysipelas. Skin bluish-red; low fever.

Gangrene: skin separated from muscles by a fœtid fluid. Black spots with red areola and dark, blackish redness of adjacent tissues.

"*Crotalus* is indicated in disease of the very lowest, the most putrid type, coming on with unusual rapidity, reaching that putrid state in an unusually short time" (KENT). (*Bapt.*)

CROTON TIGLIUM

"*Erysipelas that itches very much.*"

"Eruptions that itch very much; but cannot bear to scratch, as it hurts. A very slight scratch, a mere rub, serves to allay the irritation" (GUERNSEY).

Sensation, "Insects creeping on face."

"Cough disappears and the eruption comes; then eruption goes and cough comes back."

CUPRUM METALLICUM

Erysipelas of face disappears suddenly.

Eruptions "strike in" and cramps, spasms, convulsions supervene. To bring the eruption back, with relief.

Cramps begin characteristically in fingers and toes.

EUPHORBIUM

Vesicular erysipelas: erysipelas bulbosum.

Red inflammatory swelling, with vesicles as large as peas, filled with yellow liquid.

Red, inflammatory swelling, with boring, grinding, gnawing from gums into ear, followed by itching and tingling.

Vesicles burst and emit a "yellow humour".

Shuddering and chilliness.

Temporary attacks of craziness.

HIPPOZÆNINUM
(Nosode of Glanders)

"Malignant erysipelas, particularly if attended by *large formation of pus, and destruction of parts.* Ulcers with no disposition to heal, livid appearance" (CLARKE).

LACHESIS MUTA

Purple, mottled, puffy.

"When the cerebral condition does not yield to *Belladonna.*" *Bell.* is red: *Lach. less red and more blue.*

Especially affects the left side.

Lachesis, typically, is worse after sleep: is loquacious—suspicious—jealous.

Is hypersensitive to touch, esp. on throat: wants face free, or suffocates.

MERCURIUS

With salivation: bitter or salt taste.

With offensiveness: breath, sweat.

Erysipelas with sloughing: with "brown mortification". With burning: ulceration.

Chilliness and heat alternately: or heat and shuddering at the same time.

Creeping chilliness: in single parts: in places of pus formation, or ulceration.

Worse at night.

RHUS TOXICODENDRON

Erysipelas of the vesicular variety, accompanied by *restlessness.*

Erysipelas of face with burning; large blisters, rapidly extending: becomes very purple and pits on pressure.

Often extends from l. to r. across face.

Rhus is worse from damp: from cold: relieved, temporarily, by motion.

SECALE CORNUTUM

Gangrenous erysipelas: competes with *Ars.* The only distinguishing feature between the two remedies may be that *Secale* wants cold and *Arsenicum* wants heat.

Burning: "sparks of fire" falling on the part.

Formication: "mice creeping under the skin."

THUJA

Œdematous erysipelas of face.

Cases that occur in the much vaccinated may need *Thuja*, or cases that occur *after vaccination.*

A curious, characteristic symptom, profuse sweat only on uncovered parts.

VERATRUM VIRIDE

"One peculiar symptom I have verified in a very severe case of erysipelas, which was accompanied by great delirium, is *a narrow, well-defined red streak right through the middle of the tongue*" (NASH).

"Phlegmonous erysipelas of face and head" (CLARKE).

LESS SEVERE CASES

AMMONIUM CARBONICUM

"Erysipelas of old, debilitated persons.

Eruption faintly developed, or has seemed to disappear, from weakness of patient's vitality to keep it on the surface.

With cerebral symptoms, simulating a drunken stupor" (NASH).

"Eruption comes out, and does not give relief to the patient."

"Erysipelas of old people when cerebral symptoms are developed."

Defective reaction.

ARNICA

"Erysipelas of face, with *soreness*, and sore *bruised feeling* all over the body: you need not wait longer before prescribing *Arnica.*"

"Bed feels too hard: must move to get into a new place." "*Rhus* moves from restlessness and uneasiness, cannot lie still: *Arnica*, to ease the *soreness* by getting into a new place" (KENT).

GRAPHITES

"Eruptions oozing out a thick, honey-like fluid . . . erysipelas sometimes takes this form, and in such cases recurs again and again" (*Sulph.*).

Erysipelatous, moist, scurfy sores.

Or, "Thin, *sticky*, glutinous, transparent watery fluid" (GUERNSEY, *Keynotes*).

HEPAR SULPHURIS CALCAREA

Any trouble occurring on the skin, when there is *great sensitiveness to the slightest touch* (*Canth.*).

Extreme sensitiveness runs through the whole remedy: to the slightest draught of air: to the slightest noise: and also mental sensitiveness and irritability—almost to murder, when angered.

PULSATILLA

Erysipelas in the *typical Pulsatilla patient.*

Mild, but irritable: changeable: weeps: craves sympathy.

Craves open air: cool air: worse for heat. Not hungry or thirsty.

SULPHUR

Recurrent attacks of erysipelas (*Graph.*).

Much burning: worse from heat of bed or room. Purplish appearance (*Lach.*).

"For erysipelas, as a name, we have no remedy, but when a patient has erysipelas and his symptoms conform to those of *Sulphur*, you will cure him with *Sulph.*" (KENT).

"When symptoms agree, *Sulph.* will be found a curative medicine in erysipelas."

The typical *Sulph.* patient is hungry, especially at 10 to 11 a.m. Loves fat, "Eats anything."

Kicks off the clothes at night, or puts feet out. Craves, or hates, or is worse from fats.

His eruptions itch; are worse from heat, warm room, warm bed and from washing.

Worse at night. Skin cannot bear woollens.

The untidy ragged philosopher. Selfish.

"*Sulphur* may be given on a paucity of symptoms."

HERPES ZOSTER
(SHINGLES)

APIS

Burning and *stinging* pain, much swelling.
Vesicles large, sometimes confluent.
Come out in cold weather.
Ulcerate with great burning, stinging pain.
Worse warmth: better cold applications.

ARSENICUM ALBUM

Confluent herpetic eruptions with *intense burning* of the blisters.
Sleepless after midnight.
Nausea and prostration: weakness.
Worse from cold of any kind, better from warmth.
"Herpes having a red, unwholesome appearance."

MEZEREUM

With severe neuralgic pains.
Itching, after scratching, turns to burning.
Worse from touch: in bed.
Vesicles form a brownish scab.

RANUNCULUS BULBOSUS

One has over and over again seen shingles clear up rapidly with 2 or 3 doses of *Ran. b.* in high potency—10*m*.
Vesicles filled with thin, acrid fluid.
Burning-itching vesicles in clusters.
Worse from touch, motion, after eating.
Severe neuralgic pains, especially intercostal.

RHUS TOXICODENDRON

"Probably no remedy more often found useful in herpes zoster. Especially when it occurs after a wetting.

VARIOLINUM

BURNETT said *Variolinum* had wiped out the condition, pain and all—and one has seen this also.

MEASLES

ACONITUM NAPELLUS

Catarrh and high fever: before rash clinches diagnosis.
Redness conjunctivae: dry, barking cough.
Itching, burning skin: rash rough and miliary.
Restless, anxious, tossing: frightened.

BELLADONNA

Rash bright-red: skin hot and dry—such cases as suggest scarlet fever.

EUPHRASIA

Cases with great catarrhal intensity.
"A wonderful medicine in measles. When symptoms agree will make a violent attack of measles turn into a very simple form. . .
"Streaming, burning tears; photophobia; running from nose; intense, throbbing headache, dry cough and rash" (KENT).
Copious *acrid* lachrymation, with streaming, *bland* discharge from nose (rev. of *Allium cepa*, which has acrid discharge from nose, but bland from eyes).

GELSEMIUM

Chills and heats chase one another. Sneezing and sore throat: excoriating nasal discharge.
Severe, heavy headache: occipital pain.
Thirstlessness is the rule with *Gels.* (*Puls.*).
Drowsy and stupid. Lids heavy: eyes inflamed.
Face dark-red, swollen, besotted look (*Bapt.*).

KALI BICHROMICUM

"Is like *Puls.* only worse." Follows *Puls. Puls. in the mild cases.*
It has a rash like measles, with catarrh of eyes.
Measles with purulent discharge eyes and ears. With pustules on cornea.
Salivary glands swollen: catarrhal deafness.
Kali bich. has stringy, ropy discharges.

MORBILLINUM

Prophylactic for contacts.

PULSATILLA

"If much fever, *Puls.* will not be the remedy."
Catarrhal symptoms: profuse lachrymation.
Dry mouth, but seldom thirsty.

SULPHUR

"Measles with a purplish appearance. *Sulphur* to modify the case when the skin is dusky and the rash does not come out."
"The routinist can do pretty well in this disease with *Puls.* and *Sulph.*, occasionally requiring *Acon.* and *Euphrasia*" (KENT).
Convalescence slow, and the patient is weak and prostrate.

Tardy or Suppressed Eruption: Brain Affected

APIS

Rash goes in and brain symptoms appear.
Stupor with stinging pains, extorting cries (*Crie cerebrale*).
Thirstless: worse from heat, hot room, hot fire.
Better cool air. Urine scanty.
A great remedy for œdema and effusions.

BRYONIA ALBA

Rash tardy to appear.
Hard, dry cough with tearing pain.
Little or no expectoration.
Or rash disappears and child drowsy: pale, twitching face, chewing motion of jaws (*Zinc.* grits teeth).
Any motion causes child to scream with pain.
Mild delirium, "Wants to go home," when at home.
Or, instead of rash, bronchitis or pneumonia, with *Bry.* symptoms.

CUPRUM METALLICUM

Symptoms violent. Starts up from sleep.
Spasms: cramps: convulsions.
Cramps of fingers and toes, or start there.

HELLEBORUS NIGER

"When entire sensorial life is suspended, and child lies in profound stupor."

STRAMONIUM

Rash not out properly. Child hot, bright-red face. Tosses, cries as if frightened in sleep. Convulsive movements.

ZINCUM METALLICUM

Where child is too weak to develop eruption.
Rash comes out sparingly. Body rather cool.
Lies in stupor gritting teeth. (*Bry.* chews.)
Dilated pupils: squinting and rolling eyes.
Fidgety feet.

MUMPS

PILOCARPUS MYCROPHYLLUS
(Jaborandi)

Dr. Burnett's homœopathic remedy for mumps seems to surpass all the rest, i.e. PILOCARPUS. It acts very quickly, and also relieves the pain.

Moreover, *Pilocarpus* has a reputation for the metastases in which mumps excels, whether to testes or mammae; when the swelling suddenly subsides, as the result of a chill, and worse troubles supervene. *Pilocarpus* also acts as a prophylatic.

ACONITUM NAPELLUS

For the *Acon.* fever with restlessness and anxiety.

BARYTA IODATA or MURIATICA

In the *Baryta* child: backward—shy—"deficient".

BELLADONNA

Inflammation of *right* parotid with bright redness and violent shooting pains.
Glowing redness of face. Sensitive to cold.

BROMIUM

Parotids, especially *left* affected: especially after scarlet fever.
"Swelling and hardness of left parotid: warm to touch."
Swelling of all glands about throat.
Slow inflammation of glands, with hardness.
Brom. especially helps those who are upset by being overheated: but when attack comes on, sensitive to colds and draughts.
Worse damp, hot weather.

CARBO VEGETABILIS

Parotitis. Face pale, cold. Involvement of mammae or testes.

LACHESIS MUTA

Especially *left* side parotid, enormously swollen: sensitive to least touch; least possible pressure—severe pain; shrinks away when approached: can scarcely swallow.

Throat sore internally. Face red and swollen. Eyes glassy and wild.

There is not the offensive mouth and dirty tongue of the *Mercs.*, but more throbbing; with the usual *Lachesis* horrible tension.

LYCOPODIUM

Begins *right* side, and goes to left.

It has not the offensive mouth and salivation of *Merc.*

Desires warm drinks.

MERCURIUS

Mumps, especially *right* side. Offensive salivation.

Foul tongue, and offensive sweat. (*Merc. corr.*)

PHYTOLACCA

Inflammation of sub-maxillary and *parotid* glands with stony hardness.

Pain shoots into ear when swallowing.

Worse cold and wet.

PULSATILLA

Lingering fever, or metastases (*Carbo veg.*; *Abrot.*).

If in mumps the patient gets a cold, the breasts swell in girls, the testicles in boys.

RHUS TOXICODENDRON

Parotid and sub-maxillary glands highly inflamed and enlarged.

Mumps on *left* side.

Worse cold: cold winds: cold wet.

"Always with herpes on lips."

SCARLET FEVER

Belladonna for scarlet fever affords an excellent example of homœopathy in the common cases of epidemic scarlet fever, and shows startling results, not only for the disease (when properly prescribed, i.e. when the symptoms agree), but also as a prophylactic.

Chief Remedy

BELLADONNA

Bright red, hot face. Glossy, scarlet skin: intense heat: "burns the hand."

"In the true Sydenham scarlet fever, where the eruption is perfectly smooth and truly scarlet."

Eyes red; injected: pupils later very dilated.

Lips—mouth—throat, red, dry, burning.

Strawberry tongue.

For eruptions like roseola and scarlet fever, with fever, sore throat, cough and headache.

Twitching, jerking; possibly wild delirium.

(*Apis* wants to be cool, uncovered: *Bell.* wants to be warm. *Bell.* also has more thirst.)

Cases where it has been used as a prophylatic, or used suitably on its indications, abort, or run a very mild course, leaving no sequelae, and are practically (as so many report), not even infectious.

Sequelæ

Hahnmeann wrote:

"*Belladonna* displays a valuable and specific power in removing the after-sufferings remaining from scarlet fever. . . . ***Most medical men have hitherto regarded the consequences of scarlet fever as at least as dangerous as the fever itself and there have been many epidemics where more died of the after-effects than of the fever*.**"

And he gives one interesting hint, "where ulceration has followed scarlet fever and where *Belladonna* is no longer of service," *Chamomilla* "will remove in a few days all tendency to ulceration: and the suffocating cough that sometimes follows the disease is also removed by *Chamomilla*, especially if accompanied by flushing of the face, and horripilation of limbs and back." (*Lesser Writings.*)

Other Remedies

AILANTHUS

Scarlet fever; plentiful eruption of bluish tint.

Eruption slow to appear, remains livid.

Irregular, patchy eruption of a very livid colour.

Throat livid, swollen, tonsils swollen with deep ulcers.

Pupils widely dilated (*Bell.*).

Semi-conscious, cannot comprehend.

Dizzy: can't sit up. Restless and anxious: later, insensible with muttering delirium.

Tongue dry, parched, cracked.

"Malignant scarlet fever."

AMMONIUM CARBONICUM

Malignant type (*Ail.*) with somnolence.

Body red, as if covered with rash.

Dark red and putrid throat. External throat swollen.

As if forehead would burst.

State like blood poisoning: great dyspnœa; face dusky and puffy.

APIS

Thick rose-coloured rash, feels rough. Or,

When rash does not come out, with great inflammation of throat, with scarlet fever in family.

Throat sore, swollen, œdematous: with stinging pain.

Convulsions when rash fails to come out (compare *Bry.*, *Cup.*, *Zinc.*, as given, under Measles).

Worse from heat: wants covers off: a cool room: (reverse of *Bell.*, wants warmth).

LACHESIS MUTA

Advanced stages: malignant scarlet fever.

Purple face.

Worse for heat (reverse of *Bell.*).

Bursting, hammering pains in head.

Throat worse left side: may extend to right.

Jealousy and suspicion suggests *Lach.*

Impelled to talk: loquacious delirium.

Lach. sleeps into an aggravation.

MERCURIUS

May follow *Bell.* for sore mouth, throat, tonsils, with ulceration and excessively foul breath.

Perspiration which aggravates the symptoms.

RHUS TOXICODENDRON

"Useful in scarlet fever with coarse rash. Or rash suppressed with inflammation of glands and sore throat" (KENT).

"You may rely on *Rhus* whenever acute diseases take on a typhoid form, as in scarlet fever, when no other remedy is positively indicated" (FARRINGTON).

"*Rhus* supplants *Bell.* when child grows drowsy and *restless.*"

Fauces dark-red, with œdema (*Apis*).

Tongue red (? smooth) with triangular red tip.

TEREBINTHINA

Albuminuria and uræmia following scarlet fever.

Toxic: confused: better profuse urination.

Often indicated in dropsy after scarlet fever.

Hæmaturia: urine cloudy and smoky.

"Hæmaturia: dyspnœa: drowsiness."

Tongue dry and glossy.

N.B.—*Acidum nitricum*, *Phosphorus*, or one of many other drugs might be needed in difficult cases, or in cases first seen later on in the disease and with complications; according to the symptoms and make-up of the patient.

For SUPPRESSED OR RECEDING eruption, see under MEASLES.

SMALL-POX

ACONITUM NAPELLUS

To modify first stage and early second stage.

High fever: great restlessness. Fear of death.

ANTHRACINUM

Gangrenous cases, with severe burning.

ANTIMONIUM TARTARICUM

Long held by homœopaths to be specific for small-pox.

Pustules with red areola, like small-pox, which leave a crust and form a scar.

Pains in back and loins.

Violent pain in sacro-lumbar region: slightest movement causes retching and cold sweat.

Violent headache: < evening; < lying; > sitting up; > cold.

Variola; backache, headache; cough with crushing weight on chest; before or at beginning of eruptive stage; diarrhœa, etc. Also when eruption fails.

LILIENTHAL says: "Tardy eruption with nausea, vomiting, sleeplessness, or suppression of eruption. Putrid variola with typhoid symptoms (*Bapt.*).

APIS

Erysipelatous redness and swelling, with stinging-burning pains, throat and skin.

Absence of thirst.

Urine scanty—later suppressed.

ARSENICUM ALBUM

Great sinking of strength.

Burning heat: frequent small pulse.

Great thirst. Great restlessness.

Rash irregularly developed with typhoid symptoms.

Hæmorrhagic cases, or when pustules sink in, and areolae grow livid.

Metastasis to mouth and throat.

Worse cold. (*Apis* worse heat.)

BAPTISIA

Typhoid symptoms: fœtid breath.

Pustules thick on arch of palate, tonsils, uvula, in nasal cavities; but scanty on skin.

Great prostration with pain in sacral region.

Drowsy; comatose; limbs feel "scattered".

BELLADONNA

First stage; high fever and cerebral congestion.

Intense swelling of skin and mucous membrane.

Dysuria and tenesmus of bladder.

Delirium and convulsions. Photophobia.

CROTALUS HORRIDUS

Pustular eruptions. After vaccination.

Eruptions, boils, pustules, gangrenous conditions, when fever is low and parts bluish.

Hæmorrhagic cases.

CUPRUM SULPHURICUM

Cerebral irritation, where eruption fails to appear. Convulsive phenomena.

HAMAMELIS VIRGINICUS

Hæmorrhagic cases oozing of dark blood from nose; bleeding gums; hæmatemesis, bloody stools.

HIPPOZÆNINUM
(Nosode of Glanders)

Low forms of malignant ulcerations, especially where nasal cartilages are affected.

Confluent small-pox.

Pustules and ulcers spread extensively over body till hardly a part remains free.

HYOSCYAMUS

Eruption fails to appear, causing great excitement, rage, anguish, delirium in paroxysms. Wants to get out of bed, and uncover

LACHESIS MUTA

Hæmorrhagic cases.

Worse after sleep.

Dusky or purplish appearance, with excessive tenderness to touch.

MALANDRINUM

(The nosode of "grease"* in horses.)

CLARKE says: Homœopaths have found in *Maland.* a very effectual protection against infection with small-pox and vaccination.

MERCURIUS

Stage of maturation: ptyalism. Tendency of blood to head.

Moist swollen tongue with great thirst.

Diarrhœa or dysentery with tenesmus, especially during desiccation.

PHOSPHORICUM ACIDUM

Confluent, with typhoid conditions.

"Pustules fail to pustulate; degenerate into large blisters, which leave raw surface."

Stupid: wants nothing: not even a drink.

Answers questions but does not talk.

Subsultus tendinum: restlessness. Fear of death.

Watery diarrhœa.

PHOSPHORUS

Hæmorrhagic diathesis. Bloody pustules

Hard dry cough: chest raw.

Hæmorrhage from lungs.

Back as if broken: faintings. Great thirst.

RHUS TOXICODENDRON

"Eruption turns livid and typhoid symptoms supervene."

Dry tongue. Sordes lips and teeth.

Wants to get out of bed. Great restlessness (*Ars.*)

Confluent: great swelling at first, afterwards eruption shrinks, and becomes livid.

* *"Grease" in horses was, or is believed to be identical with pustules occurring on the udders of cows, which affected the hands of milkmaids and rendered them immune from Small-pox: it was from this observation that inoculation and later vaccination (from "cow-pox") arose.*

SARRACENIA PURPUREA

(Drug of the North American Indians) seems to have done marvellous work in aborting and curing small-pox.

SULPHUR

Tendency to metastasis to brain during suppuration.

Stage of desiccation: or occasionally inter-current remedy where others fail.

THUJA

Which will cause the pustules of vaccination to wither and abort, should be one of the remedies of small-pox also.

LILIENTHAL says: "Pains in arms, fingers, hands, with fullness and soreness of throat.

"Areola round pustules marked and dark red.

"Pustules milky and flat, painful to touch. Give especially during stage of maturation, it may prevent pitting."

VARIOLINUM

Probably the most potent of all, having the complete picture of the disease from which it is prepared.

Dullness of head.

Severe pains in back and limbs, which became quite numb.

Chills, followed by high fever.

Violent headache.

White-coated tongue.

Great thirst.

Severe pains and distress in epigastric region with nausea and vomiting, mostly of greenish water.

In many cases profuse diarrhœa. In some, despondency.

Small-pox pustules on different parts of the body, mostly abdomen and back. Pustules perfectly formed, some umbilicated, some purulent.

"Given steadily the disease will run a milder course. It changes imperfect pustules into regular ones, which soon dry up. Promotes suppuration and desiccation. Prevents pitting" (LILIENTHAL).

TYPHOID AND TYPHOID CONDITIONS IN FEVERS

ARNICA

Says she is "So well!" when desperately ill.

Can be roused, answers correctly, then goes back into stupor (*Bapt.*, *Phos. a.*).

"I am not sick: I did not send for you; go away!"

Foul breath—stool. Hæmorrhagic tendency.

"Bed feels so hard" (*Bapt.*, *Pyrogen*).

"So sore", can only lie on one part a little time: restlessness *from this cause.*

Involuntary and unnoticed stools and urine.

ARSENICUM ALBUM

Rapid sinking of strength: great emaciation.

Least effort exhausts.

Great restlessness: constantly moves head and limbs: trunk still, because of extreme weakness. Tongue dry, brown, black.

Face distorted, hippocratic, sunken, anxious.

Rapid sinking of forces: extreme prostration.

ANXIETY: RESTLESSNESS: EXHAUSTION.

Thinks he must die. (*Arn.* says he is "not ill".)

Worse 1–2 a.m. and p.m.

Cadaveric aspect: cadaveric smelling stools.

Thirst for cold sips.

BAPTISIA

Typhoid fever. Typhoid conditions in fevers.

Rapid onset. Rapid course.

Abdomen distends early.

Odour horrible. Delirium.

Besotted condition: purple, bloated face.

Answers a word or two, and is back in stupor.

Feels there are two of him. Is scattered.

Tries to get the pieces together (*Pyrog.*).

In typhoid, "*Bapt.* vies with *Pyrog.* and *Arn.*"

BRYONIA ALBA

A most persistent remedy: develops slowly.
Lacerating, throbbing, jerking headache.
Nausea and disgust, whitish tongue.
Bitter taste. Thirst for large draughts of cold water (*Phos.*).
"Nervous, versatile or cerebral typhoid."
Sluggishness, then complete stupefaction.
When roused, is confused: sees images.
Thinks he is away from home and wants to be taken home.
Irrational talk: *prattles of his business:* worse after 3 p.m.
Delirium apt to start about 9 p.m.
Wants to be quiet. Pain, limbs, when moving.
Tongue dry.
Easily angered.
Faint if sits up.

CARBO VEGETABILIS

"A sheet-anchor in low states of typhoid, in the last stages of collapse; where there is coldness, cold sweat, great prostration; dyspnœa —wants to be fanned. Cold tongue."
"Desperate cases. Blood stagnates in the capillaries."
Blueness—coldness—ecchymoses.
Can hardly breathe, air-hunger. Says "Fan me! Fan me!"
Hæmorrhages, dark, decomposed, unclotted (*Crot. h.*).
Indescribable paleness face and body.

CROTALUS HORRIDUS

Typhoid with decomposition of blood and hæmorrhages—anywhere.
Intestinal hæmorrhage; blood dark, fluid, non-coagulable.
Tongue fiery-red, smooth, polished (*Pyrog.*), intensely swollen.
Yellowness of skin is an indication for *Crot. h.*
"*Lach.* cold and clammy: *Crot. h.* cold and dry."
Attacks that come on with great rapidity (*Bapt.*, *Hyos.*).
Rapidly increasing unconsciousness. Besotted appearance (*Bapt.*).
Typhoid when it becomes putrid.
"Diseases of the very lowest, the most putrid type, coming on with unusual rapidity."

HYOSCYAMUS

Fevers rapidly develop the typhoid state (*Bapt.*, *Crot. h.*).
Sensorium clouded.
Staring eyes: Carphology. Picks bedclothes.
Teeth covered with sordes.
Tongue dry, unwieldy, rattles in mouth, so dry.
Involuntary stool and urine (*Phos.*, *Arn.*).
Subsultus tendinum.
Mutters, or says no word for hours.
Mentally very suspicious: refuses medicine, thinks you will poison him (*Rhus.*, *Lach.*).
Jealous (Lach.). Alternately mild and timid, then violent. Will scratch, and try to injure.
Exposes person (*Phos.*). Wants to be naked.
Talks to imaginary people: to dead people.
Illusions: hallucinations; talking, with delirium, then stupor.
Early can be roused: later complete unconsciousness.

LACHESIS MUTA

Loquacity: delirium with great loquacity.
Face puffy, purple, mottled.
Much rumbling in distended abdomen.
Clothing cannot be tolerated: must not touch abdomen or throat.
Tongue swells (*Crot. h.*): difficult to protrude.
Suspicious. "Trying to poison her!" (*Rhus.*).
Worse after sleep: sleeps into aggravation.
Cold, clammy (*Crot. h.* cold, dry).
Stool with dark blood.

MURIATICUM ACIDUM

"Also one of our best remedies in typhoid."
Tongue dry, leathery, shrunken (*Hyos.*, *Ars.*).
Muscular prostration comes first, mind remains long clear (reverse of *Phos. acid*).
Lower jaw drops. Slides down in bed from excessive weakness (*Phos. acid*).
Cannot urinate without the bowels also moving.
"Nearer to *Carbo veg.* than any other remedy."

PHOSPHORICUM ACIDUM

"One of our best remedies in typhoid."

Simultaneous depression of animal, sensorial and mental life from the start.

Slowly increasing prostration.

Advanced typhoid.

Lies in stupor, unconscious of all that goes on: but if roused is fully conscious.

Glassy stare, as if slowly comprehending.

Prostration. Tympanitic abdomen.

Dry brown tongue. Dark lips. Sordes.

Bleeding; nose, lungs, bowels (*Crot. h.*).

Jaw drops: "as if must die of exhaustion."

PHOSPHORUS

Abdomen distended, sore, very sensitive to touch (*Lach.*).

Worse lying left side: better, right.

Stools offensive, bloody, involuntary. *The Anus appearing to remain open* (*Apis.*).

Burning in stomach: burning thirst for cold water. Desire for ice cream.

Fear alone: in the dark: of thunder.

Especially useful in typhoid pneumonias.

Suspicious (*Lach.*).

PYROGENIUM

(BURNETT's great remedy for typhoid.)

Bed feels hard (*Bapt.*).

Great restlessness: must constantly move (*Rhus*), to relieve soreness of parts (*Arn.*).

Tongue clean, smooth, fiery-red; or dry and cracked.

Horribly offensive diarrhœa (*Bapt.*).

Sense of duality (*Bapt.*).

Pulse quick; or out of proportion to temperature.

RHUS TOXICODENDRON

"Fevers take on the typhoid type: triangular red-tipped tongue and restlessness."

Cannot rest in any position (*Pyrog.*).

Slow and difficult mentation. May answer correctly. Talks to himself.

Refuses food and medicine. Fears poison (*Hyos.*, *Lach.*).

Dreams of strenuous exertion.

TARAXACUM

Restlessness of limbs wth tearing pain. "Like *Rhus* only *mapped tongue.*"

TEREBINTHINA

Tongue bright-red, smooth, glazed (*Pyrog.*).
Extreme tympanites (*Phos. acid.*, *Phos.*).
Thick scanty urine: mixed with blood, or cloudy, smoky, albuminous.
Diarrhœa with blood intermixed.
Fresh ecchymoses in great numbers (*Arn.*).

ILL-EFFECTS OF VACCINATION 166

Homœopathy has a very great *antidote to vaccination, and remedy for the after-effects of vaccination, in* THUJA.

Numbers of persons date their ill-health, their years of headache, asthma, epilepsy, etc., from vaccination. It is just the cases that do not "take" that seem more particularly liable to chronic ill-health.

THUJA

A direct antidote to the vaccinial poison.

In acute cases, wipes out the fever and eruption, and causes the pustules to disappear.

In chronic diseases, it may be impossible to cure many conditions without *Thuja*. Where symptoms improve to a point, and then always recur, while the disease can be traced back to a vaccination, or vaccinations, *Thuja* will generally supply the deep stimulus that leads to cure.

OTHER REMEDIES

ARNICA

Must not be forgotten. It does not destroy the vaccination like *Thuja* and *Maland.*, but it has amazing power of taking away pain, swelling, and general malaise, while the process goes on to completion.

MALANDRINUM

Nosode, prepared from "grease" in horses. Very like *Thuja* in symptoms and effects.

CLARKE says: "Burnett's indications are—Lower half of body: greasy skin and eruptions. Slow pustulation, never ending."

SILICA

The *Sil.* patient is feeble, lacks "grit", shrinks from responsibility.
Is chilly: sensitive to draughts, but enervated with very hot weather.
Head sweats at night. (*Calc.*) Sweaty, offensive feet.

SULPHUR

Warm patient. Hungry for everything: for fats.
Intolerant of clothing and weight of clothes.
Kicks off bedclothes: puts feet out. Eruptions of every kind.

WHOOPING-COUGH

ANTIMONIUM TARTARICUM

Cough when child gets angry, and after eating. Ends in vomiting. "Chest full of rattles." Thirstless: coated tongue.

ARNICA

"A wonderful whooping-cough remedy."

Violent tickling cough if child gets angry: *Begins to cry before cough* (*Bell.*): knows it is coming and dreads it.

BELLADONNA

Weeping and pains in stomach before coughing. Feels head will burst.

Dry spasmodic cough, worse at night; lying.

"Spasms of larynx which cause cough and difficulty of breathing" (KENT).

Kent says, "The *Bell.* cough is peculiar. As soon as great violence and great effort have raised a little mucus there is peace, during which larynx and trachea get dryer and dryer and begin to tickle, then comes the spasm and the whoop, and the gagging." Especially after exposure to cold.

BROMIUM

With sensation of coldness in throat.

Larynx as if covered with velvet, but feels cold.

"Whooping cough in spring, towards hot weather." Worse hot weather.

BRYONIA ALBA

"Child coughs immediately after eating and drinking and vomits, then returns to the table, finishes his meal, but coughs and vomits again" (LILIENTHAL).

"Dry spasmodic cough; whooping cough, shaking the whole body." Cough makes him spring up in bed—even *Bry*.

CARBO ANIMALIS

With feeling of coldness in chest.

Severe dry cough, shakes abdomen as if all would fall out; must support belly (*Dros.*).

CARBO VEGETABILIS

Cough, mostly hard and dry: or sounds rough: apt to occur after a full meal.

Every violent spell brings up a lump of phlegm, or is followed by retching, gagging and waterbrash.

Pain in chest after cough: burning as from a coal of fire.

Craving for salt. (This determined the remedy in a case that promptly recovered.)

"One of the greatest medicines we have in the beginning of whooping-cough. Gagging, vomiting and redness of face" (KENT).

Paroxysms of violent spasmodic coughing: with cold sweat and cold pinched face after attack.

CINA

Becomes rigid, with clucking sound down in oesophagus as paroxysm ends.

Not relieved by eating: stomach bloated, yet hungry. Grits teeth.

COCCUS CACTI

Worse at night, when hot in bed.

Better lying in cool room without much covering: wants room cold.

If mother can get to it quickly enough with a drink of cold water she can ward off the paroxysm.

Child holds its breath to prevent coughing.

"Wakes in morning with paroxysm of whooping-cough, which ends in vomiting ropy mucus, which hangs in long strings from mouth—great ropes. Here *Coccus c.* will cut short the disease." ("*Kali bi.* stringy but yellow: *Coccus c.* clear" or white.)

CORALLIUM RUBRUM

Smothered sensation before cough. Exhaustion after.

CUPRUM METALLICUM

Better by swallowing cold water.

Uninterrupted paroxysms till breath completely exhausted. Gasps with repeated crowing inspirations till black in the face. Mucus in trachea and spasms in larynx.

Cramps beginning in fingers and toes.

Thumbs tucked in during cough.

DROSERA

Impulses to cough follow one another so violently, that he can hardly get his breath.

Oppression of the chest, as if something kept back the air when he coughed and spoke, so that the breath could not be expelled.

When he breathes out a sudden contraction in hypogastrium makes him heave and excites coughing.

Crawling in larynx which provokes coughing.

On coughing he vomits water, mucus and food.

When coughing, contractive pain in the hypochondria. Cannot cough on account of the pain, unless he presses his hand on the pit of the stomach.

The region below the ribs is painful when touched and, when coughing, must press his hand on the spot to mitigate the pain.

Spasmodic cough, with retching and vomiting, caused by tickling or dryness in throat.

IPECACUANHA

Stiffens: goes rigid, loses breath: grows pale: then relaxes and vomits phlegm with relief.

Convulsions in whooping-cough, frightful spasms especially of left side.

KALI CARBONICUM

Convulsive and tickling cough at night.

Cough so violent as to cause vomiting.

Cough at 3 a.m., repeated every half-hour.

Bag-like swellings between the upper lids and the eyebrows; often puffy face also.

"Dry, hard, racking, hacking cough."

KALI SULPHURICUM

Whooping-cough, with retching, without vomiting. Yellow, slimy expectoration.

Tongue coated with yellow mucus.

Hot and sweating. *Hates* cough and weeps. (*Bell.*)

Looks "fair, fat and forty" even a child.

LOBELIA

Cough ends with violent sneezing.

MAGNESIA PHOSPHORICA

Violent spasmodic attacks of cough, with face blue and turgid. Ends in a whoop.

MEPHITIS

Whooping or any violent cough: very violent, spasmodic, as if each spell would terminate life.

Frequent paroxysms especially at night.

Desire for salt (*Carbo veg.*).

Worse lying down. Child must be raised.

WITH INDICATIONS

SEE SECTION ON FEARS, ETC.

Sulphur .. *The ragged philosopher.* Untidy: and full of theories (*Cann. ind.*).

"Not disturbed by uncleanliness, but after a dose of *Sulph.* he puts on a clean shirt."

But he is over-sensitive to filthy odours.

Dwells on religious or philosophic speculations: anxiety about soul's salvation: indifference about the lot of others. Answers irrelevantly.

Foolish happiness and pride: thinks he is possessed of beautiful things: even rags seem beautiful. Fantastic illusions. Too lazy to rouse himself: too unhappy to live.

Wants to touch things. Children dread being washed. (See p. 40.)

China .. Broken down from exhausting discharges.

No desire to live; lacks courage for suicide (*Nux, Rhus*).

Apathetic, indifferent, taciturn.

Extreme sensitiveness: noise or excitement unendurable. Extreme irritability of nerves.

Nux moschata Drowsiness and sleepiness: stupor and insensibility: unconquerable sleep.

Absence of mind. Cannot think. Great indifference to everything.

Appears to be dazed. Automatic.

Complete loss of memory.

Performs all her duties in a dream.

A doctor after bad bouts of influenza; used to go into a state of indifference and ineptitude. He would carry his letters about unopened. At last *Nux mosch.* ended the trouble.

She was at death's door after a cerebral thrombosis: so drowsy and comatose that it was almost impossible to get her to swallow anything. Could not be roused. A dose of *Nux mosch.* rapidly brought back life and animation, and (at eighty years of age) she made a good recovery. *Nux mosch.* was the turning point of the illness. A unique, powerful and rapidly-acting remedy in such conditions.

Silica	Mental weakness, embarrassment, dread, yielding. Hates disputes and arguments. Dreads to appear in public (*Lyc.*, *Arg. nit.*, *Gels.*). Worn out by prolonged effort or mental work. Nervous exhaustion from brain-fag. Never the same since some great mental effort. "Anything for a quiet life." *Dread of failure*: that he will fail with his mental effort—yet does it well (*Lyc.*). Irritable: retiring: wants to shirk everything: mild, gentle, tearful. "*Puls.*—only more so." Dreads undertaking anything. Chronic of *Puls.* (*Kali sulph.*).
Lycopodium ..	Mind tired: forgetful: worried business men when times have been difficult: can't think. Aversion to work: to undertaking new things. Apprehension before the event: that he will forget something: make mistakes:—yet goes through it fluently; i.e. a public speech. No self-confidence (*Sil.*). Conscientious scruples. Distrustful: suspicious: fault-finding. Fear of men (*Nat. c.*, *Plat.*, *Puls.*, etc.). Aversion to company; yet dreads solitude. Wants to be alone with someone in the next room. Doesn't want to talk. Weeps at least joy: weeps when thanked. Worse afternoon, especially 4-8 p.m. Not worse morning, except "wakes ugly." (P. 44.)
Manganum ..	"Anxiety and fear. Great apprehensiveness. "Something awful is going to happen. "Cannot think. Business difficulties because he cannot do good thinking. "The queerest thing is how he gets relief. *He lies down, and it all passes away.* "His very life is excited, tired and anxious: he lies down and says, 'Why didn't I think of that before?'" (KENT).
Phosphoric acid	"Mental enfeeblement." Mind tired (*Lyc.*). From prolonged business worry: of feeble overtaxed school children. Answers slowly, or not: looks at the questioner. "Don't talk: let me alone: I'm tired." Mental prostration: profound indifference.

Ambra grisea — Loss of comprehension (*Aeth.*) : reads a sentence over and over again, and then does not understand it. Thinking powers impaired.
Asks question after question, never waiting to have them answered.
The presence of others, even the nurse, unbearable during stool, or during urination (*Nat. mur.*).
Presence of another person aggravates symptoms.
Mind runs on unpleasant fancies, diabolical faces and sights. Melancholy.

Baryta carb. .. Mentally and physically dwarfish.
Cannot grasp ordinary ideas.
Great aversion to strangers. Shy.
Cannot be taught because cannot remember.
Development suspended.

Coca—Cocaine — Bashful : timid : ill at ease in society.
Want of will-power : shakiness and depression.
Fear of falling when walking (*Gels.*, etc.).
Sensation as of small foreign bodies or of worms under the skin ("*cocaine bugs*").
(Cures of various conditions, as rheumatism, recorded, where this symptom was present.)

Picric acid .. Great indifference : lack of will power.
Brain-fag : mental prostration after least intellectual work (*Phos. acid*).
Disinclined for mental and physical work.
From the least study, burning along spine (comp. *Phos.*, *Zinc.*).
Useful in neurasthenia ; pernicious anæmia.
Burnett verified a characteristic symptom :—
Sensation of coldness, male genitalia.

Aethusa cyn. .. "*Fool's Parsley*," Clarke's great remedy for examination funk (*Arg. nit.*). He gives cases. *Inability to think, or to fix the attention.*
Loss of comprehension (*Ambra*) as if a barrier were between the senses and external objects.
In delirium sees cats and dogs : tried to jump out of bed : out of window (*Bell.*).

Natrum carb. .. Nervous exhaustion : physical exhaustion : weakness of mind and body.
Forgets what he reads. " Memory will not hold out from beginning to end of sentence."
Bookkeepers lose the ability to add up figures.
Confusion of mind : brain-fag.
Worse from sun : ailments after sunstroke. (See p. 43.)

Phosphorus .. Very sensitive to external impressions (*Nux*).
Better after sleep (*Sep*.). Long sleep. Better rubbed.
Sympathetic (*Puls*. craves sympathy).
Imaginations to clairvoyance (? *Acon*.) and ecstasy.
Feels as if in several pieces; cannot set the bits properly together (comp. *Bapt*., *Raph*., *Pyrog*.).
Fear ; in the dark : alone : of thunder : that something will happen : of death.
Strange faces look from the corner.
Indifferent to loved ones, friends (*Sepia*).
May uncover and expose person (*Hyos*., *Stram*.).
Maniacal attacks with extreme violence. (See p. 45.)

Tuberculinum .. Kent gives many mental symptoms, observed and cured (by his own preparation).
Hopelessness, in many complaints.
Anxiety *evenings* (*Puls*.), ***till midnight***.
Anxiety and loquacity (*Lach*.) during fever.
Thoughts, tormenting, persistent, intrude and crowd upon each other during the night.
Persons gradually running down, never finding the right remedy. Constant desire to change, to travel, to go somewhere, do something different, to find a new doctor.
" The cosmopolitan desire to travel belongs strongly to one who needs *Tub*."
Persons on the borderline of insanity.
Intellectual and lung symptoms interchangeable.
Desire for air. Suffocates in warm room (*Puls*.).
" When at every coming back of the case, it needs a new remedy."
Especially helpful for persons with T.B. history.

Ailanthus gland.	Since the poisoning all incidents of past life are forgotten, or remembered as things read about, or belonging to another.
Glonoin ..	Could not remember which side of street her house was on. Well-known streets strange. Loss of location: loses himself in streets that he has traversed for years. All right in regard to everything else. Disinclined to speak: would scarcely answer. Recognized no one: repulsed husband and children: raved, screamed, wished to rush from house, to jump from window. For bad effects of excitement, fright, fear, injuries (*Acon.*) and their later effects. Broods on old unhappiness. Fear of death: has been poisoned (*Rhus*, etc.).
Camphor monobromide	Felt he was journeying in one direction, when he was actually moving in the opposite. Sensation of going in wrong direction, but numbers on houses showed he was going the right way.
Kali bromatum	Loss of memory, had to be told word before he could speak it (*Plumb.*). Dull: torpid: perception slow: answers slow. Delusions: pursued by police: will be poisoned (*Rhus, Lach., Glon.*): is selected for divine vengeance: that her child is dead. Hands constantly busy: walks the room groaning: full of fear. Fearful delusions. "Life threatened by members of his family." Fear to be alone: at night: under the impression that they have committed, or are about to commit some great crime and cruelty. Religious delusions, feeling of moral deficiency. Indifference: almost disgust for life. Night terror of children (*Calc. carb.*): cannot recognize or be comforted by their friends: may be followed by squinting.
Eupatorium purpureum	Dull, stupid. Various delusions. *Homesick at home* (*Bry.*).

Conium .. *A gradually increasing state of imbecility.* Unable to sustain any mental effort, or to rivet the attention.

A delirium, not constant, and without fever.

Forms of insanity that are slow and passive.

Great unhappiness *recurring every fourteen days.*

Cannot endure the slightest alcoholic drink.

Characteristic, *Sweat during sleep.* (See p. 43.)

Plumbum .. *Slow of perception.* Loss of memory: while talking, unable to find the proper word (*Kali br.*).

Apathy: intellectual torpor to coma.

Language extravagant. Searching about on the floor.

People in the ward seemed as small as dolls (comp. *Plat.*), and the opposite wall of room seemed to be sunk 40 ft. below his own level.

Illusions of vision, saw castles, palaces.

Fiends that pursued him and sought his life.

Abused the doctors, tried to strike and bite the nurses (comp. *Bell.*).

Waits before answering: answers rationally, then is off the track again: talk a mixture of sense and nonsense: bursts into laughter.

Violent delirium, impelled to tear themselves and bite their own fingers.

Violent delirium succeeded the epileptic spasm.

In delirium his life was in danger from assassination or poisoning; everyone about was a murderer (comp. *Ars.*).

Greatly increased muscular strength.

Zincum .. Enfeeblement. *Mind slow: weak and tired.*

" Repeats all questions before answering."

Waits a moment, looking blank: then face lights up and he answers.

Torments everyone with his complaints.

" Not the mentally deficient: but the mental enfeeblement of disease."

(Brain trouble: spinal meningitis, etc.)

" *When the reflexes are abolished, Zinc. comes in.*"

(In paralysis from cerebral thrombosis, one has seen reflexes restored by *Zinc.* and recovery rapid thereafter.) (See p. 39.)

Pulsatilla .. Mild, gentle, tearful: yet remarkably irritable.
Bursts into tears when spoken to, or giving symptoms (*Sep.*).
CHANGEABLE, mentally and physically.
Pleasure in nothing. Vexed about "nothing".
May have aversion to marriage; thinks company of opposite sex dangerous: Abhors women (*Raph.*).
Lachrymose. Peevishness. Slow, phlegmatic.
Worse warm room: better cool open air; walking slowly out of doors. (See p. 45.)

Raphanus .. Aversion to all women: weariness, disgust and rage at approach of women (*Puls.*, *Lach.*).
Aversion to children: especially to little girls.
Attracted to all men without distinction.
Moral feeling completely extinct (*Absinth.*).
Extreme anxiety and fear of death. (See p. 30.)

Cimicifuga, Actea rac. Thinks she is going crazy. Fear of death (*Acon.*).
Sensation of a heavy cloud settling over her.
All dark and confused, with weight on head.
Loquacity: goes from subject to subject (*Lach.*).
Grieved, troubled: sighing (*Ign.*): next day joy.
Mind disturbed by disappointed love (*Nat. mur.*, *Ign.*, etc.): business failures.

Ignatia .. "The sighing remedy." Remedy of silent grief. Sobbing: utterly absorbed in grief.
Unable to control emotions and excitement.
Effects from long-continued grief; bad news.
Unhappy love: misplaced affections (*Nat. mur.*).
The remedy of MOODS, of changeable moods.
Delights to bring on her fits and make a scene.
You cannot depend on her being reasonable or rational: what you say will be distorted.
Does unaccountable and unexpected things.
Thinks she has neglected some duty.
The remedy of contradictions: of the unnatural: the unexpected.
Can't stand contradiction or fault-finding.
Over-sensitive to pain (*Cham.*, *Acon.*).

N.B.—*Ign.* cannot stand past worries and grief; *Staph.* past annoyances. (See p. 39.)

Natrum mur. Easily weeps : grieves for no cause. Consolation aggravates—angers her. The remedy of unrequited affections, misplaced affections. (*Cimic.*: *Nat. m.* is the chronic of *Ign.*). (See p. 41.)

Psorinum .. Sad : hopeless. All dark.
Business a failure : going to the poor-house.
Sinned away his day of grace (*Stram.*, *Lach.*).
No joy : despair of recovery. (See p. 40.)

Sepia .. Propensity to suicide from despair about his miserable existence. Resigned despair.
Aversion to ones occupation and family, great indifference to those they love best (*Phos.*).
Sad about health and domestic affairs ; discontented with everything.
Did not care what happened : no desire to work : inattentive, absent-minded, indolent.
Causeless weepings (*Nat. mur.*, *Apis*, *Puls.*, *Sul.*, etc.). Passionate. Irritable.
"*Sepia* seems to abolish the ability to feel natural love" (i.e. can restore it).
"Absence of all joy : things seem strange ; no affection for the delightful things of life."
Face shows no sharp lines of intellect.
Symptom-complex, "gnawing hunger, 'dragging down,' constipation and indifference." (See p. 44.)

Natrum sulph. Depressed : tearful : music makes her sad.
Irritable in a.m., hates to speak or be spoken to.
Satiety of life : must use self-control to prevent shooting himself.
After injuries to head. With chronic lung affections, with green discharges. Hypersensitive to warm and WET COLD.

N.B.—"*Aur.*, wants to kill himself : *Nat. sul.* wants not to."
Nat. sulph., lungs affected : *Aurum*, heart.

Nitric acid .. Satiety of life with fear of death.
Anxious about his illness : thinks of his past troubles : mind weak and wandering.
Nervous : excitable : discontented with himself. Fits of rage, despair, cursing, maledictions. Typical *Nit. ac.* craves fats and salt.

Aurum .. The greatest among the suicide remedies, and a remedy of the deepest depression.

Melancholy: imagines he is unfitted for the world: filled with intense delight when he thinks of death, so that he longs to die.

Meditates on death: on suicide: wants to get out of the world, to destroy himself. Has no love for his life, which he thinks worthless.

Morose: indisposed to talk. Sulky.

Sits apart in deepest melancholy. The slightest contradiction excites anger and he forgets himself; with quarrelling.

Discontent with his circumstances: with himself: hopeless: "people find him no good."

Great anxiety felt in the precordium.

Feels hateful and quarrelsome: anxious palpitation with desire to commit suicide.

"Among the causes of the *Aurum* mental state of insanity, grief and hopelessness, syphilis is a common one; loss of property is another." —KENT.

Lack of gold has driven many to suicide: potentized gold has brought many back to life and hope. (See p. 46.)

Drosera .. Dejected about the malice of others; disheartened and concerned about the future.

Extremely uneasy, sad disposition: imagined he was being deceived by spiteful, envious people.

Anxiety as if his enemies would not leave him quiet; envied and persecuted him.

Anxiety, especially in the evening; impelled to jump into the water to take his own life—not impelled to any other mode of death.

Takes insults resentfully. Trifles excite him so much that he is beside himself with rage.

Restlessness: reading, cannot stick long to one subject—must always go to something else.

"Curative reaction of vital powers,—happy, stedfast disposition: dreads no evil because conscious of having acted honourably."

Particularly useful where there is a T.B. history. *Dros.* breaks down, and therefore enhances resistance to tubercle. (See p. 46.)

Lyssin: Hydrophobinum

Something terrible going to happen to him: impelled to throw child which he carries through the window, and the like.

Insane ideas, to throw glass of water into someone's face; to stab him with the knife he is holding.

Mental faculties in state of excitement; with quick perception, amazing acuteness of understanding and rapidity of answers.

Or, range of ideas very limited: occupied continuously with the same thing, brings out same ideas always in the same manner.

Energetically protect themselves against fancied attacks and insults.

See objects, animals and men, not present.

Fear of becoming mad.

Cannot sleep: driven from bed by indescribable anxiety. Can only sit and walk—and pray.

(Hering gives cases of persons bitten by dogs, with symptoms of hydrophobia, quickly cured by *Lyssin* 200.)

Hearing water or seeing it, becomes irritable, nervous, with desire for stool, involuntary urination and other ailments.

Driven incessantly about without definite aim.

Felt the same rheumatic pain his brother complained of.

A curious symptom, "copper, in his room, makes him restless and full of pain."

Curious exalted senses: on a watch held to epigastrium, he sees the hour and minute hands.

Can see hands on dial-plate of church clock.

Can hear what is spoken in next room, and counting of coppers in the room below.

Linen dipped in sugar water, put on pit of stomach, gives a sweet taste in mouth.

The sight of water, a looking-glass or white substance, renews pain, distress, or convulsions.

Current of air, bright light, sight of any shining object, slight touch, even conversation nearby, may throw him into violent agitation, or bring on a convulsion. (See p. 35.)

Medorrhinum .. Time moves too slowly. Dazed far-off sensation, as if things of to-day occurred a week ago (comp. *Cann. ind.*).

Is in a great hurry (comp. *Lil. tigr.*, *Arg. nit.*) when doing things, in such a hurry that she gets fatigued.

Is always anticipating : feels things before they occur and generally correctly.

Seems to herself to make wrong statements.

Thinks someone is behind her, hears whispering (*Rhodium*) : sees faces that peer at her from behind bed and furniture. One night saw large people in room : large rats running; felt a delicate hand smoothing her head from front to back.

Sensation as if all life were unreal, like a dream.

Suicidal. Wild, desperate feeling, as of incipient insanity: gloom, relieved by torrents of tears.

Fear of the dark.

Had committed the unpardonable sin and was going to hell (*Psor.*, *Lil. tigr.*, *Kali ph.*, *Rob. Kali. br.*, *Chel.*, etc.).

Very impatient. Very selfish (*Puls.*, *Sul.*). Intense selfishness and self-pity.

< sunrise to sunset (*Luet.* sunset to sunrise). (See p. 37.)

Rhodium .. In the evening a constant whispering heard (*Medorrh.*), as if caused by human beings, makes him look to see if there were somebody near causing the whisper.

Indigo .. Illusions of sensation : it constantly seems to her as though she had a large goitre, which was very prominent ; she was constantly obliged to look down and feel whether it was so (comp. *Zincum*, *Sabadilla*).

(N.B.—Such sensations have given us valuable remedies, as in *Silica* and *Arnica* : i.e. *Indigo* should be a remedy to be considered in goitre. *Indigo* has also " pressure in ball of eye ".)

Sabadilla .. Imagines strange things : that his body had shrunk like that of dead persons ; his stomach was corroded, his scrotum swollen, etc. Knows it is all fancy, yet continues to imagine it (comp. *Indigo*).

Secale .. *Frightful anxiety: anxiety and fear of death.*
Delirium bordering on mania. Raving, with an attempt to jump into the water (*Dros.*, etc.).
Impression that there were two sick persons in the bed (*Bapt.*, *Pyrog.*, *Petrol.*), one of whom recovered and the other did not.
The room gave the impression of water, agitated like the "foaming of a troubled sea".
"Must have something to relieve her, or will die." Or, all the senses benumbed. (See p. 29.)

Crotalus cascavella Magnetic state. Hears nothing; sees the spectre of death, as a gigantic black skeleton. Hears a strange voice to left and behind her; follows it; throws herself against closed doors and scratches them with her nails.
Attempts to throw herself out of the window.
Fancies her eyes are falling out: hears groans. Thoughts of death. Clairvoyant (*Acon.*, etc.).

Anacardium .. LOSS OF MEMORY.
Everything strange: nothing real (*Med.*). Things have no reality: as if in a dream.
Thinks he is double (*Bapt.*, *Petrol.*, *Pyrog.*).
Fixed ideas: mind and body separated. about redemption of soul and the devil: stranger is at his side: strange forms accompany him, one to his right and one to his left.
Has a devil in his ear whispering blasphemy.
A demon sits on his neck telling offensive things
In one ear a devil, in the other an angel prompts to murder or acts of benevolence.
Contradiction between reason and will.
Her husband not her husband, her child not her child: now fondles, now pushes them away.
Disposed to malice: bent on wickedness.
Irresistible desire to curse and swear (*Stram.*).
Plug sensations. Hoop sensations.
"Wants to swear"—a mental disease in a minister, with "plug" and "band" sensations, was cured by *Anac.* (See p. 42.)

Osmium .. Thoughts of accidents which have happened: grow on him, till he thinks of doing the same injuries to others.

Aconite .. Terror: ANXIETY. Agonizing fear:—of death.
Frantic with pain (*Cham.*).
Palpitation with great anxiety.
Inconsolable anxiety and piteous howling.
Complaints and reproaches about trifles.
Pains are intolerable ; drive him crazy (*Cham.*).
Restlessness, agony, internal anxiety : does things in great haste. Must move often.
Screams at slightest touch : screams with the pain (*Coloc.*, *Mag. phos.*). Cannot bear light.
Slightest noise intolerable : music intolerable, goes through every limb.
Excessive tendency to be startled. Extremely cross.
Clairvoyant. Predicts the day of his death. Bids friends good-bye.
Fear of some misfortune happening to him.
Remote effects of fear, fright ; (esp. jaundice): (but jaundice from a fit of anger, *Cham.*).
Ailments from shock ; fright ; exposure to cold dry winds ; operation. (See p. 29.)

Arsenicum .. " INTENSE ANXIETY : RESTLESSNESS : PROSTRATION : with BURNINGS."
"*Anxiety* with fear ; impulse ; suicidal inclinations ; with sudden freaks : with mania."
Weary of life : loathes it : wants to die.
A remedy of suicidal tendencies (AUR., but *Aur.* has not the restlessness of *Ars.*).
Thoughts of death ; " incurable ! "
Fear: alone; things will injure him (*Arn.*) if alone.
Dread of death when alone, or going to bed.
Worst sufferings from 1 to 2 a.m. and p.m. : after midnight : from midnight on.
Melancholy : dread of death when alone : " going to die and wants someone with him."
Despair of recovery—after midnight.
" Anxiety as of one who has committed a murder " (*Rob.*, *Chel.*, *Thuja*). Officers coming to arrest him."
Fear that something terrible is going to happen.
Very chilly. Very particular : " The gentleman with the gold-headed cane."
Fastidious : exacting : fault-finding : violent. (See p. 31.)

Rhus .. .. Great RESTLESSNESS : anxiety, apprehension (*Acon.*). Great fear at night (*Acon., Ars.*).

Fear of poison (*Lach., Hyos., Bell., Kali br., Phos.*).

Despondent. Mental prostration.

Disgust of life and thoughts of suicide.

Wants to die, but lacks the courage (*Nux, China*).

Wants to drown himself, but fears death. (See p. 40.)

Hyoscyamus .. *Suspicious* (*Lach., Phos.*, etc.). Says medicine is poisoned (comp. *Lach., Rhus, Bell., Kali br.*).

Non-inflammatory cerebral activity.

Jumps out of bed : tries to escape (*Bell.*).

" In delirium midway between *Bell.* and *Stram.* Lacks the fever and congestion of *Bell.* and rage and maniacal delirium of *Stram.*"

Of the three, *Bell.* has most fever, *Hyos.* least. *Stram.* is the most violent, *Hyos.* the least.

All three have fear of water (*Lyssin*).

Wants to uncover : to go naked (*Phos.*)

Invol. stool, from excitement—jealousy. (P. 30.)

Belladonna .. Remarkable quickness of sensation, motion.

Excitement : delirium. Raves. Spits.

Wants to bite, injure, strike, escape (*Crot. h.*).

" The Mental symptoms active, never passive."

" Delirium better by eating a little light food."

Heat, redness, burning, with the fever and delirium. Sees ghosts, hideous faces, black animals (*Aeth.*) : things on fire (*Calc., Hep., Puls.*).

Twitches and screams out in sleep. (See p. 32.)

Stramonium .. Young people, hysterical, praying (comp. *Opuntia*) and singing.

Fear alone, in the dark : or cannot bear light.

" *Stram.* stands alone among deep-acting remedies in its violence of mental symptoms."

The mind in an uproar, cursing, tearing clothes, violent speech, frenzy, exposes person (*Hyos., Phos., Sec., Tarent., Verat., Phyto.*).

Screams day and night. Violent laughter. Queer notions: dogs attacking him (*Bell.*, etc.) Sees animals, ghosts, angels, devils. Has sinned away her day of grace (*Psor.*, etc.).

Exhorts people to repent : prays. (See p. 34.)

Camphora .. Agitation. Indescribable wretchedness.

Afraid of the mirrors, lest he should see himself in them. So excessive was this fear in the night that he would have got up and broken them, *only he was still more afraid to get up alone in the dark.*

Screaming " I shall not faint! for if I do I will have fits and never come out of them."

" I am dead. No, I am not dead! but indeed I must be dead!

" The external world existed for me no longer. My thoughts were gone. I sat up in bed, but all about me had disappeared. I was alone in a great universe, the last of all things. My ideas of the world, God, and religion now seemed to have existed only in my imagination. . . No feeling in my soul, but of hopeless, endless damnation . . . believing that I was the spirit of evil in a world forsaken of God. . . . The Infinite, like His works, had ceased to be. . . . What soul could paint to itself my everlasting dwelling as the Evil One, alone in a vast universe without faith or hope, and my heart forever broken by unimagined tortures."

" Horror! my hand no longer perceived resistance, my whole body was insensible and dry as marble. In evergrowing terror I sought to recall sensation, even pain, and tore the skin of face and hands. . . . Since that time, I have been subject to these attacks of terror at night when alone: constrained to this agonizing self-contemplation."

(Years ago, a patient came with just such terrible nights. She was continually taking Camphor—a doctor had told her to, for her " attacks ". Discontinued, and *Phos.*, as an antidote, put her right). (See p. 43.)

Elaps. .. .. Irresistible desire to scream at top of her voice (*Calc., Lil. tigr., Sep.*).

Desires to be alone.

Dread of being alone.

Excessive horror of rain. (See p. 41.)

Veratrum alb. .. Violence and destructiveness. Wants to destroy, tear (*Cup.*). Tears off clothes.

Religious frenzy. Preaches, prays (*Stram.*, *Opunt.*). Despair of salvation (*Ars.*, *Arn.*, *Lach.*, *Lil. tigr.*, etc.): of recovery. Attempts suicide. (See p. 9.)

Cold sweat on forehead with anguish and fear of death.

Curses: groans: howls: kisses.

Silent: or talks of faults of others. Scolds (*Nux*) and calls names.

Attacks of pain, driving to madness (*Acon.*, *Cham.*, etc.).

Head cold: forehead wet and cold. (See p. 41.)

Opuntia .. Desire to be at prayer; then, in a minute or two, desires to go and "tidy up"; soon went on an errand downstairs, then up again to prayer (comp. *Stram.*).

Involuntary, blasphemous mood (comp. *Stram.*).

Petulance: anger at near relatives: swearing on disappointment of plans: cannot get over injuries done by friends (*Staph.*, *Ipec.*).

Cuprum .. "*Mental and bodily exhaustion* from over-exertion of mind, or loss of sleep." (FARRINGTON.)

The great remedy of spasms: begin in fingers and toes, and spread.

Remedy of violence. (In many ways like *Bell.*)

Mania with biting, beating, tearing things.

Foolish gestures of imitation and mimicry.

Full of insane, spiteful tricks (*Tarent.*).

Illusions of imagination.

Does not recognize his own family. Attacks end in sweat.

Bellows like a calf during delirium. Shrill screams.

Tongue darts forth and back with great rapidity, like a snake. (See p. 31.)

Viscum alb. .. Incoherent talk and spectral illusions.

Inclined to be violent.

Feels as if going to do something dreadful.

Keeps waking, thinking horrible things.

Stupor: roused by noise: answers questions, then relapses into former condition (*Bapt.*).

Bryonia .. Dread of the future: prattles of his business.
In delirium, *thinks he is away from home* (*Op.*) *and wants to go home* (*Eup. pur.*).
Irritable: wants to be left alone.
"Do not cross a *Bry.* patient: it makes him worse". (See p. 40.)

Kali carb. .. Cannot bear to be touched (*Ant. t.*, *Ant. crud.*): starts when touched ever so slightly, especially on the feet.
Great aversion to being alone. (See p. 44.)

Antimonium crud. Serious minded. No desire to live.
Over-excitable; intense; hysterical ecstasy.
"Sentimental mood in the moonlight."
Desire to talk in rhymes or repeat verses.
Fretful: peevish: child *cannot bear to be touched* (*Kali c.*) or looked at (*Ant. t.*).
Is angry at every little attention.
An intensely white tongue, no mere coating, is a curious characteristic of *Ant. crud.*

Kali phos. .. Weariness of life, and dread of death.
Melancholy. Says she is eternally and irretrievably damned (*Med.*, *Lil. tigr.*, *Verat.*, etc.). Weeps: wrings hands.
Shyness: excessive blushing.
Morbid activity of memory: haunted by visions of the past: longing after them.
Delirium tremens. Fear of drunkards.

Mercurius .. Hastiness. Hurried, restless, anxious, impulsive.
Mind won't work on cold, cloudy, damp days: it is slow and sluggish and he is forgetful.
Impulses he tries to control—in a "*Merc.* patient".
Sudden anger with impulse to do violence (*Nux*, *Hep.*).
Impulse to kill or to commit suicide.
Some evil impending, worse at night, with sweat.
But all with the *Merc.* trembling, weakness, sweat, fœtor: the aggravation at night and from heat and cold. (See p. 38.)

Nux .. Frightfully over-sensitive: (*Hep.*) to noise, light, touch, smells, draughts: to contradiction.

Lack of balance. Uncontrollably irritable.

Violent temper: cannot be contradicted or opposed. Jerks about: tears things.

Takes everything amiss: breaks into abuse. Scolds. (*Verat.* Comp. *Kali iod.*)

Anxious, zealous, fiery temperament: or malicious, wicked, irascible disposition.

Feels everything too strongly.

Driven by impulses to commit acts that verge on insanity: the destruction of others (*Hep.*).

Suicidál, but lacks courage (*China, Rhus*).

Desire, or sudden impulse to kill (*Hep., Aloe*).

Persons addicted to wine, coffee, live sedentary lives with much mental exertion. (See p. 42.)

Hepar .. The slightest thing puts him into a violent passion: could have murdered anyone without hesitation. Very cross: trifles annoy.

Frightful anxiety (evening). Thought he was ruined: so sad he could have killed himself.

Over-sensitive to impressions: to surroundings: to pain (*Nux, Acon., Cham.*).

What would be to a normal person an ache, or a disagreeable sensation, is with *Hepar* intense suffering (*Cham.*).

Extremely irritable: anything that disturbs makes him wild and abusive and impulsive.

Impulse, sudden (*Tarent.*), to kill his best friend: to stab: to throw child into fire (*Nux*), or set herself on fire; to do violent things and to destroy (*Aloe*). Mania to set fire to things.

Hyperæsthesia: mental; physical (*Nux*). (See p. 42:)

Tarentula Mental chorea. Nervous excitement.

RESTLESSNESS; cannot keep quiet in any position: worse walking (rev. of *Rhus*).

Very sensitive to music (*Nux*): better from.

Lacks control. Sudden violent actions.

Sudden violent impulse to do harm (*Hep.*).

Sudden sly destructive tendency. Changed to someone terribly self-centred and selfish.

Feigns sick, to have people around.

Chamomilla

Frantic irritability :

CANNOT BEAR IT—whatever it may be !

Hypersensitive to every impression : to PAIN.

" Excessive sensibility of nerves, so excessive that only a few remedies equal it, such as *Coff.*, *Nux* and *Opium*." (KENT.)

Driven to frenzy by the pains (*Acon.*).

Inability to control temper. Cross, uncivil.

Wants something new every minute, and hurls it away (*Staph.*, *Cina*). Cannot keep still.

Angry at the pain. Scolds (*Nux*).

Complaints that come on after anger (*Coloc.*) : uterine hæmorrhages; jaundice; convulsions.

9 a.m. fevers : many complaints worse 9 p.m.

One cheek red and hot.

Vomiting after MORPHIA — uncontrollable retching ; " *Cham.* will stop that instantly." (After CHLOROFORM, *Phos.*)

Pains so violent, especially at night, cannot keep still : Child must be carried : adult must get up and walk.

Numbness with the pains (*Plat.*).

A remedy for teething, rheumatism, and indeed for any condition—*with these mentals*.

Cina

Children wake in a fright ; jump up, see sights, scream, tremble, talk about it. Pitiful weeping.

(Very like the *Cham.* child, must be rocked, carried, dandled constantly : or—must not be touched, and you must not come near. Desires many things, which it refuses. Throws away things, cries about nothing. (*Cham.*, *Staph.*))

Exceedingly cross, cries and strikes out.

Can't be quieted, proof against persuasion and caresses.

" Troubles cause a constant desire to rub, pick or bore into nose" (*Ail.*). Children with dilated pupils ; night terrors and WORMS.

Antimonium tartaricum

Wants to be let alone (*Bry.*).

Child will not allow itself to be touched. (*Ant. crud.* to be looked at or touched.)

Peevish and quarrelsome.

Magnesia phos. — Laments all the time about her pain: screams out (with abdominal pain).

Talks to herself constantly: or sits in moody silence: carries things from place to place and then back (comp. *Opuntia*).

Pains: stab, shoot, ***paroxysms unbearable, drive patient to frenzy*** (*Acon.*, etc.). Rapidly change place.

Colocynth .. "Pains due to a very singular cause, viz. anger with indignation (*Cham.*).

"Anger will be followed by violent neuralgia, in head, eyes, down spine, in intestines.

"Screams with the pain (*Mag. phos.*).

"Friends irritate him: wants to be alone.

"He has all he can do to stand those terrible pains . . . often the result of ***anger with indignation***." (KENT.) (Comp. *Staph.*, *Cham.*)

> pressure and heat: worse when still: if abdominal, better bending double and pressing hard.

Staphisagria .. Suppressed anger: suppressed indignation. Controls it, then suffers from it. (*Ipec.*, etc.).

Great indignation about things done by himself or others (*Opuntia*).

Ailments from indignation or vexation.

Sufferings from pride, envy or chagrin.

If *Staph.* has to control himself, goes all to pieces; loses voice—sleep—ability to work.

Broods over old slights or injuries.

Whole mind and nervous system in a fret.

Children ill-tempered: cry for things which they throw away (*Cham.*, *Cina*).

Ailments from chagrin, indignation, quarrels.

Ipecacuanha .. Peevish: irritable: impatient: morose, scornful.

Despises everything. Scorns everything, and desires that others shall not appreciate or value anything.

Ailments from vexation (*Cham.*), and reserved displeasure (*Staph.*, *Opunt.*).

But the great characteristic of *Ipec.* is NAUSEA —nausea unrelieved by vomiting. Nausea and vomiting with a clean tongue.

Aloe
Easily excited, angry, revengeful: brooks no opposition: wants to destroy objects of wrath (*Hep.*, *Nux*).
Better for tea, or mild stimulant.
(Action centres on rectum. A strange symptom, strains in vain for stool, then a large stool slips out unnoticed.)

Kali iodatum
A strong degree of irritability, cruelty and harshness. Harsh with family and children: abusive (comp. *Nux*).
Nervous: better in open air (*Puls.*): walking (*Ferr.*, *Puls.*); can walk long distances without fatigue; back in house, weak, tired, exhausted. *A nervous and mental exhaustion comes on from resting* (comp. *Iodum*, *Puls.*).

Absinthium ..
Brutality: mental dullness.
Great terror: terrifying hallucinations.
Stupefaction with dangerous violence.
Walks about in distress, seeing all sorts of demons (comp. *Anac.*, *Bell.*, etc.). (See p. 32.)

Phytolacca ..
Great loss of personal delicacy: a total disregard of all surrounding objects: no disposition to adjust their persons under any circumstances (comp. *Hyos.*, *Phos.*, *Stram.*).
Sense of entire indifference to life.
Irresistible desire to bite teeth together.

Bufo ..
Feeling of intoxication; intoxication a pleasure.
Paroxysms of fury, cease when he sees anyone.
Defiance, duplicity, spitefulness (*Tarent.*): bites (*Bell. Stram.*).
Enfeebled intellect: apathy: stupidity.
Pronounces badly: angry when not understood.
Aversion to strangers: desires solitude: yet fear of being alone and dying forsaken.
Moral depravity (*Selen.*). "Sexual epilepsy."

Baryta mur. ..
In every form of mania, as soon as the sexual desire is increased.
Idiocy.

Robinia .. Mental alienation and craziness: furious motions or laughter, buffoonery, jumping and dancing (*Croc.*).
Always under the impression that he will be disgraced :- has committed a crime (*Ars.*, *Thuja*, etc.).
Dread of everything that is sombre and black.
Bacchanalian, erotic, or religious mania.
Love and excited passions lead him to the grossest excesses, even to homicide.
Disposition to be obscene, to gormandize, and for all kinds of orgies. (See p. 39.)

Cantharis .. Great amativeness: amorous frenzy.
IRRITATION: mental and physical.
Anger: paroxysms of rage.
Constant, complete, almost frenzied delirium.
The characteristic symptom, leading to the use of *Cantharis* in almost any disease,—***violent burning, cutting pains, before, with and after urination: violent pains in bladder; intolerable tenesmus.***

Agaricus mus. One of the delirium tremens remedies.
Constant raving: tries to get out of bed.
Sings, talks, does not answer questions.
Extraordinary fancies and delusions, as "commanded by a mushroom to commit suicide".
Ecstasy: makes verses (*Ant. crud.*), prophecies.

Oenanthe crocata Disturbances of intellect: mad and furious.
Extreme restlessness, approaching mania.
Furious delirium. Hallucinations.
Delirium like delirium tremens. Constantly moved from place to place; talked without cessation, without knowing what they said.
Grasped at imaginary objects.
Epileptic insanity: sudden furious attack.

Cicuta virosa .. Does rash and absurd things.
Frightened, suspicious, distrustful, moans, howls.
Is violent in all his actions.
Strange desires, to eat coal, etc. (*Alum.*, etc.).
Spasms and convulsions *of great violence.*
Head retracted. (See p. 37.)

Lilium tigr. .. Crazy feeling in head: as if she would go crazy.
Hurry: aimless hurried motion (*Arg. nit.*).
Wants to walk. Must keep busy to repress sexual excitement.
Tormented about her salvation (comp. *Med.*, *Lach.*, *Stram.*, *Psor.*).
Imperative duties, and cannot perform them.
Depressed: weeps: indifferent (*Sepia*, *Phos.*, etc.).
Pelvic symptoms, also, are those of *Sepia*.
But *Sep.* is chilly and indifferent, while *Lilium* feels the heat, and is full of rush and torment. (See p. 35.)

Argentum nit. .. Greatest remedy for ANTICIPATION.
When ready for church, opera, interview, gets diarrhœa (*Gels.*, *Phos.*, etc.). Diarrhœa from anticipation. " *Exam. funk.*"
Hurried, anxious, irritable, nervous.
Must walk fast—faster: so hurried! (*Lil. tigr.*).
Disturbances of memory: of reason.
Irrational: does strange things: has strange obsessions: fear of passing a certain corner: of bridges and high places: he might have impulse to jump off; to jump into river.
Sight of high houses makes him dizzy and stagger: houses might approach and crush him.
Craves sweets which disagree: salt. (See section " Fears ".)
"A fool beyond hope for this world." (See p. 36.)

Borax .. Great fear of downward motion (*Gels.*, *Cup.*, p. 31).
Afraid to go downstairs; can't swing, ride, use a rocking chair, such is the fear of downward motion.
Children wake, scream, grasp sides of cradle.
Easily startled by sudden noise.
Nervous: fidgety: sensitive.
Anxiety increased till 11 p.m.
" When thinking at his work, nausea. Strong nausea."
One of remedies of sea-sickness, "When boat went down, felt everything inside me come up."

Gelsemium .. Bad effects of great fright or fear (*Acon.*, *Opium*).
Stage fright: fear of appearing in public: anticipation brings on diarrhœa (*Arg. nit.*).
Involuntary discharges from fright, or surprises.
Fear of falling (*Bor.*, *Cup.* p. 31, *Stram.* p. 34, *Lac. c.* p. 33).
Tremor: wants to be held. Lack of courage.
Wants to be quiet: to be let alone.

Arnica .. In serious illness, says there is nothing the matter with him (*Opium*). Or
Horrors in the night (*Acon.*).
Horror of instant death, with cardiac distress at night. "Send for the doctor at once!"
Restlessness, because everything he lies on is too hard. Must move for ease.
Everything coming towards him is going to hurt him (*Ars.*, *Stram.*, *Valer.*, p. 34). Fears approach—being struck.
Great desire to scratch, will scratch wall, bed, his head, etc. (See p. 29.)

Opium .. Tells you she is not sick (*Arn.*).
Says she is well and happy: wants nothing: has no symptoms: (when desperately ill).
Talkative: mental activity (*Coff.*).
Much affected by sound—light—faintest odours.
Not at home sensation (*Bry.*, *Eup. pur.*).
Most of the complaints are painless.
Wants a cool room: kicks the clothes off.
Dullness, insensibility, to deep coma.
Again—rouses from stupor with a look of awful fear or anxiety.
Complaints from fear, when the fear remains.
Sees frightful images: black forms: ghosts, devils, etc. (comp. *Bell.*).
Complaints from joy (*Coff.*), anger (*Cham.*), shame (*Staph.*) sudden fright (*Acon.*). (P. 32.)

Hura brazil .. Sensation of floating.
Imagines she sees a dead person and cries.
Sensation of falling to the ground: as if hanging three feet from the ground.
Imagines she is alone in the world.
Impatient: because her ideas flow too slowly.
Sadness: despair: feels abandoned.

Baptisia ..	In delirium, imagines he is in pieces and scattered about the bed. Cannot get himself together (*Petrol.*, *Pyrog.*, *Phos.*). Cannot sleep, because she cannot get herself together. Thought she was three persons and could not keep them covered (comp. *Anac.*, *Valer.*, *Sec.*, *Petr.*, *Pyrog.*). Stupor: falls asleep while being spoken to. Indisposed to, or want of power to think.
Petroleum ..	Did not know where she was in the street. Thinks another person lies alongside of him; or that one limb is double (comp. *Bapt.*, etc.). That another baby is in bed and needs attention. That she has a third leg which would not remain quiet. Little time left to make his will.
Pyrogen ..	Loquacious: thinks and talks faster than ever before. Sees a man at the foot of the bed. Feels she covers the whole bed. Knows her head is on the pillow, but not where her body is (comp. *Bapt.*, etc.). Feels crowded with arms and legs. Is one person, when lying on one side, and another when she turns over. Hallucinations of wealth: during fever.
Valeriana ..	Nervous irritation: cannot keep still. Feels as if floating in the air: legs floating in the air (*Sticta*, *Phos. ac.*). Hysteria. Hallucinations, especially at night; sees figures, animals, men, etc. Ideas: that she is someone else. Moves to edge of bed to make room (comp. *Sec.*, *Bapt.*, *Petr.*, *Pyrog.*). Imagines animals lying near her that she fears she may hurt. "Raving, tearing, swearing mania (*Stram.*). Worse evening: worse when still: sleepless in early night: all like *Pulsatilla*, but temper decides." Suddenly changeable mood and symptoms (*Croc.*, *Puls.*). (See p. 37.)

Crotalus horridus	Loquacity with desire to escape (*Bell*, etc.) from bed. Stupid: cannot express herself. Makes ridiculous mistakes. Torpid: sluggish: incoherent: hesitating. Snappish temper.
Sticta pulmonaria (*Lung wort*)	Great desire to talk about anything and everything—whether anyone listens or not: feels cannot keep her tongue still (*Lach.*). Felt light and airy: legs as if floating in air (*Valer.*, *Phos. ac.*). (Ancient remedy for larynx, chest, rheumatism.)
Veratrum viride	Loquacity (*Lach.*, *Sticta*, *Crot. h.*, etc.), with exaltation of ideas (comp. *Lach.*). Exalted opinion of her ideas and powers (*Plat.*). Everything seems clear: clearly understands formerly mysterious things. Wants no medicine, as that may restore her former condition. Talks: laughs: pays no attention to what is said to her. Will not answer questions: nothing must be said that she cannot hear. Characteristic tongue, white or yellow, with red streak down middle, or no coating sides.
Platina ..	" Represents the woman's perverted mind." Arrogant, proud, contemptuous, haughty. Over-estimates herself. Contemptuous. FEELS TALL: other people and things small, and persons physically and mentally inferior. " The prim old maid gone insane." Any disturbance to pride brings on symptoms. Fears death and loathes life. Amativeness: madness: hysteria. Characteristic, *Numbness with pain* (*Cham.*). (See p. 43.)
Atropinum ..	Rambling speech: fits of idiotic laughter. Spectral illusions. Speaks with imaginary beings. In talking, has to stop and ask what she is talking about. Says her blood does not circulate. " Feet must be in hot water or she will die."

Thuja .. Many strange symptoms and fixed ideas.
Thinks she is followed : so delicate, as if made of glass, and will break : someone walking beside her : body and soul separated : is pregnant : something alive inside (*Croc.*).
Violent irritability, jealousy, quarrelsomeness. Can control herself with strangers (*Sep.*).
Disposition to cheat.
Walks room in a circle (*Bell.*)—unable for simple work. Mental symptoms after vaccinations. (See p. 37.)

Lachesis .. From slightest exertion of mind or emotions, extremities become cold.
Self-conscious. Conceit, envy, hatred.
Revengeful : cruel. An improper love of self.
JEALOUSY. SUSPICION. Impulsive insanity.
People talking about her : trying to injure her : poison her : put her into an asylum.
Thinks, or dreams she is dead : of death.
Thinks she is somebody else : is under superhuman control.
Compelled to do things by spirits : hears voices : hears commands that she must obey.
Confesses what she has never done.
Religious insanity : full of wickedness : has committed the unpardonable sin (*Psor.*, *Med.*, *Arg. nit.*).
Is going to die, and going to hell.
LOQUACITY (*Sticta*, etc.). Impelled to talk continuously (*Cann. ind.*).
Jumps from one idea into another.
SUSPICION : JEALOUSY : LOQUACITY. (See p. 30.)

One remembers a woman, frantically jealous of her husband : always peeping to see if he was not flirting with their shop-girl : with all sorts of delusions : even suicidal. *Lach.* completely cured her in a short time : and she became her own rosy and sunny self.

Apis .. .. Jealous and suspicious (*Lach.*, *Hyos.*).
Sad, constant weeping without cause.
Mental, and all symptoms, worse in warm room
Premonition of death (*Acon.*).
Stupor, with sudden shrill, sharp cries.
Alternately dry and hot, or perspiring.

Coffea .. Unusual activity of mind and body.

All senses more acute. Over-sensitive.

Excitable and over-active (rev. of *Nux mosch.*).

Sleeplessness from mental activity.

Full of ideas.

Over-sensitive to noise. Pains of extremities aggravated by noise.

Pains insupportable (*Cham.*).

Effects of violent emotion, especially joy.

All senses more acute, sight, hearing, smell, taste, touch (*Bell.*, *Cham.*, *Opium*, *Nux*).

A great sleep remedy.

She had been very ill : doctor suggested a cup of strong coffee. That night absolutely sleepless : quite cheery and happy, but hour after hour, wide awake. At last she got a dose of *Coffea* 200, and was asleep in a few minutes.

Crocus .. Jumping, dancing, laughing, whistling : very affectionate : wants to kiss everybody.

Alternations of excessive happy affectionate tenderness, and rage.

" *Hysteria, all changes in mood she rings,*
She loves and she kisses and jumps and sings,
Then cries and abuses and rages ; and then
Starts loving and whistling and dancing again."

Sings involuntarily, on hearing even one note sung : laughs at herself, but soon sings again, in spite of her determination to stop.

Feels something alive in her, jumping about (*Thuja.*).

Cannabis indica Very forgetful : cannot finish a sentence : forgets what he was about to say.

Time seems long : spaces and distances immense. (Characteristic.)

Thoughts crowd on the brain (*Coff.*).

Laughs immoderately at trifles.

Excessive loquacity (*Lach.*, *Hyos.*), constantly theorizing (*Sulph.*).

Horror of darkness, of approaching death.

Fixed ideas. In constant fear he would become insane. (See p. 35.)

SECTION 2

SOME DRUGS OF FEARS AND ANXIETIES: WITH THEIR DREAMS

Aconite .. " Fear is depicted on his countenance " (*Op.*, *Stram.*, *Lac. c.*, etc.).

Fear of Death :—" no use, I am going to die."

Fear of ghosts (*Ars.*, *Manc.*, *Phos.*, *Puls.*, etc.) : of the dark (*Phos.*, etc.).

Fear of death with great loquacity, or great anxiety in the region of the heart (compare *Lyss.*, *Med.*, *Rhus*).

Extreme fearfulness.

Dread of some accident happening.

Fear lest he might stagger and fall.

Fear to go out alone after dark.

" Intense fear : awful anxiety, and great restlessness." Not only fear, but ailments from fear : remote effects of fright (*Op.*), especially jaundice.

Anxious DREAMS with anxiety in chest.

Frightful dreams. (See p. 13.)

Secale .. Anxiety. Great anxiety. Frightful anxiety.

Great anguish : wild with anxiety.

Constant moaning and *fear of death : with strong desire to live.* (See p. 12.)

Variolinum *Fear of death :* wild excitement, begs to know if he is to die, and before answer, drops into a heavy sleep. Morbid fear of smallpox.

(Mental and neurasthenic conditions in persons who have, even years ago, had smallpox.)

Arnica .. Hypochondriac anxiety. " No doctor any use."

Violent attacks of anxiety.

Apprehension of future evils.

Horror of instant *death* (*Plat.*, comp. *Cann. ind.*).

DREAMS that she is overwhelmed with reproaches. Can hardly realize it has been a dream.

Fearful dreams of large black dogs (*Bell.*), cats.

Of men being flayed : about frightful objects : of lightning having struck : of graves.

Typically, *Arn.* feels bruised and sore. (See p. 24.)

Raphanus .. Extreme anxiety and *fear of death.* Believes she has an unrecognized *disease* (*Lil. tigr.*).
Raph. has distension: accumulation and retention of flatus. (See p. 7.)

Hyoscyamus .. Excessive *fear of death.* Wishes to run away (*Bell.*).
Fear: being left alone: being bitten: poisoned, or sold: betrayed: injured.
Remarkable fear that he had been devoured by animals.
Dread of drinks: of water. (*Lyss.*, *Stram.*). (See p. 14.)

Lachesis .. Religious monomania: fear she will be damned. (*Psor.*, *Med.*, *Arg. nit.*). Is in the hands of a stronger power.
Robbers in the house (*Nat. mur.*, *Ars.*), wants to jump out of the window (*Aeth.*, *Bell.*).
Pursued by enemies: tries to leave the room, as if frightened by visions behind him.
Afraid to go to bed. *Dread of death. Afraid to sleep* lest he die before he wakes.
Fear of being poisoned (*Rhus*, *Hyos.*).
Fear of suicide (*Ars.*, *Merc.*, *Nat. s.*).
Nightly attacks of anxiety: cramps in calves from fear. Ailments from fright (*Acon.*).
Sleepless from anxiety: short naps with frightful dreams: springs up with terror and suffocation (*Spong.*) and palpitation.
Dreaming; frequent waking: again and again dozing and dreaming. (See p. 27.)

Lueticum .. *Terrible dread of night* (of *sleep*, *Lach.*): the mental and physical exhaustion on waking. It is intolerable: death is preferable.
Fears to prepare for night, is in abject fear of suffering on waking. Always worse as night approaches: leaves her at daylight, which she prays for. (How often has one seen this "worse at night" relieved by *Luet.*)

Sambucus .. A dread of some undefined danger: that the horse might run away: or the wagon break.

Anthemis nobilis Fear out of doors: exceedingly afraid of being run over.

Arsenicum .. Fixed idea that he and his family will die of starvation (*Sepia*).

Fear drives him out of bed: he hides in a closet: runs about at night looking for thieves (comp. *Lach.*, *Nat. mur.*, *Psor.*).

Says little, but complains of fear (*Acon.*).

Fear of being left alone.

Fear of death (*Acon.*) when alone, or going to bed.

Anxiety and restlessness; worse after midnight.

Excessive anxiety: drives out of bed: must jump out of bed.

Anxiety like that of one who has committed a murder: driven from place to place.

ANXIETY: with restlessness: yet cannot rest anywhere. Fears something may have happened to his relatives (comp. *Sulph.*, *Phos.*).

Sees all kind of vermin on his bed: throws handfuls of them away: tries to escape from them.

Imagines he sees burglars in his room: listens under the bed: is bathed in cold sweat.

Imagines space under bed, and whole house is full of thieves: sees thieves in his room, and hides under his bed (comp. *Nat. mur.*).

Sees a man who has hanged himself beckoning to him to cut him loose

Has offended people: he knows not how.

Wakes with horrible anxiety, palpitation and restlessness: fear of death.

The greatest fear and anguish: sees ghosts day and night (comp. *Acon.*, *Manc.*, *Phos.*, *Puls.*).

Anxiety and restlessness indescribable.

Fear: Deadly fear.

Afraid he will not prevent himself from killing a person with a knife (*Nux*, *Merc.*).

DREAMS of care, sorrow, fear, danger, fire, thunder, black water, darkness, death. (P. 13.)

Cuprum .. In delirium, afraid of everyone, shrinks away: tries to escape (*Bell.*): in the evening and dark.

Fears he will lose his reason.

Afraid of strangers. Shrinks from everyone who approaches.

Fear of falling: clings to nurse (*Gels.*, *Bor.*, *Coca*, *Lac. c.*). (See p. 16.)

Belladonna .. Fear of imaginary things, ***wants to run away; to escape*** (*Opium, Hepar, Cup.*).

Fear of a big black dog (*Arn.*): the gallows.

A crimson snake at foot of bed threatens to fasten on his neck (*Lac can.*).

Fear of *ghosts*, soldiers who come to take him away: of black animals, rats, dogs, wolves.

Starts in fright when approached (*Arn., Cup., Stram., Thuja*, etc.), even in the street.

Great anxiety: must flee away.

Delirium and mania; violent and furious.

"Violence runs through all the mental symptoms of *Bell.*" (See pp. 16, 17.)

DREAMS of murder; street robbers; danger from fire; of swimming; pursued by giants.

Wakes full of fright and fear: something under the bed (comp. *Ars.*) making a noise.

Jumps out of bed with fear: ***tries to run away and hide*** (*Hell., Puls., Stram.*).

Characteristically *Bell.* has a red, hot face, and big pupils. (See p. 14.)

Opium .. Sees frightful *ghosts* (*Bell.*, etc.): easily frightened.

Frenzy: ***desires to escape*** (*Bell.*). Says a regiment of horses are on his bed, and he fears to be trodden on. Told that horses are very careful, says, he will be crushed by the wagons following.

Face wears ***a constant expression of fright and terror*** (*Stram., Lac can., Acon.*).

They see frightful objects and are in great fear.

Believe themselves murderers; criminals to be executed; want to run away (*Bell., Rob.*).

After fright with fear (*Acon.*).

After fright, the fear of the fright still remaining.

Anxiety; apprehension; fear of impending death (*Arn., Acon.*, etc.).

Characteristic: contracted pupils. (See p. 24.)

Absinthium .. Fear of assassination (*Cimic., Op., Phos., Plumb., Stram.*).

Terrifying hallucinations: persons pursuing him (*Bell.*, etc.): sees animals, rats, cats of all colours: grotesque animals: is pursued by soldiers, imaginary enemies, naked women.

Lac caninum .. Fear of falling downstairs. (See *Gels.*, etc.) That she will be unable to perform duties.

Fear of *death* with anxious face (*Acon.*, *Stram.*).

Wakes distressed: must rise and occupy herself. Fear she will be crazy.

Imagines that any symptom is some settled disease: that everything she says is a lie: that she is looked down upon by everyone: that she is of no importance in life: that she is dirty: that she wears someone else's nose: that she sees spiders.

That she is surrounded by myriads of SNAKES. Some running like lightning up and down inside skin; some inside feel long and thin. Fears to step on floor lest she should tread on them, and make them squirm and wind round her legs (comp. *Arg. nit.*, *Sep.*).

Fears to look behind lest she should see snakes: *seldom troubled with them after dark.*

On going to bed, afraid to shut her eyes lest a large snake should hit her in the face (*Bell.*).

Horrid sights presented to her mental vision (not always snakes). Terror lest they show themselves to her natural eye.

Fear lest pimples would prove little snakes, and twine and twist round each other.

Feels she is a loathsome mass of disease; cannot look at any part of her body, even hands, as it intensifies the feeling of disgust and horror.

Can't bear any part of body to touch another: one finger to touch another. If she cannot get out of her body, will soon become crazy.

Feels that heart or breathing would stop; frightens herself, which makes heart palpitate. Fancies he is going out of his mind.

Looks under chairs, table, sofa, expecting some horrible monster to creep forth: feels that it would drive her mad. *Not afraid in the dark: sees them only in the light* (rev. *Luet.*).

Feels that she is going to become unconscious: wakes with sensation of bed in motion (*Bell.*).

DREAMED of a large snake in her bed (*Bell.*).

Dreams often that she is urinating: wakes to find herself on the point of doing so (*Sep.*).

Mancinella .. FEAR OF INSANITY (*Lac can.*, *Calc.*, etc.).
Fear of going crazy: of evil spirits: of being taken by the devil.
DREAMS of ghosts, of apparitions.
(Aversion to work: bashful: timid.)
Thought vanishes: forgets from minute to minute what she wishes to do.

A case. She had a terror of insanity; if heard of a case, nearly went crazy with fear. Sat apart: neglected her duties: said nothing. Lost appetite, flesh and colour. No interest in anything—only consumed with her fear.

Puls. and *Ign.* were useless. Then for the strong mental, *Mancinella* was given and quickly cured. Later, on the first slight sign of recurrence (two or three times only in some twenty years), *Mancinella* put her right promptly.

Onosmodium .. Something terrible going to happen, and powerless to prevent it.
Fear to look down, lest she fall downstairs (*Gels.*).
Fear that he might fall into the fire when walking by it, and spite of his will power, he did stagger into the fire.
Wants to think, and thinks till she forgets everything and where she is.

Stramonium .. Fears: he will *loses his senses*: that his lips will grow together: of suffocation: of falling: of everything falling on her (comp. *Arg. nit.*).
Frightful fancies: *face expresses fright and terror* (*Acon.*, *Opium*, *Lac can.*).
Sees *more horrifying images at his side than in front of him*, and they all occasion terror.
Sees frightful figures, cats, rats, mice, dogs (*Bell.*, *Abs.*). Springs away with signs of terror.
Delirium of fear as though a dog were attacking him (*Verat.*, comp. *Bell.*).
Asked her mother not to leave her, as something was going to hurt her (*Valer.*, comp. *Arn.*).
Mania for light and company: cannot be alone.
Hydrophobia (*Bell.*, *Hyos.*, *Lyssin*, *Agave*).
Child wakes terrified, knows no one, screams with fright, clings to those near (*Calc.*).
Imagines he is alone all the time: tries to escape (*Bell.*). Is afraid. (See p. 14.)

Lyssin .. Fear *of becoming mad.*

Fear that he cannot physically endure his fears much longer.

Something terrible going to happen to him. Fear of being alone.

Restlessness and anxiety *at precordia* (*Med., Rhus*), frequent change of position and sighing.

Frightened at a bird: thought it was a mouse.

When he hears water (*Bell., Hyos., Stram.,* etc.). *poured out,* or hears it run, or sees it, becomes irritable and nervous: it causes desire for stool and other ailments.

Thinking of fluids, even of blood, brings on convulsions.

Symptoms brought on by dread and fear.

DREAMS. Of influential persons to whom he is a servant or subordinate.

Of a Latin debate with law students: astonished at the facility and fluency with which he has spoken Latin: far greater than was possible to him when awake (comp. *Ign., Nux*).

Of dogs all the time (*Bell., Stram.*).

Of fighting: of high places: of insane asylum: of churches.

Exciting dreams: frightful dreams. (See p. 10.)

Cannabis indica Constant fear of *becoming insane* (*Manc.,* etc.).

Horror of darkness: of approaching death (*Arn.*).

Dread of congestion: of apoplexy, hæmorrhage, and a multiplicity of deaths.

Dare not use his voice, lest he should knock down the walls, or burst himself like a bomb.

DREAMS: delightful: delicious: prophetic: Or, of danger and dead bodies. (See p. 28.)

Lilium tigrinum Tormented about her salvation (*Lach.*).

Fear: disease incurable: that symptoms denote an internal organic disease that nobody understands.

Fear insanity: heart disease: incurable.

Frightful, laborious dreams (*Rhus*).

Frantic hurry—walks fast (*Arg. nit.*). (See p. 23.)

Argentum nitricum .. Apprehension of some serious disease.

Apprehension; when ready to go to church or opera, diarrhœa sets in (*Gels.*, comp. *Puls.*). Examination funk (*Aeth.*).

Fear, or thinking, brings on diarrhœa.

Fears to be alone, as he thinks he will die.

Fear in passing a certain corner or building that he will drop down and create a sensation: is relieved by going in another direction.

Tormented with anxiety: faint with anxiety when walking, *which makes him walk faster.*

Nervous when walking: will have a fit, or die suddenly.

Dizzy and staggers at sight of high houses: seems as if the houses both sides of the road would approach and crush him.

Often wakes his wife or child to have someone to talk to.

"Lost beyond hope for this world."

Horrible DREAMS: sees departed friends, ghosts: dreams of putrid water: of serpents, which fill him with horror (*Lac can.*, *Bell*, etc.).

Dreams: hungry: wakes with violent spasm, hunger, nausea and flatulence. Typically, loves salt; sweets, which disagree. (See p. 23.)

Digitalis .. Great anxiety; as from a troubled conscience.

Tortured by fear of death, or loss of reason.

Fear of the future: with desire to escape (*Bell.*).

DREAMS: frequent waking at night by dreams of falling from a height (*Thuja*) or into water.

Chelidonium .. Imagines she cannot think, and will lose her reason (*Calc.*, etc.): that she must die (*Acon.*, etc.).

That he has committed the unpardonable sin, and will be eternally lost (*Med.*, etc.). (P. 11.)

As if she had committed a crime (*Op.*, *Rob.*, *Chel.*); fear of going crazy with restlessness and heat.

DREAMS: corpses: funerals (*Calc.*, *Thuja*, etc.).

Vivid dreams of business matters (*Bry.*, *Psor.*).

Dreams of great lice (*Nux*) on her shoulders.

Dreams: pneumonia, falling, bloody wounds, being killed, being buried alive (*Arn.*, *Ign.*).

Medorrhinum Everything startles her : news coming seems to touch her heart before she hears it (compare *Rhus, Psor.*).

Woke with frightened sensation, as if something dreadful had happened.

Fear of the dark. Sensation of unreality (*Valer., Cic., Alum., Cann. ind., Lac. c., Lil. tigr., Staph.*).

Had committed the unpardonable sin and was going to hell (*Chel.*).

Dreadful DREAMS of ghosts, dead people. (See p. 11.)

Thuja .. Fearful anxiety, like death agony : a nameless internal ache, as if the soul were escaping from the body, with most terrible uneasiness.

Constantly tormented by groundless anxiety.

Constant anxiety as if he had committed great crime (*Ars., Rob., Ign.*). Fear of misfortune.

Frightful anxiety at night (*Acon., Ars.*, etc.).

Fear of apoplexy : with anxious perspiration.

Terrible DREAMS of the dead.

When asleep, dead persons appear to her ; distinctly sees them, feels them (*Elaps*): thinks she is talking with them.

Constant dreams of the features of a corpse.

Espec. useful after vaccinations, or inoculations.

Voluptuous dreams. Dreams of danger and death. Of falling from a height. (See p. 27.)

Valeriana .. Fearfulness in the evening when sitting in the dark, imagining that someone might hurt him (*Stram., Arn.*).

Anxiety as if objects round him had been estranged from him : rooms seem to him desolate: does not feel at home, is impelled to leave it (*Med.*, comp. *Cic.*). (See p. 25.)

Cicuta .. Everything appears strange : almost terrible.

Feels in a strange place (*Valer.*) which causes fear. Sensation of unreality (see *Med.*).

Old men fear long spell of sickness before dying.

Afraid of society : wants to be alone.

Thinks himself a young child: likes childish toys.

Disposition to be frightened. (See p. 22.)

Calcarea .. "*Calc.* has every kind of fear."
Concern about imaginary things that might happen to her.
Anxiety, as if he had done evil, or ought to apprehend reproaches. (See *Cocc.*, p. 39.)
Great anxiety with palpitation.
Uneasiness of mind. Fearful and uneasy, as if some accident or misfortune were to happen to himself, or someone else (*Ars.*, *Phos.*, *Sulph.*): As if expecting sad news. Dread and anxiety for the future.
Fear of consumption.
Fears to lose her reason. (See pp. 34, 35.)
Fears lest people should observe her confusion of mind. That they look at her suspiciously.
Fears of disease and misery, with foreboding.
Despairs of life; imagines she must die (*Acon.*, etc.); despairs of salvation (*Lach.*, etc.): wants to stab himself.
Fear about health: of an organic heart disease: that something terrible will happen.
Fear of death: consumption: that she has some fatal disease (*Lil. tig.*); misfortune; being alone.
Child afraid of everything it sees.
Fear excited by report of *cruelties*.
Easily frightened: tendency to start.
Night-terrors in children (has cured many cases).
When closing eyes, horrid visions.
DREAMS. Horrible, frightful: of sickness, death and corpses; smell of corpses (comp. *Thuja*).
Fear of fantastic dreams during sleep.
Voluptuous dreams.

Mercurius sol. Anxiety and apprehension *in the blood*.
As if he had committed a crime; done wrong. (*Rob.*).
As though he had no control over his senses.
Fearful DREAMS: of falling from a height (*Thuja*): of robbers (*Ars.*, *Nat. mur.*, etc.) of shooting: of a flood.
Excessive sweating; at night. (See p. 17.)

Ruta .. Anxious as if he had done something wrong.
If anyone opened the door, feared someone had come to arrest him (*Ars.*).

Cocculus indica Overpowered with the most frightful fearfulness.

Sudden excessive anxiety, as if he had committed a crime—done evil (*Ars., Calc., Ruta, Rob., Zinc.*).

Robinia .. Fear and confusion of conscience, as if he had committed a crime (*Merc.*). Fears disgrace.

Dread of everything sombre and black (*Ars., Verat., Stram., Tarent.*).

DREAMS full of disputes, scolding, anger, cruelties which have happened, or will.

The great feature of *Robinia* is heartburn: especially at night.

Eructations and vomiting of an intensely sour fluid: sets teeth on edge. (See p. 22.)

Ignatia .. Dread of every trifle (*Calc.*); especially of things coming near him (*Arn.*).

Fears she will have an ulcer in the stomach.

Fear of thieves on waking after midnight (*Ars., Lach., Nat. m.*, etc.).

Fearfulness; does not like to talk; prefers to be alone.

As if he had committed crime (*Ars., Merc., Rob.*).

As though something terrible had happened: cannot speak of it.

As if she had done something wrong; or as if some great misfortune were about to happen.

A state of anguish in which she shrieks for help.

DREAMS with reflections and deliberations.

Dreams full of mental exertion and scientific investigations (comp. *Lyssin., Nux*). (See p. 7.)

Zincum .. Anxiety; uneasy mood as though he had committed a crime (*Calc., Ruta, Rob., Cocc.*). On account of thieves (*Ars.* etc.), or horrible apparitions while awake.

DREAMS: being strangled: after waking, fear lest the man who strangled her would return.

Dreams of corpses (*Thuja*, etc.); horses which changed to dogs under him: of being smeared with human excrement. Quarrelsome, vexacious dreams. (See p. 6.)

Rhus .. Restlessness and anxiety about heart (*Psor.*, *Med.*), as if had committed a crime (*Ars.*, *Merc.*, *Rob.*, or of some great misfortune in store for her.

Inexpressible anxiety, *esp. at heart* (*Acon.*, *Psor.*).

Restlessness with anxiety and apprehensions that *clawed at her heart.*

Great fear at night; cannot remain in bed.

Fear and despair because of sad thoughts which she cannot get rid of.

Frightened by a trifle (*Calc.*, *Lyc.*, *Anac.*).

Fearful DREAMS: that the world was on fire (*Puls.*): of great exertion; rowing, swimming, walking, climbing, working hard (comp. *Ars.*).

Anxious dreams of business (*Bry.*, *Psor.*) (P. 14.)

Psorinum .. Anxiety: full of forebodings.

Great *fear of death: anxiety about heart* (*Acon.*, *Rhus*, *Med.*): believes stitches in heart will kill him if they do not cease.

Despair of recovery: thinks he will die (*Acon.*)

Anxiety when riding in a carriage (*Sep.*).

Fears to fail in business.

DREAMS of business and plans (*Bry.*, *Chel.*, *Nux*).

Of robbers (*Ars.*, *Nat. mur.*) travels; danger.

That he is in a closet, and nearly soils his bed (comp. *Sep.*, *Sulph.*).

In many ways a chilly *Sulph.* patient. (See p. 8.)

Sulphur .. Anxiety as if he would cease to live: fear of some great misfortune.

Great anxiety in bed at time of full moon.

Fear for others (*Ars.*, *Phos.*, *Plat.*, etc.).

Fear that he would take cold in open air.

DREAMS vivid: anxious; vexatious.

That she sat on the chamber, so passed her water in bed (*Sep.*).

DREAMS of danger from fire: water: that he had been bitten by a dog (*Stram.*, etc.); of falling (*Thuja*); disgust; and nausea. (See p. 1.)

Bryonia .. Anxiety and apprehension about the future (comp. *Psor.*): great sense of insecurity.

In DREAMS: busy about his household affairs.

Anxiety about his business (*Psor.*, *Chel.*). (P. 17).

Veratrum alb. .. If he stands, is tormented with frightful anxiety ; *the forehead becomes covered with cold sweat*, with nausea even to vomiting.

Anxiety as if he had committed a crime (*Ars.*, *Rob.*, *Chel.*, *Thuja*) ; as if he dreaded a misfortune (*Lyc.*, *Anac.*, *Nat. mur.*, etc.).

Anxiety causing crawling in the fingers.

Fear of apoplexy during an evacuation.

DREAMS of robbers : is pursued : that a dog was biting him and he could not get away (*Stram.*). Frightful dreams. (See p. 16).

Strychnine .. Like a mad woman all night : shouted, "they are coming for me" (comp. *Ars.*, etc.).

Begged piteously that I would not hurt him. (*Arn.*). Excessive anxiety and restlessness.

Feeling of dread : begged that he might not be left alone.

Afraid—weeps : asked why—" I don't know ! "

Characteristic : hyperaesthesia, and a shrinking from draughts (*Nux*, *Hep.*).

Natrum mur. Fears to lose his reason (pp. 34, 35). Startled.

Fearfulness : " Something going to happen."

Fear of robbers (see *Ars.*), of insanity: of dying.

Anxiety, as if he had done something wrong.

As if he would fall when walking.

DREAMS anxious, vivid, frightful : of conflagrations (*Rhus*, *Puls.*) : of death and battles ; of scenes of murder ; that he had been poisoned.

Of robbers in the house, and will not believe the contrary till search is made (*Ars.*, *Lach.*).

Anxious dreams : *weeps in sleep* (*Cham.*, *Puls.*).

Horrible, disgusting dreams ; reproaches himself for past mistakes, for crimes for which he must answer (comp. *Ars.*, *K. br.*, *Rob.*). (P. 8.)

Elaps .. Fear of being alone : something will happen : rowdies will break in (comp. *Ars.*, etc.).

Excessive horror of rain.

DREAMS : fighting with a galley slave : puts a dead body in a shroud and digs a knife into its wounds, then is remorseful and weeps.

Dreams of the dead and embraces them (*Thuja*, *Calc.*) : falls into pits : bites herself. (See p. 15.)

Hepar sulph. .. Frightful imaginings. Frightful visions of fire (*Rhus*, *Puls.*, *Anac.*) and dead persons (*Thuja*, *Anac.*, etc.).

Great anxiety, evenings (*Puls.*, *Phos.*, *Lyc.*).

Violent fright on slumbering, even p.c.

Starts from sleep as if about to suffocate (comp. *Lach.*, *Spong.*).

DREAMS of danger, anxiety : of fleeing from danger : expectorating blood and pus.

Hepar is chilly, with hyperaesthesia mental and physical (*Nux*). (See p. 18.)

Nux .. .. Anxiety with irritability : inclined to suicide, but afraid to die.

Great anxiety of mind with no particular cause : easily frightened.

Fears to be alone.

Fear of knives, lest she should kill herself or others (*Ars.*, *Merc.*, *Alum.*).

DREAMS, sad or frightful. Of mutilations; pursued by cats and dogs (*Stram.*, *Bell.*), etc.: about fatal accidents ; of quarrelling : about exerting the mind (*Lyss.*, *Ign.*). Amorous.

Wakes from troubled, busy dreams (*Bry.*, *Psor.*, *Chel.*), frightened as if someone were in room.

Dreams of lice (*Chel.*) and vermin.

Nux is irritable and chilly; with hyperaesthesia, mental and physical (*Hep.*). (See p. 18.)

Alumina .. Seeing blood on a knife (*Nux*, *Ars.*), horrid ideas of killing herself : abhors the idea.

Fear of losing his reason (*Ars.*, *Calc.*, *Merc.*).

Anacardium .. Fearfulness. Cowardice.

Fear of paralysis. Despair of getting well.

When walking, anxious as if pursued : suspected everything around him.

Fear of death—close at hand (*Acon.*, *Arn.*).

Every trifle might lead to great misfortune.

Characteristic, Warring wills—to evil, to good. " Devil and angel sensation " (comp. p. 25).

DREAMS vivid : recur during day as if real ; as if they had really happened.

Of smelling burning spunk or sulphur : of fire (*Puls.*, *Rhus*) : of dead bodies. (See p. 12.)

Camphora .. Very great anxiety and extreme restlessness.
Extremely fearful, especially in the dark : of being alone in the dark (*Calc.*, *Cann. ind.*, *Phos.*, etc.).
Indescribable fear of being drawn upwards.
Fear of mirrors lest he see himself in them.
"I shall faint !—I shall have fits, and never come out of them !" (See p. 15.)

Conium .. Dread of men, of their approach : yet dread of being alone (comp. *Lyc.*, *Puls.*).
Fear of thieves (*Nat. mur.*, *Ars.*, *Merc.*, *Lach.*).
DREAMS : full of shame : of threatening dangers : of anger and vexation.
Of physical mutilation : of wretched diseases.
Of dead people, and deaths of those living. (P. 6.)

Spongia .. Very easily frightened : startles : it *seemed to shoot into her feet*, which remained heavy.
Anxiety : in features : looks round anxiously.
Very timorous : starts with every trifle, which makes feet feel heavy.
Terror and fear : of approaching death : that she will die of suffocation (comp. *Lach.*).
Wakes at night in great fear (*Acon.*).

Platina .. Every serious thought is terrifying.
Deathly anxiety, as if senses would vanish, with trembling of limbs.
Satiety of life, with taciturnity and *fear of death*, great dread of death which she believed near at hand (*Arn.*, *Acon.*).
Precordial anguish, with fear of death and of imaginary forms ; ghosts (*Puls.*, etc.).
Fear of men (*Lyc.*, *Con.*, *Nat. c.*, *Plat.*, *Puls.*).
Mental disturbance after fright, grief or vexation (*Acon.*).
DREAMS amorous : of fire (*Rhus*, *Puls.*).
"Wants to go, but cannot get there." (See p. 26.)

Natrum carb. Intolerable melancholy and apprehension constant fear and forebodings.
Anxiety during thunderstorm (*Phos.*, *Sep.*): worse from music. (See p. 4.)

Sepia .. Filled with concern about health: thinks she will have consumption and die (comp. *Calc.*).
Fearfulness: dare not be alone for a moment.
Very fearful and frightened.
Fear of real and imaginary evils: evening.
Afraid to speak, or to be spoken to.
Fearful when riding in carriage (comp. *Cocc.*).
Fear of starvation (*Ars.*): full of evil forebodings. Total loss of courage.
Anxious DREAMS as if body were disfigured. As if threatened with rape: voluptuous dreams.
As if chased and had to run backwards.
Frightful dreams of murder: falling from high mountain (*Thuja*). Dreams full of dispute.
Of urinating into chamber, but was wetting the bed (*Sulph.*, comp. *Psor.*, *Lac can.*).
Of mice, rats, snakes (*Bell.*, *Lac can.*).
Of spectres outside the window.
Awakes screaming: imagines she has swallowed something; feels it lodged in her throat. (P. 8.)

Lycopodium .. Dread of men (*Aur.*, *Nat. c.*, *Plat.*, *Puls.*); of solitude (*Ars.*, etc.).
Easily frightened, starts up. Feels frightened at everything, even ringing of the door bell.
Fear lest something should happen: lest he should forget something.
Very fearful all day: fear of going to bed: on entering a room as if he saw someone: seized with fear if a door opens with difficulty.
Of frightful imaginary images in the evening.
Increasing dread of appearing in public, yet a horror at times of solitude.
Fear of appearing in public, lest he stumble and make mistakes: yet gets through with ease.
Anticipation (*Arg. nit.*, *Gels.*, *Ars.*, *Sil.*, *Thuja*).
DREAMS anxious: vivid: frightful: horrid. Of sickness: people drowning; boats capsizing.
Wakes cross: or terrified.
Children scream out suddenly in sleep: stare about and cannot be pacified (*Calc.*). (See p. 2.)

Kali carb. .. Fears about her disease: that she cannot recover.
Frightened if anything touches the body lightly.
Shocks are felt in epigastrium. (See p. 17.)

Phosphorus .. Anxious: filled with gloomy forebodings:— "About to die": about the future: during a thunderstorm. Fear of the dark.

Fear and dread: in the evening (*Calc.*, *Camph.*, *Puls.*): of death (pp. 29, 30): something were creeping out of every corner: a horrible face looking out of every corner.

Uncommon fearfulness with great fatigue.

Fear; anguish when alone, or stormy weather.

After excitement at theatre: sleepless; then full of fear, especially at piano.

DREAMS, vivid: of restless work and business (*Bry.*, *Psor.*, *Rhus*) which he could not finish.

Of fire (*Stram.*, etc.): of biting animals (*Merc.*, *Stram.*, *Puls.*, etc.); lascivious.

After a great fright 2 years before, involuntary stool and urine, especially at night; was always wet and dirty.

When threatened with a whipping would immediately soil himself from fright.

(One of the curious symptoms of *Phos.*, anus stands open, i.e., incontinence of fæces.)

(N.B.—*Hyos.* has *involuntary stool from jealousy*; verified in a cured case.) (See p. 4.)

Pulsatilla .. When evening comes he begins to dread ghosts.

Sleeplessness on account of great fear. Fear and rage in spells. Despairs of salvation.

Forebodings: anxiety from epigastrium.

Hides in a corner to escape from a little grey man who wanted to pull out her leg.

Abhors and hates women (*Raph.*). He looks upon them as evil beings and is afraid . . .

Sees the devil coming to take her (*Manc.*): the world on fire during the night (*Rhus*).

Afraid of everybody. . . . Cannot sleep on account of fear and dread. Dread of people.

Fright followed by diarrhœa (*Arg. nit.*, *Gels.*).

Anxiety worse during rest—sitting, lying; better by motion.

DREAMS. Confused. Full of fright and disgust.

All her dreams are about men: a naked man wrapped in her bedclothes under her bed, while she has only a sheet to cover her. (See p. 7.)

Iodum .. Peculiar anxiety; with a thrill that goes through body, unless he removes it by motion and change of position. The more he tries to keep still, the worse the anxious state (comp. *Puls.*).

While attempting to keep still is overwhelmed with impulses—to tear things—to kill himself—to commit murder.

Attacks come on at most unexpected times.

Violent palpitation drives him out of bed.

Worse by quiet and meditation: must be in action, in some laborious occupation.

Feels some dreadful thing is coming on (*Lyc.*).

A doctor described his experiences after taking *Iodine* :—his unbearable apprehension ;—how he awaited in terror an expected telephone ring :—his indescribable restlessness and apprehension; for no cause.

And numbers of persons are taking "iodized salt"—and other iodized preparations—with the idea, "*Iodine is good for you!*" A doctor wrote recently to the *British Medical Journal* protesting against the universal use of iodine—for wounds, etc. He had seen the harm it can do.

One patient, afraid of goitre, ate iodized salt—*till she produced one.*

Aurum .. Apprehensiveness: full of fear: a mere noise at the door makes him anxious (comp. *Lyc.*).

Fearfulness: a longing for death.

Dread of men (*Lyc.*, etc.): anxiety and dread.

Characteristically, *Aur.* is suicidal.

Feels that he is not fit for this world: that he can never succeed: that he is irretrievably lost: thought of death gives him intense joy.

DREAMED a great deal of death.

Dreaming of the dead and corpses (*Thuja*, *Elaps*, etc.). Anxious dreams, full of disputes.

Frightful dreams about thieves (*Ars.*, *Nat. mur.*), falling from a height (*Thuja*). (See p. 9.)

Dros. .. .. Anxiety at 7-8 p.m., as if impelled to take his life by drowning (*Bell.*, *Hell.*, *Hyos.*, *Lach.*, etc.).

Anxiety as if his companions allowed him no rest, but persecuted and pursued him.

DREAMS frightful: of being maltreated: of thirst, and drinking. (See p. 9.)

SOME DRUGS OF NEPHRITIS

WITH INDICATIONS

Aconite .. Incipient nephritis.

Stinging and pressing pains, kidney region.

Kidneys act but slightly: urine contains albumen and fragments of casts.

Urine hot, dark; red, with white fæces: red and clear. Bloody urine.

Also, urine *suppressed* or retained.

Renal region sensitive, with shooting pains.

Painful urging to urinate.

Aconite has FEAR: tosses about with anxiety.

Attacks are sudden, violent.

Ailments from fright, vexation, chill: cold winds (*Bry.*, *Nux*, *Hepar*).

Apis .. Pain in both kidneys (Bright's disease).

Renal pains; soreness; pressure on stooping.

Pain left kidney (*Benz. a.*, *Thuja*, *K. ars.*).

Suppression of urine.

"Acute inflammatory affection of kidneys, with albuminuria, as in scarlet fever or diphtheria: or, after these, as a sequel to acute disease." KENT.

"Inflammation of kidneys closes up the case" (Scarlet fever) "and kills off a good many in allopathic practice, never in homœopathic hands." KENT.

Typical *Apis* is thirstless: intolerant of heat.

Arnica .. In inflammation of kidneys, bladder, even pneumonia: its mental state, and the sore bruised feeling all over the body would enable you to do astonishing work.

Does not want to be touched.

Horrors in the night (*Acon.*). Horror of instant death.

Chill followed by nephritic pains, nausea and vomiting.

Piercing pains *as from knives* plunged into kidneys: chilly and inclined to vomit.

Urine difficult, scanty, dark, with thick brown sediment. *Suppression* of urine.

Terebinthinum " Congestive kidneys, with dull aching, and smoky-looking urine."

Violent *burning* and drawing pains in kidneys, bladder and urethra.

Pressure in kidneys when sitting; relieved by motion.

Stiff all over; heaviness and pains in region of kidneys.

Renal disease producing dropsy. Rapid attack with lumbar pain. Urine greatly diminished: loaded with albumen: contains casts and blood. *Suppressed.*

Urine smoky: with " coffee grounds " or thick, slimy, sediment. *Smells of violets.*

Early scarlatinal nephritis.

Tongue smooth, glossy, red (*Crot. hor.*, *Pyrog.*). Or a coating which peels in patches.

Tereb. has purpuric conditions: ecchymoses (*Arn.*).

" Hæmorrhages from all outlets, especially in connection with urinary or kidney troubles." NASH. (Comp. *Phos.*, *Crot. hor.*)

Ascites with anasarca, in organic lesions of kidneys.

Belladonna .. Stinging, *burning* pain, from region of kidneys down into bladder. *Suppression.*

" No remedy has a greater irritation in the bladder and along the urinary tract."

Bell. pains, clutch: come and go suddenly.

Bell., typically, has redness, great heat to touch: dilated pupils.

Helonias di. .. *Burning* sensation, Kidneys: can trace their outlines by the burning.

Congestion and pain in kidneys with albuminurea. Right kidney extremely sensitive. Albuminuria acute or chronic. Usually tired but knows no reason.

Burning, scalding pain when urinating (*Canth.*).

Affects the female genital organs.

Eryngium aquat. Must urinate every five minutes: urine dripping away all the time, burning like fire.

Cantharis .. The whole urinary organs and genitalia are in a state of inflammation and irritation.

Discharge of bloody urine burns like fire.

Intensity and rapidity are the features of this remedy.

Dull pressing or paroxysmal *cutting and burning* pains in both kidneys; very sensitive to slightest touch. Urging to urinate. Painful evacuation, by drops, of bloody urine, or pure blood.

Intolerable urging, before, during and after urination. *Suppression.*

Violently acute inflammation, or rapidly destructive. (Compare *Merc. c.*)

Mercurius cor. Tenesmus vesicæ with intense burning.

Urine *suppressed*, or hot urine passed drop by drop with much pain (*Canth.*).

Urine, hot, burning, bloody: contains filaments, or flesh-like pieces of mucus: albuminous: shows granular fatty tubuli, with epithelial cells on their surface also in a state of granular fatty degeneration (*Ars., Phos.*).

Patient looks pinched; shrivelled; melancholy.

A drug of violence: of inflammations with *burning* (*Canth.*) of *desperate tenesmus*: the "Never get done" remedy, in dysentery.

Mercurius .. Nephritis with diminished secretion of urine, with great desire to pass it.

Urine saturated with albumin: dark brown: mixed with blood: with dirty white sediment.

Hæmaturia, with violent and frequent urging to urinate.

Urine dark-red; becomes turbid and fetid: smells sour and pungent (*Benz. ac.*): mixed with blood; white flakes; or as if containing pus: flesh-like lumps of mucus: as if flour had been stirred in: scanty, fiery-red; very dark: With burning and scalding sensation during urination as from raw surfaces (*Canth.*).

Worse at night: worse heat and cold; profuse, oily sweat, which does not ameliorate.

Chelidonium .. Violent paroxysms of pain in kidneys, with intense headache, vertigo and syncope.

Pain and tenderness kidney regions : sensitive to pressure even of clothing (*Arg. nit.*, *Hep.*) (Compare *Lach.*)

Urine reddish, turbid, contains fibrin, flakes and sand.

Characteristics. ***Pain under right shoulder angle.*** A great liver medicine : a right-sided medicine.

Colchicum .. Pain in region of Kidneys. Hyperæmia.

Nephritis ; bloody, ink-like, albuminous urine.

Dropsy after scarlatina.

Urine like ink, after scarlatina. (Compare *Lach.*, *Kali. chlor.*)

Urine burns when it passes.

Suppression ; retention. " The kidneys manufacture no urine : scanty urine with dropsy."

" Chiefly in acute form of Bright's disease."

Characteristics of *Colch.* Smell painfully acute : nausea and faintness from smell of of cooking (*Ars.*, *Sep.*).

Loathing of food, sight and smell of it.

Urine contains clots of putrid decomposed blood, albumin, sugar.

Helleborus .. Post scarlet fever nephritis.

Congestion of kidneys with extensive effusion of serum in abdominal cavity and tissue of lower extremities.

Dropsy after scarlet fever with albumen and fibrin casts in urine.

Suppression of urine ; or urine highly albuminous, dark, no sediment ; ***breathes easier lying down*** : acute dropsies.

Urine scanty, dark, or smoky with decomposed blood with floating dark specks, like coffee grounds ; albuminous, scanty. Top part clear.

A great remedy in meningitis and hydrocephalus. Chewing motions : boring head into pillow. Automatic motion of one arm and leg.

Staring : eyes wide open : insensible to light.

Allium cepa .. Pains in renal region, and region of bladder very sensitive.

Burning pressure in bladder, then in sacrum: pain in kidney region, more left side.

Urine frothy and iridescent (*Hepar.*). Red.

Berberis .. Soreness lumbar region and kidneys. Can bear no pressure : no jar Has to step down carefully. Jar or jolt intolerable (*Bell.*).

Burning; burning stitches, loins and kidneys.

Sore kidneys with urinary disturbances; and excessive deposits.

" Little calculi form, start down ureter: pains run up kidney and down to bladder."

Berb. has bubbling sensations, and pains that radiate from a point.

" Pain in back a chief indication for *Berberis*."

Sabina .. Nephritis with retention, or discharge by drops with burning (*Canth.*, etc.).

Urine bloody and albuminous.

Pain from lumbar region to pubes.

Ardor urinæ in rheumatic subjects.

Metrorrhagia from plethora.

Benzoic acid .. Kidney pains, which penetrate the chest on taking a deep breath.

Sore pain in back: *burning in left kidney*; with drawing pain when stooping. Dull pain in kidneys; loins stiff.

Urine of a very repulsive odour (*Ocim. can.*, *Calc.*, *Ars.*, etc.). Pungent (*Merc.*). From the time of first passing it.

" Urine on clothing scents the room."

Contains mucus and pus.

Strong, hot, dark-brown urine.

Ocimum canum Kent gives this in black type for nephritis.

Used in Brazil as a specific for diseases of kidneys, bladder and urethra.

Crampy pain in kidneys.

Turbid urine: saffron coloured.

" Discharge of large quantities of bloody or thick purulent urine." HANSEN.

Urine with *intolerable odour*, like musk.

Phosphorus .. " Bright's disease, with sensations of weakness and emptiness."

Albumen and exudation cells in urine.

" Fatty degeneration (*Merc. cor.*, *Ars.*) of kidneys, liver and heart, with anæmia."

Urine contains epithelial, fatty or waxy casts.

Dropsy accompanied by diarrhœa.

Uræmia, with acute atrophy brain and medulla.

Hæmaturia : general dissolution of blood.

Thirst : craves ices : worse lying on left side : fears thunder, dark.

Phos. is a profuse, easy bleeder. (Comp. *Crot. hor.*, *Terebinth.*) Blood bright.

Hepar .. Pain, kidneys, with incessant, painful urging and voiding a few drops of ***purulent*** urine.

Emaciation : renal region sensitive to slightest touch (*Arg. nit.*).

Violent fever with unquenchable thirst : diarrhœa and night-sweats.

Croupous nephritis, suppurative stage ; fever ; chills, alternating with burning heat.

Has to wait for urine to pass : never able to finish urinating, some remains in bladder.

Urine : dark red and hot : acrid : scalding : brown-red ; last drops mixed with blood : on standing, turbid and thick : with greasy pellicle, or iridescent (*All. cepa*).

Hepar is characteristically chilly, with hyperæsthesia mental and physical.

Silica .. Suppuration of kidneys : abscesses.

" All sorts of *suppurative conditions* in the urinary tract ; catarrh of the mucous membranes.

Old inveterate catarrhs of bladder, with pus and blood in the urine."

Bloody, purulent discharge, thick or curdy.

Sil. is chilly : worse cold damp weather.

Sensitive to noise, pain, cold. Every hurt festers.

Silica headaches need heat, and wrapping up.

Foot-sweats : especially foul : ailments from suppressed foot-sweat.

Hippozæninum (Glanders) Tubercles and *abscesses* in kidneys.
Albuminuria ; also leucine and tyrosine.
" Used in a large number of cases involving low forms of suppuration and catarrh, malignant ulcerations and swellings, abscesses and enlarged glands." CLARKE.

Arsenicum .. Nephritis with stitches in renal region ; on breathing or sneezing.
Abscess of kidney (*Merc.*, *Hipp.*, *Hep.*, *Sil.*, *Crot.*).
Uræmia, with vomiting, colic.
Urine, dark-brown ; dark yellow ; turbid : mixed with blood and pus ; greenish.
Urine like thick beer ; rotten smell (*Benz. acid*, etc.).
Suppression of urine.
Albuminuria ; fatty degeneration (*Merc. cor.*, *Phos.*).
Extreme restlessness, anxiety, prostration.

Crotalus horridus Nephritis albuminosa, in toxæmia, or pregnancy.
Urine dark, smoky from admixture of fluid blood. Hæmaturia.
Urine extremely scanty, dark red with blood ; jelly-like ; green-yellow from much bile.
One of our greatest remedies for *sepsis*.
Black water fever, urine like dark bloody jelly.
Skin may be yellow to green : yellow colour of eyes.
May have hæmorrhage from any and every part of body (*Tereb.*). Dark thin blood.
Putridity.
Even the most rapid and desperate cases.

Lachesis .. Stitches in kidneys, extending through ureters.
Urine almost black : frequent, foamy, dark (*Kali ars.*).
Like coffee grounds : black, scanty after scarlatina (*Colch.*). Loaded with albumen.
Suppressed. No urine : no stool.
Lach. is cyanosed : extremely sensitive to heat and TOUCH : especially about neck and abdomen.
Sleeps into an aggravation.
Typically, loquacious, suspicious and jealous.

Kali ars. .. Tensive pain in left kidney: œdema left foot, extending to right and over whole body.
Blackish urine (*Lach.*), foams on shaking, on standing leaves a thick, reddish, slime.
Stitches, dull, or sharp in both renal regions.
Urine: the more one presses the less the flow.

Kali chlor. .. Nephritis. Frequent urging. Could only pass a few drops of bloody urine (*Canth.*, etc.). Urine black and albuminous, greenish black.
Prostration, coldness and easy hæmorrhage.
A cold day had "cooled off her blood".

Argentum nit. Touching the kidney region increases the pain to the highest degree (*Hep.*, *Chel.*, etc.).
Acute pain, kidneys, extends down ureters to bladder (*Lach.*); worse slightest touch or motion, even deep inspiration.
Typical *Arg. nit.* has apprehension. Gets diarrhœa from anticipation (*Gels.*).
Craves sweets, which disagree: salt.
Is nervous: hurried: walks fast (*Lil. tigr.*).

Cannabis indica Constant pain right kidney: sharp stitches both kidneys. Aching, *burning*, in kidneys keep him awake at night.
Pain in kidneys when laughing.
Cann. ind. (Hashish) has the most extravagant mental symptoms; with exaggerations of time and space.

Cannabis sativa Ulcerative pain in Kidney regions.
Sensation of soreness kidneys and bladder.
Gonorrhœal cases (*Thuja*).

Aurum met. .. Kidneys hyperæmic, with pressure round waist, and increase of urine (*Cardiac hypertrophy*).
Suppression or retention of urine. Hæmaturia.
In *Aur.* all the natural healthy affections are perverted: he loathes life: is weary of life: longs to die; is suicidal.
Absolute loss of enjoyment in everything.

Eupatorium purpureum	Chronic nephritis. Dull, deep pain in kidneys: cutting pain. *Suppression* of urine.
Senecio aur. ..	Recurrent attacks nephritis, especially right kidney. With intense pain, fever. Every time he passed water, cried out in anguish. CLARKE.
Sarsaparilla ..	Neuralgia; attacks of most excruciating pain from right kidney downwards. Chronic nephritis. Renal colic and passage of gravel. Much pain at conclusion of passing water, almost unbearable. "*Lyc.* has red sand with clear urine; *Sars.* white sand with scanty, slimy or flaky urine." NASH. Urine dribbles while sitting.
Lycopodium ..	Nephritis with characteristic *Lyc.* symptoms. One of the *suppression of urine* drugs. 4 to 8 p.m. aggravation of symptoms. Desire for hot drinks: sweets. Characteristics, Red sand in (? clear) urine. Urine reddens and causes eruptions if allowed to remain in contact with parts (esp. babies). A (*Lyc.*) symptom: polyuria at night only.
Bryonia ..	Inflammation and pain kidneys. "Pinkish urinary deposits: uric acid crystals." Whenever he *strains himself*, *lifting*, or unusual motion, pain in kidneys; a rousing up of congestion and long-lasting pain. "After overheating or over exertion, he gets pain in the back." KENT.
Sulphur ..	Violent pain kidney region *after long stooping*. Chronic nephritis, especially. Secretions burn and redden orifices: eyelids, anus, etc. 11 a.m. emptiness and hunger. Burning soles at night: puts them out. Theorizing: "the ragged philosopher."

Nux .. Nephritis from *stagnation of portal circulation.*
Bloating of abdomen.
Pressure, heat, *burning* in loins and kidneys.
Pains in small of back, as if bruised: so violent, he cannot move.
Hæmaturia, after abuse of alcoholic stimulants, or drugs; suppression of hæmorrhoidal or menstrual discharges. Pressure and distension in abdomen, loins, and kidneys.
Spasmodic retention of urine: discharge drop by drop.
Strangury after beer.
Nux is irritable and chilly: with hyperæsthesia mental and physical (*Hep.*).

Rhus .. Tearing pain in kidneys: œdema: *after exposure to wet.*
After exposure to much dampness, œdema of face, feet, developing into general anasarca: urine full of albumen.
Tearing pains small of back ; urine contains blood and albumen.
Urine voided slowly, paralytic weakness of bladder.
Rhus is worse for COLD: WET (*Dulc.*): washing; chill, and draught.
Worse for first moving: but better for continued motion.

Natrum mur. .. Must be considered where there has been much *malaria, and quinine.*
Tension and heat in renal regions.
Polyuria with violent desire to urinate; inability to retain urine.
Curious symptom, unable to urinate unless alone.

Thuja .. Kidneys inflamed: feet swollen.
Urine: profuse, light yellow: contains sugar: foams, scanty, exceedingly dark: deposits brown mucus.
Pain left kidney to epigastrium.
Especially useful in gonorrhœal, or "*Vaccinosis*" (BURNETT) cases.

Laurocerassus .. Urinary difficulties, with palpitation and gasping for breath, coming on by spells.
Suppressed urine: retention from paralysis of bladder. Involuntary urination.

Stramonium .. Kidneys secrete less urine or none, in acute diseases, in children, in eruptive fevers etc. Great desire to urinate, though secretion is suppressed.
Urine dribbles away very slowly and feebly.
Retention: sensation urine could not be passed, because of narrowness of urethra. After straining, a few drops are passed. Better after drinking vinegar.

Scarlatinum or *Streptococcin* As an intercurrent remedy in cases that have followed an attack of scarlet fever.

Streptococcin .. After scarlet fever, or *acute tonsillitis*.
"Scarlet fever is a well-known cause" (of nephritis) "but acute tonsillitis is eight times as common as scarlet fever as the predisposing cause." (TAYLOR'S *Practice of Medicine*.)

Urtica urens .. Burnett's great remedy for *suppression of urine*: (5 or 10 drops of the ϕ in hot water). (Dramatically verified in the case of a child dying of T.B. meningitis.)

N.B.—Consider any of the nosodes, family history, or past history suggesting them.

SOME REMEDIES OF RENAL AND VESICAL CALCULI. RENAL COLIC

WITH INDICATIONS

Berberis .. " Excellent remedy for renal calculi."

Pains shoot : *radiate* from a point (*Bell.*).

Cannot make the least motion : sits over to painful side for relief.

Sharp, darting pains following ureter and extending down into legs.

Pains run up into kidneys and down into bladder.

Formation of little calculi like pin-heads in pelvis of kidney, start to go down to bladder, with great suffering.

" You will be astonished to know how quickly *Berberis* will relieve this particular colic."

" Anything that is spasmodic can be relieved instantly."—KENT.

Burning and soreness, lumbar, in region of kidneys. Cannot bear any jar (*Bell.*) : has to step down carefully.

Urine dark, turbid, with copious sediment : slow to flow : but constant urging.

May be associated with biliary calculi.

Nux .. .. Indicated in renal colic when one kidney (especially the *right*) is the seat of the disease.

Pains extend to genitalia and down leg, with nausea and vomiting.

Renal colic, especially *when each pain shoots to the rectum and urges to stool.* (Compare *Canth.*)

" Must strain to urinate : bladder is full and urine dribbles away ; yet when he strains it ceases to dribble."

" Renal colic is caused by a stone in the ureter, which by its irritation causes a spasmodic clutching of the little circular fibres of that canal ; the proper medicine relaxes these fibres, and the pressure from behind forces these calculi out at once."—KENT.

The *Nux* patient is hypersensitive, mentally and physically : choleric ; irascible : quick and active : generally lean. Chilly.

Tabacum .. "*Pains down the ureter, with deathly sickness and cold sweat.*
Nausea with burning heat in abdomen, the rest of the body being cold. Patient persists in uncovering the abdomen.
Such sickness suggests *Tab.* in renal colic."

Ocimum can. .. Renal colic where there is considerable hæmorrhage. Urine has brick-dust sediment and considerable blood.
Clarke says, "Used in Brazil as a specific for diseases of kidneys, bladder, and urethra."
"*Renal colic with violent vomiting every fifteen minutes:* wrings the hands and moans all the time."
Urine "saffron colour; or thick, purulent, with an intolerable smell of musk".

Ipomea nil. .. For the passage of stone from kidney to bladder: with severe cutting in either renal region, *extending down ureter.* Pains excite nausea.

Nitric-acid .. Urinary calculi when the urine contains oxalic acid: and for *oxalic acid calculi.*
Fetid urine of intolerable odour; or smells like horse's urine. *May feel cold as passed.*
Typical *Nit. ac.* craves salt and fats.
Has "splinters" pains: < touch.

Benzoic acid .. Nephritic colic with *offensive urine.*
Urine deep-red, of strong odour:—dark-brown; smells cadaverous, putrid.
Urine alternately thick like pea-soup, then clear like water.
But patient feels better when urine is profuse, thick and offensive: suffers in joints—heart—when it is clear and scanty.
Highly intensified urinous odour.

Hydrangea .. "Has been used for the intense pain of gravel and calculus.
"Relieves distress from renal calculus, with soreness kidney region and bloody urine.
"The *thirstiest plant known* (diabetes)."

Belladonna .. Renal calculi with sharp, shooting pains.
Come suddenly, and radiate (*Berb.*).
Spasmodic, crampy straining along ureter, during passage of calculus.
Feverish and excitable.
" Irritation and clutching and spasm where there are little circular fibres in small canals—as in gall-stones (which see) or in renal calculi."
Bell. is red, and hot, and dry : hypersensitive, especially to jarring (*Berb.*).
Bell. pains *come and go suddenly*.

Cantharis .. " One of the best remedies during the paroxysms of renal colic."
Pain and excitement found in no other remedy.
Pains lancinating, cutting, stabbing like knives, shoot off in different directions.
Burning pain, with intolerable urging to urinate. Tenesmus. Sits and strains and gets no relief. " If he could only pass a few drops more urine (or a little more bloody stool) he would get relief : but no relief comes. Intolerable urging, before, with and after urination : violent pain in bladder " (Cystitis).
Thirst, with aversion to all fluids.
" The burning pain and intolerable urging to urinate point to *Canth.* in all inflammatory diseases of other parts."

Argentum nit. " Nephralgia from congestion of kidneys or passage of calculi."
Dull aching in small of back and over bladder.
Urine dark, contains blood, or deposit of renal epithelium and uric acid : passed often and little at a time, in drops (*Nephritic colic*).
Urine burns while passing (*Canth.*) and urethra feels swollen.
Face dark : dried-up look.
Arg. nit. craves sweets and sugar, which disagree.
Suffers from anticipation : hurry.
Flatulent dyspepsia.

Lycopodium .. Usually *right*-sided. *Pain extends along ureter and ends in bladder :* not down leg.

Back-ache, $>$ by urination.

Lithic acid in urine. *Red sand in clear urine.*

Characteristics of *Lyc.* Desire for sweets (*Arg. nit.*) and hot drinks.

All symptoms $<$ 4-8 p.m.

Hunger : but fullness after a little food.

Distension, must loosen clothing.

Pareira brava .. Renal colic. *Excruciating pain radiates from left kidney to groin : follows course of ureter.*

Excessive pain in kidneys, shoots down left ureter ; urine passes drop by drop with violent tenesmus, nausea, vomiting of bile.

Constant urging to urinate : pain extorts screams. *Must go down on all fours to urinate. Almost touches floor with forehead in order to be able to pass urine.* (Compare *Sarsa.*, *Chim.*)

With tearing, burning pains at point of penis.

Copious sediment of uric acid and blood.

Thick, stringy, white mucus, or red sand (*Lyc.*).

Sarsaparilla .. Excruciating neuralgia of the kidneys.

Renal colic. Passes gravel : vesical calculi.

Tenesmus : *extreme pain at conclusion of urination : yells with pain* (*Pareira*) :—or urine passes without sensation.

" White sand in scanty, slimy or flaky urine, or red sand in clear urine (*Lyc.*)."—NASH.

Renal and vesical calculi.

Kent says, " This medicine has many times dissolved a stone in the bladder ; it so changes the character of the urine that it is no longer possible for the stone to build up, and it grows smaller by continually dissolving off from the surface."

Curious symptom, " *Urine only passes freely when standing.*" (Comp. *Pareira.*)

Hot food and drink aggravate all the complaints ; but wants heat applied externally. After the remedy has been given there is a deposit of sand in the urine, which should not be stopped.

Chimaphila umb.	Constant pain in region of kidneys. *Fluttering sensation in kidneys.* Catarrh of bladder caused by stones. Smarting pain from neck of bladder *to end of urethra.* (Compare *Pareira.*) Great quantities of thick, ropy, bloody mucus in urine. Urine colour of green tea. Queer symptom : *feels as if sitting on a ball.* Worse damp weather : washing in cold water.
Uva ursi ..	Farrington says, " Has no equal when cystic and urethral symptoms are referable to stone in bladder." Burning ; scalding : *flow stops* as if a stone had rolled in front of orifice of urethra. Diminishes the inflammatory thickening of cystic walls and relieves suffering. *Urine ropy from mucus and blood.* Feels bruised all over.
Hydrastis ..	Dull aching in kidney region. Intense pain in left ureter. Frequent, scanty urination, with burning at the end of it. Thick, ropy, mucous sediment in urine.
Lachesis ..	Stitches in kidneys, extend down through ureters. Pain in left lumbar region. Pain and tenderness left iliac region, intolerance of pressure. Lifts clothing from abdomen. Extremely sensitive to touch : especially about throat and abdomen. Left side ailments. Worse for sleep : worse on waking : sleeps into an aggravation.
Lithium carb. ..	Kent's Repertory gives *Lith.* in black type for renal calculi. Curious symptom, " *Pains in heart when urinating :* when bending over." Heavy deposits, urine ; dark, reddish-brown. Soreness and sharp sticking pain right side of bladder.

Phosphorus ..	Dull pain in renal region. Renal calculi: congestive and inflammatory symptoms, with purulent, chalky or sandy sediment. *Phos.* craves cold food: ices: salt. Can't lie on left side. Fear of thunder: darkness.
Calcarea carb.	Gravel: urinary calculi. In a *Calc.* patient: chilly: cold *sweating* feet: sweating face: head sweats at night (*Sil.*). *Often fat, flabby and weak.* Lethargic. Longs for eggs.
Silica	Renal and vesical calculus. Involuntary discharge of urine after urination. Constant urging. Nightly incontinence (*Sep.*, etc.). *Sil.* is a weakling mind and body: "*lacks grit*". Worse cold feet: damp feet: checked sweat. Often, offensive foot-sweat: or (?) suppressed.
Sepia	Gravel. Urine leaves *adhesive sediment:* may have cuticle on surface. Urinary troubles—enuresis—extreme urging to urinate—frequency: in a *Sepia* patient. Typical *Sepia*, is indifferent: brown saddle across nose and cheeks: tiredness and downward sagging of all parts and organs.

As always, be careful to treat the past history of the patient, possible Chronic Measles, Diphtheria, Mumps, etc., besides the Venereal Diseases, T.B., etc.

SOME DRUGS THAT CAUSE AND CURE CYSTITIS WITH INDICATIONS

Cantharis .. The remedy *par excellence* of cystitis. Violent tenesmus and strangury (*Lil. tigr.*).

Painful discharge of a few drops of bloody urine with very severe pain, as if a red-hot iron were passed along urethra.

Violent burning, cutting, stabbing pain in neck of bladder.

—worse before and after urinating.

Urging to urinate, from smallest quantity urine in bladder (*Puls.*).

Must double up and scream from the pain.

Urine only drop by drop (*Apis.*) with extreme pain.

" Cures acute cystitis more frequently than all other remedies put together." (FARRINGTON.)

GUERNSEY : "*It is a singular fact, that if there be frequent micturition attended with burning, cutting pain, or if burning and cutting attend the flow, Canth. is almost always the remedy for whatever other suffering there may be, even in inflammation of brain or lungs.*"

KENT : " The most important feature of this medicine is the rapidity with which it develops a gangrenous state. . . . The patient is violently sick in a great hurry. . . . The bladder and genitals are inflamed, and the excitement and congestion often arouse the sexual instinct to sexual thoughts, and even sexual frenzy. . . . Intensity and rapidity are its features. A state of pain and excitement found in no other remedy."

Tarentula .. Cystitis with high fever, gastric derangement ; excruciating pains and impossibility to pass a drop of urine. Bladder seems swollen and hard. Great spasmodic tenesmus.

Passes by drops a dark-red, brown, fetid urine, with gravel-like sediment.

Excessive restlessness : hurried and fidgety : rolls from side to side.

Pareira brava Atrocious pains with strangury.
Constant urging : violent pain extorts screams.
Must get down on hand and knees to urinate : almost touches floor with forehead, in order to be able to pass urine. (Comp. *Chimaph.*, *Sarsa.*)
Pains down thighs in efforts to urinate.
Passes stringy white mucus, or red sand.

Apis .. Excessive pain in region of bladder.
Frequent, painful, scanty, bloody urination.
Much straining, then a few drops : dribbles a little hot bloody urine (*Canth.*).
Urine almost suppressed.
Scanty urine in little boys, with foreskin enormously distended, or hydrocele.
When call comes to urinate, will shriek, because he remembers the pain last time (*Acon.*).
Whole urinary tract irritated, like *Canth.* — "*these two, antidote one another.*"
Agony in voiding urine. Retention in nursing infants. KENT says ; " Old women knew, long before *Apis* was proved, that when the new-born babe did not pass its water, they could find a cure by catching bees, over which they poured hot water, and gave the baby a teaspoonful."
The pains of *Apis* are burning, *stinging.*
Apis is *worse from heat* : *better from cold.*
Has plenty of œdema. Is thirstless. (*Rev.* of *Acon.*)

Belladonna .. No remedy has a greater irritation of bladder and along urinary tract.
Urging to urinate constant. Urine dribbles : burns intensely along length of urethra.
Bladder sensitive to pressure : to jar.
After urination sits and strains : intense torment.
Sometimes bloody urination : or blood in bladder comes away in little clots.
Urine strongly acid. Fiery red urine.
Bell. has quick sensations and motion.
Pains come suddenly, and go suddenly.
Bell. in fever, craves lemons. Is usually hot, and red. Tends to violent delirium.

Aconite .. Inflammation of bladder and kidneys ; bloody urine. Violent burning in bladder.

Urine scanty, suppressed or retained. *From shock.*

Cystitis ; cutting, tearing pains : burning. Urine hot, dark, red ; clear or bloody.

Retention from cold. In children urging ; crying ; fear of the pain (*Apis*).

" Inflammation of bladder, in adults or infants : with the *Aconite* anxiety ; restlessness ; fear." KENT.

Acon. is thirsty : *Apis.* thirstless.

Sarsaparilla .. Unbearable pain at end of urination (*Equiset.*).

Tenderness and distension of bladder.

Cannot pass urine when sitting : it passes freely when standing. Dribbles while sitting.

Floods the bed at night ; by day can only pass it standing.

" Passes enormous quantities of sand. In one case, this mitigated the catarrh and kept bladder comfortable." KENT.

Also, " Urine passed without sensation." (See *Caust.*, p. 25.)

Terebinthina .. Violent burning and cutting in bladder, alternating with similar pain in umbilicus. *< at rest > walking in open air.* (Comp. *Puls.*)

Sensitive in hypogastrium ; tenesmus, bladder.

Spasmodic tenesmus, urging and pressing while sitting : pain streaks up to kidneys.

Hæmaturia : albuminuria : urine cloudy, *smoky.* (A great hæmorrhagic remedy.)

Smooth, glossy, red tongue (*Pyrog.*, *Crot.*).

Urine smells strongly of violets.

Tereb. has also excessive tympanites. Ecchymoses : purpura. (A less acute *Canth.*)

Equisetum .. Dull pain in bladder, as from distension.

Constant desire to urinate and pass large quantities of pale urine without relief.

HERING'S case :—" General paralysis in an old woman in whom control over stools and urine, long completely lost, was rapidly restored."

Has severe pain at end of urination (*Sarsa.*).

Lachesis .. Cystitis with offensive mucus, tending to putrescence. " The more the offensiveness, the more it is *Lach.*"

Sensitiveness over abdomen. Can hardly allow her clothes to touch her.

Urine blackish, or dark brown: foamy: or has little black spots like soot floating in it.

Feeling as of a ball rolling about in bladder or abdomen.

Ineffectual urging; Violent burning when it does pass.

No urine: no stool.

Always has to urinate after lying down: especially after sleep.

Typically *Lach.* is purple: loquacious: suspicious: sleeps into an aggravation, or is worse after sleep.

Is hypersensitive to heat and touch.

Chimaphila .. Cystitis with great quantities of ropy bloody mucus in urine: muco-purulent: foul, scanty.

Curious sensation of swelling in perineum, or near anus, " as if sitting on a ball ".

Must stand, feet wide apart to urinate. (Comp. *Sarsa.*)

" Prostatic troubles." NASH.

Acute inflammation in urinary tract.

Pulsatilla .. Wonderful tenesmus: extremely painful, bloody, burning, smarting urine: scarcely a drop collects in bladder, but it must be expelled (*Canth.*).

Cannot lie on back without desire to urinate.

Dribbling urine: on slightest provocation—coughing, sneezing (comp. *Caust.*), surprise, joy, laughing, the slam of a door (*Sep.*).

Great urgency: impossible to delay: when going to urinate, sensation as if it will gush away.

Tenesmus vesicæ: cystitis or catarrh. As if bladder too full.

Must keep mind constantly on bladder, or she will lose her urine (*Sepia*).

Flows away in sleep (*Lyc.*, *Caust.*, etc.).

In the *Pulsatilla* patient: changeable, extremely touchy and weepy. Heat and stuffiness unbearable. (Comp. *Terebinth.*)

Chamomilla .. Sticking pain in neck of bladder when not urinating: burning pain, when urinating.
Ineffectual urging, with anguish: smarting or burning in urethra when urinating.
Urine hot, scanty, turbid; red as blood.
But with the *Cham.* mentality:—
Piteous moaning, in child: because he cannot have what he wants.
Wants this and that, then pushes it away.
Snappish: uncivil: irritable: impatient.
Oversensitive to pain: "cannot bear it."

Staphisagria .. KENT says, "*Staphisagria* is very comforting to the young wife."
Frequent and painful urging to urinate: urine bloody, involuntary, acrid and corroding, with burning: worse from motion.
Burning during and after urination.
NASH says, "our only remedy for burning all the time, between the acts of urinating."
A remedy of strong mentality: ailments from indignation about acts of others—or his own.

Arnica .. Bladder affections after mechanical injuries.
Constant urging, while urine passes involuntarily by drops.
Frequent attempts to urinate: has to wait a long time for urine to pass.
Urination involuntarily during sleep: when running.
Hæmaturia from mechanical causes:
Urine thick, with much pus.
Urine very acrid, with increased specific gravity.
With *Arn.* the body feels sore and bruised, and the bed too hard.
Fear of touch: of approach.
A curious symptom: says she is well, when very ill.

Petroselinum .. Such pain when he passes urine, as to cause him to shiver and dance round the room in agony.
Sudden agonizing desire to urinate.

Mercurius cor. Tenesmus vesicæ with intense burning in urethra ; discharge of mucus and blood with urine or after it.

Micturition frequent : urine in drops with much pain. Scanty: hot; burning; bloody (*Canth.*, *Apis.*).

Stools also hot, scanty, bloody, with great straining, not relieved by stool. (Dysentery.)

Ptyalism, with salty taste.

Skin cold, pale, dripping with sweat.

A remedy of violent conditions.

Dulcamara .. Cystitis, or catarrh of bladder : from changes in the weather : from hot to cold : especially to damp cold.

If chilled must hurry to urinate.

"Every time he takes a little cold, urine bloody, with frequency." KENT.

Constant desire to urinate, felt deep in abdomen.

Dulc. is a medicine of Autumn ; hot days and cold evenings. They bring out sweat, then suppress it.

"*Dulc.* is for affections of *damp cold*, what *Acon.* is for the same, from *dry cold*." NASH.

Causticum .. Frequent urging, day and night.

Ineffectual attempts to urinate : when a few drops passed, had violent pain in bladder.

Urging : had to wait a long time, when only a little passed : urging soon renewed, without pain.

Painful retention, brought on by cold (*Acon.*).

Catarrh of bladder.

Queer symptom, itching at urethral orifice.

KENT says, *Caust.* has two kin of paralysis of bladder : one of muscles of expulsion, when urine is retained : one of sphincter vesicae, when urine is passed involuntarily.

Again, paralysis of bladder, from over-distension ; after having to delay urination.

Post-operative retention.

Sepia .. *Sepia* also, may be compelled to keep her mind on the neck of the bladder, or she will lose her urine (*Puls.*).

Enuresis when coughing, laughing, the slam of a door, or when mind is diverted (*Puls.*).

Constant urging for a milky urine that burns like fire, and deposits a material hard to wash off the vessel.

Bloody urine, scanty and suppressed : sudden desire, and tenesmus *as if uterus would come out.*

" Sudden desire with cutting like knives, and chill all over the body." KENT.

More chronic, and in the *Sepia* patient. Indifferent : cold, mentally : no joy in life. Chilly ; sallow : brownish skin. Faint sinking at epigastrium. Wants to get away and be at peace. (Antithesis of *Puls.*)

Lycopodium .. Cystitis : turbid, milky urine, with offensive purulent sediment : dull pressing in bladder and abdomen. Heaviness in bladder.

Urging to urinate : must wait long before it will pass, with constant bearing down.

Supports abdomen with hands. (Vulva, *Sep.*)

Urging, children cry out and grasp abdomen.

" Copious red sand in urine, in acute cases : in chronic, when the patient feels best, red sand is found in urine." KENT.

Involuntary urination in sleep.

Polyuria during the night, though normal or even scanty by day.

Involuntary in sleep.

Passes enormous quantities of urine, very clear and of light specific gravity.

Red sand in the baby's diaper : the urine causes great irritation where left in contact with skin.

But in the *Lyc.* patient ; more mental than physical development. Worse 4-8 p.m.

Desire for sweets and hot drinks.

A remedy of great flatulence and fullness after eating but a little.

THE MORE COMMON REMEDIES OF ENURESIS WITH INDICATIONS

Causticum .. *Caust.* has weakness or paralysis of single parts :—paralysis of face, or of anus, or of bladder, etc. Expectoration slips back.

Or anus prolapses on coughing. Or urine spurts on coughing. Paresis of vocal cords.

" Unconscious of urine as it passes " (*Apis, Argn., Cup., Mag. m., Sars.*) (*Aloe,* of stool). Urinates so easily that he is not sensible of the tream." Useful in children who wet the bed, especially in first sleep (*Sepia, Kreos*).

Typical *Caust.* is worse for *cold dry weather and winds.* (*Rhus* and *Dulc.* worse *cold wet.*)

" Worse in clear fine weather : better in wet weather." Worse changes of the weather.

Sepia .. " *Sepia* is compelled to keep her mind on the neck of the bladder, or she will lose her urine."

Involuntary urine as soon as the child goes to sleep at night. The bed is wet almost as soon as the child goes to sleep (*Caust., Kreos.*).

Typical *Sepia* is sallow : indifferent : hates sympathy; wants to get away alone. (Comp. *Nat. mur.*)

Kreosotum .. Sudden urging to urinate : can't go quick enough (*Petroselinum*).

Sudden urging during first, very profound sleep : (*Caust., Sepia*) wets the bed.

Frequent urging : at night can't get out of bed quick enough.

Wakes with urging, but cannot retain urine, or dreams he is urinating and wets bed (*Bell.*).

Urine flows during first (*Sep.*) deep sleep, from which the child is roused with difficulty.

Apis .. .. Incontinence of urine with great irritation of the parts. Worse night and from coughing.

(It may have, also, incontinence of stool, as if anus were constantly open. *Phos.*)

Typical *Apis* is apathetic, indifferent, joyless, jealous. Its pains burn and *sting.*

Intolerance of heat. Thirstless (*Puls.*).

Pulsatilla .. Involuntary micturition : urine *dribbles* while sitting (Compare *Nat. mur.*) or walking while coughing (*Caust.*), passing wind : at night in bed, especially in little girls.

As " Enuresis noctura for 2 years in a girl of 5½, of mild disposition, fair, frequently changing colour."

Especially after measles ; worse in autumn.

Typical *Puls.* is changeable and fickle : touchy and weepy. Loves fuss and sympathy. Worse heat : stuffy room : fat and rich food. Better moving about in the open air.

Belladonna .. " No remedy has greater irritation in bladder and along urinary tract than *Bell* " (*Staph.*).

Constant urging : *dribbles* : burns (*Staph.*) like fire along whole length of urethra.

Spasmodic retention, or involuntary passage.

During sleep, dribbling of urine.

Dreams of passing urine, and involuntarily passes it (*Kreos.*).

Dribbling when standing or walking : or from mere motion, urine spurts (*Puls.*). (Reverse of *Rhus.*)

When cold or chilled, they lose their urine (*Dulc.*, *Rhus*, *Caust.*).

Starts in sleep, and wets the bed.

Staphisagria .. Teasing and tearing all night long : bloody urine : involuntary urine, acrid and corroding; with burning (*Bell.*). Worse from motion (reverse of *Rhus*). In young women after marriage : in old men with prostatic troubles, continued teasing with *dribbling* (*Bell.*).

After urination feels bladder not empty, for urine continues to dribble away.

Staph. is a great remedy of sphincters : for sphincters stretched during operations.

Also the great remedy of suppressed anger, suppressed feelings. Irritable bladder after suppressed wrath ; after insults.

" Great indignation about things done by others or by himself."

Hypersensitive spots and areas ; little points.

" Whole mind and nervous system are in a fret."

Lycopodium .. *Involuntary urination during sleep.*
"A marked feature of *Lyc.* is *polyuria during the night.* Passes enormous quantities of clear urine: by day, quantity normal."
Urine dribbles away, afternoon and evening, after 4 p.m.
Urine reddens and irritates skin: especially babies,—if left in contact.
Another leading symptom, RED SAND IN URINE: on child's diaper.
Typical *Lyc.* craves sweets, sugar; hot drinks; has afternoon or evening aggravation of symptoms: especially 4-8 p.m.
Lyc. is more alive mentally than physically.
"Ugly on waking", otherwise better in the mornings. May have the curious symptom, weeps when thanked.

Equisetum .. Enuresis day and night; profuse, watery urine: especially enuresis from habit.
Has many urinary troubles. Pain in bladder as from distension: tenderness.
Constant desire to urinate and pass large quantities of pale urine without relief.
"Rapidly restored control over stools and urine in an old woman with general paralysis."

Argentum nit. .. Urine passed unconsciously and uninterruptedly.
Spasmodic enuresis at night: (by day too).
Typical *Arg. nit.* craves sugar—which disagrees: craves salt; cool, open air: is worse in high places.

Hepar .. .. "Urine passes very slowly, drops perpendicularly, is not voided with force. If with this you find wetting of the bed at night, *Hepar* is the remedy."

Cina . .. Urine copious and involuntary: with worm symptoms and ravenous appetite.
Typical *Cina* is cross and "ugly": wants to be carried: or won't be looked at or touched. Wants things and throws them away.
Bores into nose with fingers.
Urine turns milky on standing.

Natrum mur. ..	Involuntary escape of urine while walking, coughing or sneezing (*Caust.*, *Puls.*).
	Violent desire and inability to retain urine (*Sulph.*).
	Whenever he sat down urine came away (Compare *Puls.*) ; day and night ; necessitating very frequent change of clothing and bed-clothes : continual craving for salt.
	Has to wait long for urine to pass (*Lyc.*) especially if others are near by.
	Morbid appetite for salt (*Phos.*, *Nit. a.*, etc.).
	Typical *Nat. mur.*: mapped tongue : herpes about lips : crack middle lower lip.
	Better alone : hates sympathy : maddening headaches.
	After malaria and much quinine.
Sulphur ..	Constant desire to urinate : a few drops pass involuntarily.
	Nocturnal enuresis.
	Sudden, imperative desire, if not gratified, urine passes involuntarily (*Thuj.*, *Nat. m.*, *Kreos.*).
	Irresistible desire to urinate on seeing water running from a hydrant (*Canth.*, *Lyssin*).
	Must rise at night to urinate : rushes away from work to relieve bladder, or wets clothes.
	"Enuresis in pale, lean children, with large abdomen, who love sugar and highly-seasoned food, and abhor to be washed" (*Psor.*).
	Hungry at 11 a.m. Won't be covered at night.
Thuja	Involuntary urination at night or when coughing (*Caust.*).
	Got up at least six times nightly : saturated the bed frequently : urine highly coloured, strong odour.
	Incontinence of urine (*Sulph.*, *Nat. mur.*, *Kreos.*, etc.) : sudden desire, unable to retain it without grasping penis.
	Cannot hold urine when riding, or during a long walk (*Bell.*).
	Chronic incontinence from paralysis of sphincter.
	After vaccination. From tea-drinking.
	Drops in sleep : worse onions. (? Warts, etc.)

Dulcamara .. *If chilled must hurry to urinate.*

Bladder troubles better in summer: worse in winter.

Involuntary urination after wading in cold water.

Typically: worse *cold wet* weather; suppressed discharges, sweat, etc. (Comp. *Rhus*; rev. *Caust.*)

Rhus .. Urine involuntary at night: *when at rest* (reverse of *Bell.*).

Weakness of bladder in girls and women, with frequent desire to urinate.

Constant *dribbling* in boys.

Dribbling of urine *in cold air*, and on becoming very cold. (Compare *Dulc.*)

May be violent tenesmus of bladder, with dribbling of bloody drops.

Typical *Rhus* is much affected by *damp and cold*: by washing (*Sulph.*, *Psor.*). Better for heat. Relieved by motion (*Puls.*).

Nux moschata Incontinence of urine.

Typical *Nux mosch.* is worse from COLD: (*Dulc.*, *Rhus*, *Ars.*) from cold winds, draughts, drinks, bath.

Is indifferent, apathetic, automatic, drowsy. with dry mouth and no thirst.

Arsenicum .. Involuntary micturition, and bed-wetting.

Typical *Ars.* is nervous and *anxious*: *restless*: *fastidious* (*Nux*). "Will get out of bed to put a chair straight." Very *chilly*.

Its worst hour, 1-2 a.m.—thereabouts.

Phosphorus .. Involuntary urination in children of the *Phos.* build, who grow too rapidly.

Typical *Phos.* craves salt: cold drinks: ices. Fears the dark, being alone, ghosts, thunder.

The *Phos.* build is tall and slender: fine hair.

May pass copious, watery, colourless urine.

Psorinum .. Vesical paresis. Obstinate cases of enuresis: wets the bed: during full moon.

Typical *Psor.* is chilly. Dreads washing (*Sulph.*): is greasy and "offensive to sight and smell"

SOME USEFUL REMEDIES IN RETENTION* OF URINE WITH INDICATIONS

Aconite .. *Retention from shock.* In the new born it is the principle remedy. The child cries and is restless.

Retention from cold, especially in children, with much crying and restlessness.

Retention or suppression with pressure in bladder, or stitches in kidney region.

Painful, anxious urging to urinate.

Retention, with agonized tossings and extreme anxiety (*Ars.*). *Ailments from chill, fright, injury, operation.*

Apis .. Retention of urine in nursing infants. "It is queer how the old women knew, long before *Apis* was proved, that when the little new-born baby did not pass its water they could find a cure by going out to the bee-hive and catching a few bees, over which they poured hot water, and of which they gave the baby a teaspoonful. . . . it is consistent, because it is just like what we give *Apis* for." KENT.

Retention or suppression—with thirstlessness. Characteristics: pains stinging: with *thirstlessness and intolerance of heat.*

Opium .. Urine retained from fright (*Acon.*).

Bladder full.

Urine suppressed: passes with difficulty.

Cannot strain to urinate: retention. Acceleration muscles are in a state of paresis (see *Caust.*, *Con.*, etc.).

Paralytic atony of bowels and bladder after laparotomy (*Acon.*, *Arn.*).

Strangury and retention from excessive use of tobacco.

Guiding symptoms may be:—

Great fear, and the fear remains.

Placid: *says nothing ails him* (*Arn.*).

Imagines that parts swell, and that he is going to burst (*Pareira*).

* *For Suppression see also Nephritis.*

Arnica .. Retention of urine from *over-exertion*.
Frequent attempts to urinate.
Has to wait a long time for urine to pass.
Bladder affections after *mechanical injuries*.
Urine retained *after labour*. (Compare *Acon.*)
Bladder feels overfilled, ineffectual urging.
Arnica is bruised: sore: weary. "Bed too hard."

Causticum .. "Has two kinds of paralysis of bladder: one affects the muscles of expulsion and urine is retained, the other the sphincter, when urine is passed involuntarily."
Paralysis of bladder after urine has been *too long retained*, with inability to pass it.
"*Rhus* and *Caust.* are the two great remedies for paralytic weakness of the muscles from being overstrained, or overstrained and chilled." KENT.
Typical *Caust.* is better on warm, wet days.

Nux .. Urine retained in the bladder after drinking beer. Spasmodic retention: discharged drop by drop.
Painful, ineffectual urging to urinate.
Paralysis of bladder .. urine dribbles.
Nux is excitable; irritable: oversensitive. Chilly if he uncovers or moves.

Lycopodium .. Retention of urine: flows in fits and starts.
Violent pain in back every time before urinating: retention, gets into position to pass urine, but waits a great while before it comes. (*Lyc.*) accompanied by characteristic pain in back, which ceases when the water flows.
Inability to pass urine, with constant bearing down: supports abdomen with hands.
In children, urging with inability to pass water: they cry and grasp abdomen.
Often, brick dust or red sand in urine.
Children wake "ugly"; cross and crying.
The *Lyc.* cravings are for sweets, for hot drinks.
Afternoon aggravation of symptoms.

Natrum mur. .. Slowing down of action of bladder. Must wait before urine will start (compare *Lyc.*); then it comes slowly, dribbles.

If anyone is present cannot pass his urine: cannot pass it in a public place.

Typical *Nat. mur.* can weep easily—but no one must see. Irritable with sympathy (reverse of *Puls.*). Often a craving for salt; and not well at the seaside.

Conium .. Intermittent flow of urine with cutting after micturition.

The urine *stops and starts.* Strains to expel urine, gets tired and stops. Stream stops, and without pressure starts again—two or three times during urination. Irregular muscular action while passing urine.

Belladonna .. Suppression or retention: or urine passes drop by drop.

Much difficulty in passing a small quantity.

Urine flows in a feeble stream, or in drops. Spasmodic retention or involuntary passage.

Retention after shock, parturition, in congestion of brain. (Compare *Arn.*; *Aconite*, with anguish and tossing; *Bell.*, twitching and dry heat.)

When a little urine has collected, a sudden, painful, violent urging, with clutching at neck of bladder.

Belladonna burns and throbs: has intense dry heat. (Typically) pupils dilated; thirst for cold drinks, especially lemonade: starts and jerks in sleep: can't stand least jar.

Arsenicum .. Atony of bladder: no desire to urinate and no power to do so. Seems to have lost all control over power to emit. (Comp. *Caust.*)

Paralysis of bladder: atony in old persons; or, great desire but passes no urine.

Urination scanty: passed with difficulty, with burning during discharge.

Probably with the *Ars.* chilliness, restlessness and anxiety.

Pareira .. Great desire to pass urine: fancies quarts will come away, but the greatest difficulty to pass any. *Must get on knees*, pressing head against floor, and remain, forcing, till sweats profusely: then, in ten to twenty minutes, urine dribbles away with great pain.

Strangury with bursting feeling in bladder.

Stramonium .. Retention, sensation that urine could not be passed for narrowness of urethra.

Better after drinking vinegar.

Kidneys secrete less or no urine: especially in acute diseases, and of children.

Great desire, though secretion suppressed.

Rigor during urination.

"An absolute stand-by for renal convulsions."

Cantharis .. Retention of urine, causing pain.

Retention: passes none or only a drop or two.

Constant tenesmus: sits and strains without relief.

Urinary organs and genitalia are in a state of inflammation and irritation: even to threatened gangrene.

The intensity and rapidity are the features of this remedy. KENT.

Tarentula .. Cystitis: high fever: gastric derangement: excruciating pain and inability to pass a drop of urine: or passes drop by drop a dark-brown, fetid urine with gravel-like sediment.

Restless, fidgety, hurried. Jerking and twitching.

Hysterical: lacks control.

"Keeps hands busy."

Terebinth .. Spasmodic retention of urine (? gonorrhœa).

Suppression of urine.

Retained urine from atony of bladder.

Violent burning and cutting in bladder.

A feature of *Terebinth* is the haemorrages from kidneys and bladder.

Spasms from any attempt to urinate.

SOME REMEDIES OF VERTIGO*

WITH INDICATIONS

Conium .. A very great remedy of vertigo—*of its kind.*
Vertigo, *turning or moving head, turning eyes.*
Sensation of turning in a circle.
Lying, *as if bed turned in a circle.* Vertigo on turning eyes when lying.
Vertigo turning in bed : looking round :—
When rising from a seat :—
When watching moving objects.
Cannot endure the slightest alcoholic drink.
Curious symptom : sweats, day and night, on closing eyes.

Sanguinaria .. Dizzy : *cannot turn quickly* without fear of falling.
Vertigo with long-continued nausea and headache : then spasmodic vomiting.
With sensation of some hard heavy substance in stomach.
Vertigo on quickly turning head : looking up : lying down : during sleep.
Rush of blood to head with dizziness; feels sick and faint : would fall if she rose from sitting.
(One of the "sick-headache" remedies.)
Vertigo in cold weather.

Aconite .. Vertigo : *on rising up from lying* ; red face becomes deathly pale ; or, becomes dizzy, falls : and fears to rise again ; with nausea.
Vanishing of sight, or unconsciousness.
Vertigo, from fall or concussion : after a fright : anxious as if dying : must lie down.
Vertigo from congestion, as in the sun (*Bell.*) : on stooping : staggers to right.
Ailments with anxiety and restlessness.
"*Aconite is a great storm and soon over.*"
"A woman runs up suddenly against a dog and becomes violently dizzy. Vertigo that comes on from fear : from sudden fear."

N.B.—Manipulation of neck—atlas—will often cure vertigo.

Bryonia .. Vertigo, rising; from a seat, or from lying.
Dizzy and faint on raising head.
Worse from least motion.
Vertigo and confusion on least motion.
Typically, tongue dry: constipation with hard dry stools.
Thirst for large drinks. White tongue: irritable. Better left alone.
Curious symptoms, sinking with, or through bed. (Comp. *Thuja.*)
Tendency to run backwards. (Comp. *Camph. monobrom.*)

Nux Vertigo: *rising from seat or bed* (*Acon.*, etc.): or raising head (*Bry.*).
Vertigo with vanishing of sight and hearing:
At night, wakes him from sleep.
After stooping: when looking up: must clutch something to avoid falling.
Objects seem to move round him.
Falls forward—to one side—backward.
As if brain turning in circle: room whirling.
Reeling in a.m.; after dinner; red, hot face, vision obscured: staggering.
From digestive disturbances; constipation; sedentary habits; alcohol; smoking, smell of flowers, gas; from mental over-exertion. (Comp. *Phos.*)
Nux, typically, is irritable: oversensitive: drowsy p.c. Chilly if uncovers or moves.
Better for sleep. Red face.

Belladonna .. A remedy of *suddenness*: of *violence.*
Has quickness of sensation: of motion.
Pains come and go suddenly.
Blood goes to head, with vertigo.
Vertigo with pulsations in head, dilated pupils, nausea.
As if being rocked: when lying down: *as if bed bounced her up and down.*
When stooping: at night: turning in bed: with every change of position.
As if sinking with, or through bed (*Bry.*, comp. *Thuja*).
Tends to fall to left, or backwards.
Objects sway to and fro.

Phosphorus .. Vertigo: *looking upwards, downwards.*
On rising from a seat: on moving head.
Sensation, as if looking down.
Chair seems to rise with him.
Sensation, as if would fall forwards.
Staggers while walking. Everything turns.
Worse lying on left side.
Worse mental exertion: smell of flowers (*Nux*).
Typical *Phos.* tall, thin; craves cold drinks: ices: salt.
Fears thunder, the dark: being alone.

Natrum muriaticum .. Vertigo *with flickering before eyes.* Objects turn round.
Tends to fall forward.
After coffee, tea, alcohol, tobacco (*Nux*).
From straining eyes or close study.
Typical *Nat. mur.* weeps, but no one must see: sad, reserved. Craves salt.

Opium .. Great vertigo *compels him to lie down.*
As if *all went round in a circle with him.*
Giddy intoxication: staggers hither and thither.
Vertigo from injuries to head: after fright.
As if flying or hovering in air (rev. of *Bry.*, etc).
Fainting turns with vertigo, rising from bed: with return of animation on lying down.

Secale .. VERTIGO: constantly increasing: stupefaction.
Reeling: inability to stand upright.
Head, esp. occiput, feels light (*Gels.*, rev. of *Tabac*). Unsteady gait.
Typical *Secale* is emaciated, withered, wrinkled; with unhealthy skin.
Externally icy-cold; yet burns internally.
Numbness; tingling; crawling; cramping.

Onosmodium .. *Fears to look down,* lest she fall down (Comp. *Gels.*) that she might fall into fire: "in spite of all his will power, did fall into fire."
Inco-ordination. Misjudges distances.
Staggering. Feels as walking on cotton.
Curious symptom: *headache worse in the dark.*

Camphor monobromide — *Feels he is journeying in one direction when actually moving in the opposite.*
Imagines that he is turned round, going north instead of south.
Feels he is going in wrong direction: though house numbers show he is not.

China .. Dizziness and fainting after loss of blood.
Vertigo, head tends to sink backwards: worse moving and walking: better lying down.

Salicylicum acidum .. Vertigo, tends to fall to left side, while surrounding objects seem falling to right.
Auditory nerve vertigo. (Menière's disease.)
Comes and goes from no known cause.
Noises in ear. (?) deafness.

Lycopodium .. Nausea: *everything turning round*: dreads falling.
Vertigo while drinking: *in hot room* (*Puls.*): rising from seat: from bed. Reels back and forth.
Gets hot, face reddens, eyes dim and watery.
Flatulence and distension: has to loosen clothing about waist. Worse cold drinks.
Lyc. has the 4-8 p.m. aggravations.

Dulcamara .. Momentary vertigo, with darkness before eyes.
At noon, before eating, while walking, giddy, *as if all objects remained standing* before him, and as if it became black before eyes.
On rising, almost fell: with weakness and trembling.

Tabacum .. Vertigo: *excessive heaviness of head* (rev. of *Secale*).
Qualmishness stomach: deathlike paleness of face: weakness, to loss of consciousness.
Better in open air, and by vomiting.
Vertigo on rising, and looking upwards.
From immoderate smoking of cigars (*Nux*).
Excessive vertigo *with copious* (*cold*) *sweat.*
Deathly nausea with violent vomiting: worse least movement. Worse opening eyes.

Gelsemium .. *Head feels light and large,* with vertigo.
Dizziness with blurring of vision: gradually increasing. Spreads from occiput over head: pupils dilated (*Bell.*); sight dim: from heat of sun, or summer.
Seems intoxicated when trying to move.
Worse from smoking (*Nux*).
Giddiness, with loss of sight, chilliness, quick pulse: double sight.
Muscles refuse to obey will: giddy: confused; loss of co-ordination.
Sensation of falling. Child clings to nurse, or crib: screams with fear of falling (*Borax*).
(Case: child with this fear of falling: must hold to something firm—not even to her mother.
After *Gels.* she was climbing trees.)

Ferrum .. Face fiery red (Comp. *Bell.*), feet cold: with vertigo *worse rising from lying or sitting* (*Acon.*).
From walking over a bridge, or by running water, or riding in car or carriage.

Argentum metallicum .. Crawling and whirling in head, as if drunken.
When *looking at running water,* is giddy.
Or when crossing running water. (Comp. *Con.*)

Argentum nitricum .. Vertigo *looking at high buildings.*
Has great fear of high places.
Craves sugar and sweets, which disagree.

Pulsatilla .. Excessive -violent vertigo like intoxication: as if one had turned round in a circle a long time: with nausea.
Worse sitting; lying. *Better walking in open air*:—or the opposite, "as a secondary or alternating state" (rev. of *Sulph.*).
Vertigo caused by indigestion: with vomiting p.c.
Vertigo when turns eyes upwards: as if would fall: as if dancing. Better in cold room.
Stooping: could scarcely raise herself again.
Typical *Puls.* is changeable, weepy, exacting, irritable—the *wind-flower.*
"A remedy of many uses (polycrest)."

Ceanothus am. Violent vertigo, on lying down and then turning over to right side.

Everything turning violently to right: has to cling to sides of bed.

Chelidonium .. Vertigo: with bilious vomiting: with pain in liver.

With confusion: stumbling, as if to fall *forwards*.

On closing eyes, as if *everything turned in a circle*. (Comp. *Con.*, *Apis.*) On sitting up in bed.

With shivering, upper part of body.

On attempting to rise. Keeps him in bed.

Giddiness on waking, with indigestion.

Typical *Chel.* has *pain under angle rt. scapula.*

Tongue coated thickly yellow with red edge: tooth-notched.

Desire hot drinks: hot milk. (*Phos.* cold.)

Apis .. Vertigo *on closing the eyes*: worse sitting than walking, extreme when lying and closing the eyes (*Chel.*).

Typical *Apis* is intolerant of heat: thirstless: has relief from cold.

Ailments from jealousy, fright, rage.

Silica Vertigo: to fainting: with nausea.

Vertigo *creeping up spine into head.*

Tends to *fall forward*: worse motion: looking up. Staggering.

Worse closing eyes (*Chel.*, *Apis*): lying on right side (*Phos.* worse lying on left).

Vertigo *during sleep*.

On closing eyes all things turn with him: passes off on opening them.

Vertigo as if moving to and fro in head.

Vertigo with retching: water comes from mouth.

Better riding in open air: worse back in room.

" As if head were teeming with live things whirling around it."

Silica patients lack " grit "—" Sand ".

Are worse for cold: head and feet sweat—ailments from suppressed foot-sweat (? foul).

Sulphur .. Much troubled with dizziness. When *he goes into the open air*, or *when he stands* any length of time, he becomes dizzy.

On rising in the morning his head feels stupid, and on getting on his feet he is dizzy.

Not rested by sleep: "things go round". "Takes time to establish an equilibrium."

Worse from sleep and from standing.

Vertigo lying on back.

After lying a quarter of an hour, whirling vertigo, as if would faint.

Typical *Sulphur* is the "ragged philosopher": unkempt: argumentative.

Agaricus .. "Vertigo and confusion of mind are mixed up."

Vertigo when walking *in open air* (*Sulph.*): reeling: great sensitiveness to cold air.

Objects whirling: tends to fall forward.

Better by quickly turning the head (rev. *Con.*).

Cannabis indica .. Vertigo on rising, with *stunning pain back of head*, and he falls.

Heavy pressure on brain, must stoop.

(Typically) *Cann. ind.* has exalted sensations: with exaggeration of time and distance.

Sensation of calvarium opening and shutting: as if brain boiling over and lifting cranium like lid of tea-kettle. (Comp. *Cocc.*)

Cocculus indicus .. Vertigo: *things go round*: *whirl from right to left*; with confusion; with nausea.

Whirling vertigo: worse *rising from lying.*

Nausea to fainting with severe vertigo.

Sick-headache with vertigo and nausea: from riding in carriage, boat, train, car.

(Sea-sickness *Tab.*)

Head, abdomen, chest "empty and hollow".

Hot, flushed face.

Extreme aversion to food: nausea from smell of food (*Colch.*, *Sep.*, *Ars.*) but with hunger.

Inco-ordination: tremor: prostration.

"Occiput opens and shuts" (Comp. *Cann. ind.*).

Petroleum ..	Vertigo: *in occiput*: as if intoxicated: like sea-sickness. *Obliges him to stoop*: more violent when standing than sitting (Comp. *Puls.*). Goes all over him, makes him numb and stiff.
Digitalis ..	Vertigo from cardiac weakness (*Ars., Hydrocy. acid, Camph., Verat.*). Severe vertigo *with very slow pulse*. With anxiety, as if she would faint. On rising from sitting: limbs weak. Constant dizziness with ringing in ears. "As if heart would stop if she moved" (*Gels.* must move to keep it beating). Pulse full, irregular, slow and weak; intermits.
Cyclamen ..	A curious "*transparent vertigo*"—to coin an expression. On waking in a.m., or on rising, looking ahead, any object—say a wardrobe—is seen whirling unsteadily, and flickering away to the side (? right side); while all the time, through the whirl, the same object is seen standing solid and immovable. *Cycl.* has promptly cured. Sensation of brain moving within cranium. Vertigo: *objects turn in a circle*, or about her, or make a see-saw motion: when walking in open air. "Visual effects, or vertigo."
Baptisia ..	A *rapid* septic state. Stupid: prostrated: looks besotted. Swimming sensation: worse stooping and noise. Confusion as if drunk. Vertigo with paralysis of eyelids. Feels scattered about: can't get the pieces together (*Pyrog., Petr.*).
Ailanthus ..	Dizzy: face hot: cannot sit up: drowsy but restless and anxious. In malignant scarlet fever, diphtheria, etc.: with stupidity and mottled skin.

SOME COMMON REMEDIES FOR HEADACHE

Natrum muriaticum

" One of our best remedies for chronic headaches."

" The headaches are awful: dreadful pains: bursting, compressing as in a vice: as if skull would be crushed in."

" Little hammers in the head as soon as moves: on waking in a.m."

May begin at 10 or 11 a.m., last till 3 p.m. or evening.

Periodic, every day, or third or fourth day.

Better sleep: must go to bed and be perfectly quiet (*Bry.*). Intermittent fever headaches, *after much malaria and quinine.*

Relief from sweating: or relief to all but head from sweating. (*Gels.* has > from copious urination.)

May begin with fiery zigzags (*Sep.*).

Beware of *Nat. mur.* when acute and violent: it may needlessly increase the suffering: give its " acute " *Bry.*: and after the paroxysm, *Nat. mur.*

Characteristics. Weepy (*Puls.*) but no one must see. Emotional to pathetic things, books, plays. Worse, or anger from consolation. Aversion to bread, fats: desire for salt. A crack in middle of lower lip (*Sep.*).

Sepia .. ..

Headaches nervous, bilious, periodic, violent.

Better lying and quiet: often cured by sleep, even a short sleep (*Phos.*).

Relief from lying down, or from violent motion (slow *Puls.*). Long walk in open air that warms her, relieves.

Worse stooping, coughing, jarring, light, thinking. Better hard exercise or a tight bandage, or applied heat: but worse hot room.

Occipital headaches, loathing of food: then nausea and vomiting: then sleep and wakes without it. Headache with nausea: worse smell of food. Fiery zigzags (*Nat. mur.*).

In the *Sepia* patient: characteristically sallow with brown patches. Indifferent: wants to get away and be at peace. Hates fuss.

Aconite .. " The headaches can scarcely be described, they come with such violence.

" Tearing, burning in brain, in scalp, *with fear. with fever, with anguish.*"

Fullness and heaviness in forehead, as if an outpressing weight there: as if all would be forced out at the forehead. (Compare *Sulph.*, *Bell.*, down one nostril *Borax.*)

Throbbing in left forehead with strong beats in right side by fits.

Skull constricted by a ligature (*Sulph.*).

Acon. is sudden: wild: worse from cold winds; with restlessness, anguish, fear.

Belladonna .. Headaches of great violence.

Congestion: red, hot face: dilated pupils.

Violent throbbing in brain . . . and carotids.

Violent shoots and cutting stabs.

Jerking headache: worse walking, going up stairs. At every step jerked downwards like a weight in occiput.

Cutting knife-stabs and shoots.

Bursting pain: as if brain would be pressed out: worse stooping, as if brain would fall out, push forward: or eyes would drop out.

Worse noise, jar, motion, light, lying: better pressure.

Rush of blood to head.

Violent headaches, *better for drawing head back.*

Headache with dizziness: worse stooping.

Headache from washing the head.

Bell. headaches come suddenly, last an indefinite time, and depart suddenly.

CASE.—A little maid would come down at night, " Oh! my head! my head!"—frantic with pain: her hands held out quiveringly before her. A dose of *Bell.* and, in a few minutes, suddenly, " It's gone!" and off she would go happily to bed. (A case of cerebral tumour, as it turned out: but showed the wonderful palliative action of *Belladonna.*)

Another case:—boy, after exposure to a very hot sun, got a terrific headache, with very high temperature. *Bell.*: and well by next day. (Compare *Glon.*)

Glonoin .. Very like *Bell.*: perhaps " more so ".
Upward rushes of blood (*Bell.*).
Waves of terrible, bursting, pulsating headache. (" A tempestuous remedy.")
Worse bending head back (*reverse* of *Bell.*).
A great remedy for sunstroke (*Bell.*).
Worse for having hair cut (*Bell.*, head washed).
Can't bear heat about head.
Throbbing head: holds it with both hands.
Brain too large: full: bursting: throbs at every jar, step, pulse (*Bell.*).
Head hot: face flushed—purple or bright red.
" Skull too small: brain will burst it."
Waves of pain: and brain seems to move in waves.

CASE.—Youth, after an appalling smash (motor bicycle) skull fractured: terrific, unbearable pain in head for which he implored morphia. Got *Glonoin* instead, and never asked for morphia again. Its effect was magic.

Melilotus .. Congestion to brain equal to *Bell.* and *Glon.*
Intense redness of face: throbbing carotids.
Better for profuse epistaxis.

Lachesis .. Violent congestion to head: with vomiting and loss of sight. Almost delirious with headache.
Throbbing, bursting pains in head (*Bell.*, *Glon.*) as if all the blood of body had gone to head.
Sun-headaches, of the more chronic type (*Bell.*, *Glon.* for the very acute violent "sunstroke" headache). Chronic headaches whenever exposed to the sun. Worse heat.
Pressure on vertex: relieved by pressure: often extending to root of nose.
Sleeps into the headache: dreads to sleep, as wakes with such a distressing headache (*reverse* of *Phos.* and *Sepia*). Headaches from suppressed discharges—nasal, uterine, etc. Relief from their reappearance.
Characteristics. Loquacity; or great slowness. Intolerance of pressure, especially on throat and abdomen. Left-sided ailments; may cross to right side.

Cocculus ind. .. Headache as if skull would burst: or like a great valve opening and shutting.

Sick-headaches with vertigo.

Thought or smell of food nauseates (*Ars.*, *Sep.*, *Colch.*): makes the patient gag.

"Train sickness" with nausea and vertigo.

Effects of night-nursing and loss of sleep.

On motion, eyes as if being torn from sockets: or head empty and hollow: or constriction.

Pulsative pains, vertex or temples.

Headache, occiput and nape, pain as if opening and shutting like a door.

Worse eating, drinking, sleeping: better rest indoors.

Slow in answering.

Least jar unbearable (*Bell.*, etc.).

Crotalus cascavella .. Skull compresses brain like an iron helmet.

Something alive walks in a circle in the head.

Head and chest compressed by iron armour.

A red-hot iron stuck into vertex.

Acute lancinations right temple (many of the pains are lancinating).

Shocks in head, almost throw her off balance.

Headache after sleep (*Lach.*).

Headache, epistaxis and great excitement, caused by starting from sleep.

Great coldness: icy feet.

Crot. casc. has peculiar hallucinations.

"This terrible serpent . . . whose poison acts with frightful intensity."

Gelsemium .. Congestive headache: most violent in occiput.

Every pulsation, "a hammering base of brain".

Lies high, exhausted and paralysed with pain.

Later, whole head congested. One grand pain too dreadful to describe; lies bolstered up in bed, eyes glassy, pupils dilated, face mottled, extremities cold.

Or, neuralgic headache, temples and over eyes, with nausea and aggravation from vomiting.

Relieved by copious urination, i.e. urine, scanty, becomes free, and headache subsides.

A great influenza medicine.

Phosphorus .. Congestive and throbbing headaches.
Better from cold: worse from heat. Worse motion; better rest; but worse lying down.
Phos. is chilly and worse from cold; yet needs cold for his stomach and head: craves ices or quantities of ice-cold water.
Headaches most violent; with hunger, or preceded by hunger. With red face: scanty urine.
Violent neuralgic pains also; darting, tearing, shooting.
Periodic headaches: from mental exertion: with stiffness of face and jaws.
Worse noise; light; becoming heated.

Pulsatilla .. Throbbing, congestive headaches.
Head hot, better for cold applications.
Better slowly walking in open air.
Headaches connected with menses: or from suppressed menses.
Periodic sick headache: vomits sour food.
Headache from over-eating: from ice cream.
Thirstless: easily weeping: changeable.
Must have air; better motion. Worse heat.

Apis .. .. Pain, occiput, with occasional sharp shrieks.
Pains like bee-stings, with the thrust and the the burning pain following.
Brain affections of children with sudden sharp shriek (*Crie cerebrale*). Bends head back, or bores in pillow.
Thirstless: sweat without thirst: scanty urine: piercing screams sleeping or waking.
" Bruised all over," sensitive to touch.
Worse heat: warm room: hot bath. Better cold room: cold air: cold applications.
" Alternately dry and hot, then perspiring."

Chamomilla .. A little headache seems an enormous thing.
Congestive headaches.
Pressing, bursting pain, worse thinking of it.
Irritable: capricious: over-sensitive to pain. "*Cannot bear it.*"
Face red and hot on one side, pale the other.

Mercurius .. Congestion, head: feels it will burst: fulness of brain: constricted by a band: as if in a vice, with nausea: worse at night.

Burning in head, especially left temple: worse at night.

Headache over nose and round eyes, as if tied with a tape, or tight hat pressing.

Sensitive to air: worse cold, damp: violently worse in a draught.

Better in room: worse in cold or warm room.

Wants to be covered, but worse from heat.

Dirty offensive tongue and mouth: offensive sweat.

Catarrhal, rheumatic or syphilitic headaches.

China .. .. Congestive headaches: extremities covered with cold sweat.

Stitches from temple to temple.

Pain from one temple to the other: from occiput over whole head.

Intense throbbing headache;

Brain beats in waves against skull (compare *Glon.*). " As if head would burst " (*Glon.*).

After loss of fluids, hæmorrhages, etc.

Ringing in ears.

Worse draught; open air; sun; touch; better from hard pressure.

Nux vomica .. Headaches connected with gastric, hepatic, abdominal or hæmorrhoidal troubles.

" Congestive and abdominal headaches."

A nail driven into brain (*Thuja, Ruta*): stitching pains with nausea and sour vomiting.

" As if skull would split " (*Cocc.*).

Headaches on waking: on rising: after eating: in open air: on moving eyes.

Headaches of sedentary persons: after coffee.

Irritable, vehement disposition.

Oversensitive and touchy.

Better head wrapped up: covered: lying down: warmth and heat (Compare *Sil.*): warm in bed: in damp warm weather.

Iris versicolor .. "One of our best remedies for sick-headache."
Sick-headaches of gastric or hepatic origin: always begin with a blur before eyes.
Nausea and vomiting: burning of tongue, throat, œsophagus and stomach.
Profuse secretion of ropy saliva. (Compare *Kali bich.*)
Vomit ropy, hangs like strings from mouth.
Watery stools: anus feels on fire.
Vomiting spells *every month or six weeks.*

Sanguinaria .. Sick-headaches (*Iris.*).
Pain starts occiput, spreads over head to right eye (*Sil.*; *Spig.*, left) with nausea and vomiting.
Periodic sick-headache: *every seventh day* (or third).
Sun-headache, starts morning, increases all day, lasts till evening.
With chills, nausea, vomiting of bile.
Feels head must burst (*Merc.*, *Chin.*, *Glon.*, *Bell.*).
Better lying down in the dark: better sleep.
Vomits bile, slime, yesterday's food, then relief and sleep.
Palms and soles burn: puts feet out of bed (*Sulph.*, *Puls.*, *Cham.*, *Medorrh.*).
Circumscribed redness of cheeks.

Sulphur .. Burnings: vertex: palms: soles. Everywhere.
Heaviness in head, stooping, moving, even when sitting and lying.
"Tight hat" sensation. And headache from pressure of hat: better head uncovered.
Throbbing, beating, hammering: rush of blood to head, and pressure, as out of eyes.
Periodic sick headaches: congestive: with stupefaction, nausea and vomiting.
Sick-headache once a week or two weeks—the characteristic *seven-day aggravation.*
"The Sunday headache of working men."
Worse motion, eating, drinking.
Red engorged face, eyes red, engorged.
The characteristic *Sulph.* patient is hungry: starving about 10 a.m.; loves fat: cannot stand long; untidy: argumentative.

Cedron .. Attacks of headache occur with *clock-like regularity.*

Head felt as if swollen.

Sick-headache every other day at 11 a.m.

Arsenicum .. *Periodic headaches:* every other day—every fourth day—seventh day—fourteenth day. Malarial headaches.

Ars. is very chilly and needs warm clothing, but *with congestive headache* wants body warm and head bathed in cold water; "blankets to the chin, and head out of the window" (Compare *Phos.*)

But *Ars. neuralgic headaches* need to be wrapped up and kept warm.

Head, and physical symptoms alternate.

Congestive headaches, throb and burn, with restlessness and anxiety: hot head and relief from cold.

Headaches with nausea and vomiting. Sick-headaches of the worst sort; with thirst for little and often.

Dreadful occipital headaches; stunned and dazed: they start after midnight, or from excitement.

With head symptoms, head in constant motion.

Ars. is *restless: anxious; prostrate,* and characteristically, very fastidious (*Nux*).

Argentum met. *Precisely at the hour of noon* many troubles come on. Headaches, etc.

Violent neuralgias one side at a time, deep in brain, involving one half of brain.

Painful sensation of emptiness in the head.

Pressing, burning pain in skull, *every day at noon.*

Gradually the pain gets more violent, then *ceases suddenly.* (*Bell.* sudden onset and sudden cessation.)

Often, old history of suffering from heat of sun (*Nat. sul.*).

"All the nervous excitement that is possible in remedies comes up in this remedy."

Spigelia .. " Sun-headaches." Start every morning with sunrise: get worse till noon: gradually decrease till sun sets:—this even on cloudy days.
Pains from occiput to eyes, especially left, which waters (*Sang.*; *Sil.*, to right).
Worse from all movement (*Bry.*): noise: jar.
Stitching, shooting, burning pains: like hot needles (*Ars.*).
Very violent neuralgia, followed by soreness.
Very violent heart-action is characteristic of *Spigelia*.
Intolerable pain in eyeballs: feel too large for orbits (*Lycopersicum*); sensitive to touch.
Stitching pains.

Bryonia .. *Worse from any motion.* Cannot bear any disturbance, mental or physical.
Cannot sit up in bed.
Bursting, or splitting, or heavy crushing headache: worse any movement.
Fronto-occipital headache.
Nausea or faintness rising or sitting up: better lying still.
Irritable: thirsty: dry lips and mouth.
Vehement and quarrelsome.
Pain in head from coughing: grasps head when going to cough. Worse straining at stool.
Headache after washing with cold water when face was sweating:" from ironing ".
Rush of blood to head. Epistaxis.
Worse from slightest motion: after eating.

Eupatorium perf. Sick headache: on waking: lasts all day.
Pain and weight occiput: must use hand to raise head. " Terrible sick headaches."
Pains throbbing, shooting, darting, thumping.
Painful soreness of eyeballs.
Malarial and influenzal headaches, with aching and breaking sensations in bones and joints.

Eupatorium promptly cured a case of influenza, with soreness in bones and a headache so intense that she dared not move a hand, as the slightest movement made the pain intolerable (*Bry.*).

Silica .. .. Chronic sick-headaches with nausea, even vomiting.

Begins nape of neck, goes forward over vertex to eyes, especially right eye (left, *Spig.*).

Better pressure : better lying : *wrapping head up warmly* : tying head up tightly. *Better applied heat.* Better profuse urination. (*Gels.*)

Silica is chilly, yet sweats much, especially face and feet. Offensive foot sweat.

Calcarea .. *Icy coldness in and on head :* on vertex.

Heaviness in forehead.

Stunning, pressive pain in forehead.

Tearing headache above eyes down to nose.

Semilateral headaches with empty risings.

Head numb, as if wearing a cap (*Sulph.*).

But in the *Calc.* patient "Fat blondes who sweat easily : especially head, neck, chest, during sleep."

Cold, damp feet (*Sep.*).

Chilly : lax muscles.

Profuse head-sweats during sleep (*Sil.*).

Worse milk.

Veratrum alb. .. *Head feels as if packed in ice. Feels as if ice lay on vertex and occiput.*

Troublesome neuralgic headaches of great violence.

Violent pains drive to despair : great prostration, fainting, cold sweat and great thirst.

CASE.—Elderly woman with violent, unendurable pains in head. Almost out of her mind : utterly changed in appearance and mentality. Sensation of *ice on vertex* suggested *Verat. alb.*, which gave rapid relief and cured.

Heloderma .. Very violent headaches : pressure as if skull too full (*Bell., Glon., China, Merc., Sang.*) : as of a tumour forming and pressing inside skull.

Burning in brain : or sensation of a cold band round head.

Characteristic. *Intense, arctic coldness* : internal coldness, *as if being frozen to death from within outwards.* Coldness at heart, as if being frozen to death.

Cold rings round body : cold waves.

Arnica .. .. Burning in head—in brain, the rest of the body being cool.

Aching pain over eyes, to temples; as if integuments were spasmodically contracted.

Great shoots in head from coughing, sneezing.

Cutting in head, as from a knife; then coldness.

Effects of injuries to head; of concussion.

After cerebral hæmorrhages.

Arn. feels ***bruised and beaten***; says " bed too hard ".

Epiphegus .. Headache when " tired out ". Better for a good sleep (*Phos.*, *Sep.*).

Characteristic: constantly wants to spit: saliva viscid.

Argentum nit. Constitutional headaches from brain fag.

Hemicrania. Feeling of expansion, as if head were enormously enlarged.

Better tied up tight.

Wants cold air, cold drinks, cold things.

Craving for sweets: sugar, which disagree.

Strange notions and impulses.

Psorinum .. Always hungry during headache. (Compare *Phos.*), but the antithesis of *Phos.* in appearance.

" *Hungry headaches* " may alternate with cough.

If goes without a meal, has a headache.

Fulness vertex as if brain would burst out.

Not room in forehead for brain, in a.m.; better after washing and eating.

A chilly edition of *Sulph.* Typically, looks dirty: " offensive to eye and smell ". " No amount of washing will make him look clean."

Anthracinum .. Headache, " as if a smoke with a heating pain was passing through head" (***Fumee de douleur chaude***).

Head is affected in an indescribable manner.

Dullness: confusion: dizziness: loss of consciousness.

If conscious complain of great pain in head.

Rhus .. .. Headache, as if stupified: as if intoxicated.
As if brain loose and falls against skull.
Weight in head: stooping, a weight falls forward into forehead, drawing head down.
Must hold head up straight to relieve this.
On waking and opening eyes gets violent headache: first occiput then occiput-temples.
Brain loaded, loose, torn, fluctuating; as if much blood shot into it when stooping.
Worse from wetting head (*Bell.*), *from cold; damp: getting wet when perspiring* (*Dulc.*).

Thuja .. .. As if a nail were driven into vertex: into right parietal bone: into left frontal eminence (*Rumex*).
Severe stitches in left temporal region.
Boring-pressing in head.
Pulsation in temples.
Heaviness in head: cross and disinclined to speak.
Dull, stupifying headache: worse stooping: better bending head back.
Worse from tea: from onions.
Has cured the most severe and chronic headaches, after repeated *vaccinations.*

Always remember the nosodes of previous (*acute*) *or family illnesses.*

Remember also manipulation of neck.

THE MORE COMMON REMEDIES IN APOPLEXY

WITH INDICATIONS*

Arnica .. " Chief remedy, because of its great power to produce absorption of extravasated blood."
Stupor with involuntary stool and urine.
Paralysis—especially left side.
Pulse full and strong.
Head and face hot : body cool.
Falls into a deep stupor while answering.
Sore, as if bruised. Restless because bed feels so hard. Bedsores form rapidly.
Characteristic symptoms. Horror of instant death, especially at night (*Acon.*).
Says he is "well" when desperately ill (*Opium.*).
Fear of being touched.

Aconite .. Congestion, often apoplectic. Apoplexy.
Head hot. Pulsation of carotids. Pulse full, hard, strong (*Arn.*).
Especially after fright or vexation : or in cold dry weather (high barometer).
Dry hot skin. Arterial tension.
Often, one cheek red and hot, the other pale and cold. Looks frightened (*Stram.*).
Burning headache, as if brain agitated by boiling water. Fullness, as if everything would push out of forehead.
If conscious, terror, anxiety, agonizing fear.

Glonoine .. " Throbbing headache *seems to arise from neck* is characteristic : no mere sensation—visible in carotids. The vessels are full to bursting, and if walls unhealthy, there is danger of apoplexy."—NASH.
" Violent pulsations, upward rushes of blood. Waves of terrible bursting pulsating pain in head."—BOGER.
Worse heat : shaking : jar (*Bell.*).
Throbbing in front of head.
Pressure and throbbing in temples.
" Skull too small : brain trying to burst it."

* *Grouped for intensity or for comparison.*

Belladonna .. Apoplexy : flushed, hot, bloated face : dilated pupils ; a fixed, threatening look. Nausea. Threatening apoplexy : rush of blood to head (*Glon.*). Pulsation of cerebral arteries : THROBBING inside head.

The pain worse leaning forward, better bending back. Worse stooping : light : JAR.

" Head will burst ! "

Pressure, especially in forehead : eyes as if starting from their sockets.

Pain comes suddenly, lasts indefinitely, ceases suddenly.

First stage apoplexy where severe congestive symptoms are present ; or later, when extravasation causes inflammatory reaction. Violent delirium with intense redness, burning. Especially in plethoric, vigorous intellectuals.

" The more congestion in *Bell.*, the more excitability : the more the congestion in *Opium*, the less the excitability." KENT.

(*Bell.* craves lemons, *Stram.*, > vinegar.)

Opium .. Comatose sleep, with rattling and stertor.

Red, bloated face.

Eyes blood-shot and half open. Jaw drops.

Skin covered with hot sweat.

Cheeks blown out with every expiration.

There is no response to light, touch, noise or anything else, except the indicated remedy, which is *Opium*. NASH.

Characteristics: Abnormal painlessness. (Compare *Arn.*, *Stram.*)

Bed feels so hot, cannot lie on it. (*Arn.*, bed so hard.)

Veratrum viride Congestive apoplexy : cerebral hyperæmia.

Sudden cerebral congestion. Intensely congestive headaches.

Becomes stupid : thick speech ; slow, full, *hard* pulse.

Convulsions from intense congestion of brain.

Ringing in ears : bloodshot eyes : dim vision, with nausea and vomiting.

Millefolium .. All the blood seems to ascend to head.
Nose bleed; excessive congestion to chest and head.
Confused: especially in evening: knows not what he is about.
At night a stream from chest to head, like a gust of wind, with nose bleed.
Apoplexy.
Violent headache: strikes head against wall.
Worse stooping. (Compare *Bell.*)
Red face (? without heat).

Bryonia .. Rush of blood to head: heat in head.
Fullness, heaviness, forehead, as if brain were pressing out.
Worse moving head, or eyes: better closing eyes: *better pressure.*
Vertigo and confusion on slightest motion.
Nose bleed.
Apoplexy.

Natrum sulph. As if forehead would burst: especially p.c.
Brain feels loose, when stooping: as if it fell towards left temple.
Base of brain as if crushed in a vice: something gnawing there.
Especially after injuries to head.
Indescribable pain vertex, as if it would split.
Worse from damp.

Natrum carb. Head feels too large: as if forehead would burst (*Nat. sul.*).
Headache from slightest mental exertion.
Worse from sun: heat.
Chronic effects of sunstroke.

Strontium carb. Threatened apoplexy with violent congestion of head. Thickened arteries.
Hot, red face every time he walks.
Exertion increases circulation towards head.
Smothering sensation, heart.
Cannot rest.
Better wrapping head, cannot bear least draught of air.
Headache, better wrapping head warmly (*Sil.*).

Nux .. Apoplexy in drunkards: of high livers. Falls unconscious: tends to fall backwards.

Face pale: head hot: automatic motions of right hand to mouth.

Whole left side paralysed and motionless (*Lach.*, *Arn.*).

Mouth distorted: loss of speech: stertor.

Jaw drops. Legs cold, without sensation.

Attack preceded by vertigo: buzzing in ears: nausea, urging to vomit.

Attacks after a hearty dinner; abuse of liquor or coffee: of high livers, leading an easy life.

Paralysis, especially of lower limbs.

When spoken to opens eyes, stutters, and sinks again to sleep. Eyes muddy, with purulent matter in canthi.

Pulse quick, hard: or full, sluggish.

Organs of deglutition and lower limbs completely paralysed. Maxilla right side relaxed.

Crotalus horridus Apoplectic convulsions.

Apoplexy in hæmorrhagic or broken down constitutions; or in inebriates.

Softening of brain, etc., or apoplexy following toxæmic states.

Fevers from septic absorption.

Hæmorrhages from every part of body.

Yellow colour of whole body.

Broken-down constitutions.

Occipital ache, in waves from spine. (Comp. *Glon.*)

Right side, and worse lying on right side.

ıesis .. *Purple, puffy face*, with convulsive movements. Blowing expiration (*Op.*).

Paralysis *especially of left side.*

Preceded by absence of mind: rushes of blood to head: throbbing, burning: worse vertex.

Face spotted, or purple: eyes engorged: looks suspicious (*Hyos.*).

Suffocation and strangling: cannot bear touch on throat, or anything near mouth.

Rouses from sleep with suffocation, dyspnœa, violent pain back of head. Worse heat, *worse sleep*, loquacity, suspicion, belong to *Lachesis*.

Cocculus .. Headache as if skull would burst : or like a great valve opening and shutting. (Comp. *Actea.*)

Pain as if opening and shutting in occiput and nape.

Apoplexy : violent headache, from vertex to left forehead and nose.

With nausea and inclination to vomit.

Whirling vertigo.

Inco-ordination. Numbness.

Loathing of food—thought, smell of food.

" Attack preceded by vertigo, nausea, convulsive motions of eyes, paralysis, especially of lower limbs, with insensibility."

Actea racemosa Brain as if too large : pressing from within outwards.

Rush of blood to head : brain feels too large for cranium.

An opening and shutting sensation, when moving head and eyes. (Comp. *Cocc.*)

Top of head as if it would fly off, worse going upstairs.

" Vertex opens and lets in cold air." (Comp. *Cocc.*).

Aurum met. .. Rushes of blood to head with violent palpitation.

Sparks before eyes : glossy, bloated face.

Intense pain in head : especially in syphilitic patients.

The *Aurum* patient looks on the dark side : is weary of life : loathes life : suicidal.

Absolute loss of enjoyment in everything.

Ipecacuanha .. " Apoplexia nervosa et serosa : vertigo : drooping of lips : impaired speech ; dribbling of saliva : paralysis of extremities.

" Headaches, as if bruised all through bones of head, down to root of nose, and roots of teeth, with nausea and vomiting.

" Nausea, distressing, constant ; not relieved by vomiting.

" Loose rattle in chest.

" No thirst.

" *Ipec.* is a great stopper of bleeding." KENT.

Phosphorus .. Apoplexy: suddenly fell unconscious. Life apparently extinct: pulse and resp. lost.
Face red, but, like body, cool to touch.
Irresponsive to all stimuli.
Apoplexy: grasps at head: mouth drawn to left.
Heaviness, dulness, confusion in head.
Hyperæmia of brain: heat, vertex: buzzing and throbbing in head: swelling under eyes.
Congestion up spine to head: burning, stinging, pulsations; begin in occiput.
Thirst for cold drinks.
Worse lying left side: alone: in twilight and in the dark.
Sees "things coming out of corners".

Stramonium .. Apoplectic seizures: paroxysms of syncope, with stertor. Bloody froth at mouth. Dark brown face. Lies on back with open, staring eyes. Fetches breath with great difficulty. Paralysis after apoplexy: spasmodic drawing of head to either side. One side twitches, the other paralysed. (Compare *Hell.*)
"An absolute stand-by in renal convulsions."
"*Stram.* has more violent delirium. *Hell.* is more stupid."

Helleborus .. Stupor complete or partial. Unconsciousness.
Lies on back, eyes partly open: or wide open and insensible to light.
Rolling head: bores into pillow.
Automatic motion of one arm and leg. (Compare *Stram.*)
Answers slowly, if at all. Appears semi-idiotic.
Greedily swallows water: bites the spoon.
Chewing motions of mouth.
Apoplexy followed by idiocy.

Isemium .. Threatened or actual apoplexy with stupor, coma, and nearly general paralysis.
Intense passive congestion to head.
Headaches with nausea, giddiness, staggering.
Brain tight: eyelids and limbs heavy.
Great weight and tiredness, body and limbs.
Face purple, mottled. "The trembling remedy."
Speech incoherent, stupid, forgetful.

Pulsatilla .. Throbbing, pressive headache, worse pressure. (Better pressure, *Bry.*)
Congestion of blood to head: stinging pulsation in brain, especially when stooping (*Bell.*).
Puls. is worse from heat: craves fresh cool air.
Weeps. Craves sympathy.

Sulphur .. An old homœopathic doctor, who had recovered from several cerebral hæmorrhages, used to say, "Mind! first *Arnica* and then *Sulphur*, for apoplexy." The *Sulphur* patient is lean, lank, hungry, dyspeptic.
Rush of blood to head: burning vertex with cold feet.

Nux moschata Stupor and insensibility. Comatose condition.
Apoplexy: A case: woman of 80. Comatose condition for nine weeks, after thrombosis. Coma increased till it was almost impossible to feed her. *Nux mosch.* 200, promptly brought back consciousness; she went on to complete recovery—and lived another five years, in full possession of her senses.

Zincum .. Followed *Nux mosch.* in the above case, and seemed to quickly re-establish the reflexes, and restore motion to the paralysed limbs.
Kent says; "When reflexes are abolished then *Zinc.* comes in."

Causticum .. "Paralysis from apoplexy: not for immediate results, but for remote symptoms when, after absorption, paralysis persists on opposite side of body."

Baryta carb. .. Complaints of both ends of life.
Especially adapted to apoplexy of old people, or tendency thereto. Mental and physical weakness. In persons addicted to alcohol.
Serous apoplexy, loss of speech, trembling limbs
Absent minded.
Has no clear perception.

(A tip—one doctor gives *Diphtherinum* for all paralytic cases.)

SOME COMMON REMEDIES FOR SLEEPLESSNESS WITH INDICATIONS.

Aconite .. Restlessness: excitement: tossing: fear: anguish: fear of death. Sudden chill in cold, dry weather.

Especially useful after chill: shock: fright: operation. But in any illness the *Aconite* condition may come on at night, when *Acon.* will give peace and sleep.

Chamomilla .. Sleepy, but cannot sleep (*Bell.*). Restless.

If he sits down by day, wishes to sleep, but if he lies down, is unable to sleep.

Pain that comes on at night, so violent that he cannot keep still: in a child, it wants to be carried: an adult, gets up and walks the floor.

Pains that drive him out of bed at night, with twitchings of limbs.

As soon as bedtime comes, is wide awake: is sleepless and restless, especially early night.

Chamomilla is irritable; capricious; uncivil. Frantic with " cannot bear it! "—in adults and *teething babies.*

Staphisagria .. " Doctor, if I ever have a dispute with a man, I come down with nervous excitement, sleeplessness: headache."

Child wakes, pushes everything away, and wants everybody to go away: restless, as from frightful dreams; calls for mother often.

ılcarea .. Sleepless from many thoughts crowding mind: or mind turning on same thought: from mortification at trifles.

The same disagreeable idea always rouses the sick as often as they fall into a light sleep.

Cold feet at night in bed.

Head sweats in sleep, wetting the pillow.

" Especially helps the real leucophlegmatic constitutions, with large head, large features, pale skin with chalky look and, in infants, open fontanelles:" (and delayed dentition).

Coffea .. The kind of lively sleeplessness some persons experience after drinking coffee.

Sleeplessness from coffee :—also :

Simply wide awake. Unusual activity of mind and body. Full of ideas, i.e. cannot sleep.

From sudden emotions, pleasant surprises, exciting or bad news. (Comp. *Cypreped.*)

Cyprepedium .. Sleeplessness : with desire to talk, or with crowding of pleasant ideas.

Children wake and are unnaturally bright and playful, with no desire to go to sleep again.

Pulsatilla .. " Sleep before midnight is prevented by a fixed idea : as a recurrent melody."

Wide awake in the evening, does not want to go to bed ; first sleep restless : sound sleep when it is time to get up. (Compare *Nux.*)

Sleepless from orgasm of blood : after late supper, or eating too much ; from ideas crowding in mind.

Weeping because she could not go to sleep.

Characteristic : Sleeps with arms over head.

The *Pulsatilla* patient is changeable : weepy : mild and yielding. (Reverse of *Nux.*)

Nux .. Insomnia after mental strain : abuse of coffee, wine, alcohol, opium or tobacco.

Sleeplessness from excessive study late at night.

Sleepy in the evening, hours before bedtime : awakes at 3 or 4 a.m. ; ideas crowd on him : then falls into a dreamy sleep at daybreak from which he is hard to rouse : wakes tired.

All complaints worse from morning sleep.

Nux is irritable and hypersensitive.

Sulphur .. Irresistibly drowsy by day : wakeful at night.

Sleepy in evening ; but nights full of unrest.

Tosses, nervous, excitable ; orgasm of blood.

Cannot go to sleep for great flow of thoughts with inclination to perspire.

Wakes at 3, 4, 5 a.m., and cannot sleep again. If does sleep later, cannot be roused. Gets his best and soundest sleep late in morning.

Soles burn at night : puts feet out (*Cham.*, *Puls.*, *Med.*). Worse warmth of bed (*Merc.*).

Arnica .. Too tired to sleep.
Bed feels too hard : and part laid on too sore ; must move to try for relief.
After exertion and strain, physical or mental.

Cocculus .. From vexation, grief, anxiety, and prolonged loss of sleep.
Worn out and exhausted, and when the time has come for sleep cannot sleep.
Ill-effects from long nursing and from night watching. Slightest loss of sleep tells on him.
Extreme irritability of nervous system.

Rhus .. Restless at night : has to change position frequently. (Comp. *Arnica.*)
Sleepless : could not remain in bed.
Sleepless *from pain* : has to turn often for ease.

Arsenicum .. Sleeplessness after midnight.
Sleeplessness with restlessness and moaning.
Tossing : uneasiness : anguish (*Acon.*).
Attacks of anxiety drive him out of bed.
Despair of life : fear of death : thinks it near.
Sleepless from anguish, restless : tossing : worse after midnight.
From climbing mountains, or other muscular exertion : want of breath, prostration, cannot sleep.
Nocturnal sleeplessness, with agitation and constant tossing.
Ars. is anxious, restless, usually chilly ; fastidious. Constant thirst for small sips.

Thuja .. Persistent sleeplessness.
Restless sleep, with frequent rising from bed, and much talking. < by moonlight (*Sil.*).
If he slumbers for a moment he dreams about dead people.
Sees apparitions on closing eyes, disappear when they are open, reappear as soon as they are closed (*Spongia.*).
After vaccination, or re-vaccination

Spongia .. Very short sleep, with many dreams. Wakes at midnight, but cannot sleep again on account of restlessness; whenever he closes his lids the most vivid pictures would immediately arise before his vision, while waking: it seemed to him as if a battery of guns were discharged, or as if everything were in flames; again scientific objects forced themselves upon his mind: in short a mass of subjects crossed each other in his imagination, disappearing at once when he opened his eyes, but reappearing so soon as they were closed.
Awakens in a fright and feels suffocating (*Lach.*).

Lachesis .. Has some of its most characteristic symptoms in regard to sleep.
All symptoms are worse after sleep.
Afraid to go to sleep; or the mother afraid to let the child sleep (croup, convulsions, etc.).
As soon as he goes to sleep, the breathing stops; cannot go clear off to sleep, because just on the verge of it he wakes catching for breath (*Spong.*).
Sleeps into an aggravation.
Awakens at night and cannot sleep again.
Could not sleep on account of strangulation.
Persistent sleeplessness. Sleepless from anxiety.
Afraid to go to sleep for fear he will die before he wakes.
Wakes in a fright: worse after sleep.
Nothing must touch throat: bedclothes must be lifted from abdomen at night.

["I once had a very obstinate case of constipation . . . he was at last taken with very severe attacks of colic. The pains seemed to extend all through the abdomen, and always came on at night. After trying various remedies until I was discouraged, he let drop this expression: 'Doctor, if I could only keep awake all the time, I would never have another attack.' I looked askance at him. 'I mean', said he, 'that I sleep into the attack, and waken in it.' I left a dose of *Lachesis* 200. He never had another attack of the pain, and his bowels became perfectly regular from that day and remained so. I could give more cases where this symptom has led me to the cure of ailments of different kinds." NASH.]

Silica .. Sleepless from ebullitions, orgasm of blood.

Night sweats.

Somnambulism : esp. at new and full moon.

Argentum nit. Prevented from falling asleep by fancies and images.

Wakes wife or child, for someone to talk to.

Arg. nit. has irresistible desire for sweets and sugar, which disagree.

Feels the heat. Full of weird apprehensions.

Belladonna .. Sleepy yet cannot sleep.

Uneasy sleep before midnight : child tosses, kicks and quarrels in sleep. Twitches.

Restless sleep with frightful dreams.

Skin dry and hot to touch : face red. Dilated pupils. Quick sensations and motions.

Fear of imaginary things : sees ghosts, animals, hideous faces. (Comp. *Thuja*, *Spong.*)

Stramonium .. Sleep full of turmoil and dreams.

Sleepy, but cannot sleep (*Bell.*, *Cham.*, *Opium*).

Desires light and company : cannot bear to be alone : worse in dark and solitude.

Cannot go to sleep in the dark : but soon falls asleep in a lighted room.

Hyoscyamus .. Intense sleeplessness of excitable persons from business troubles ; often imaginary.

From nocturnal, spasmodic cough : < lying down, > sitting up. Diseases with increased cerebral activity, but non-inflammatory.

" The sleep is a great tribulation to this nervous patient : times of sleeplessness : then again, profound sleep."

Sleepless ; or constant sleep. . . .

Lying on back suddenly sits up, looks all round, wonders what terrible thing he has been dreaming about. Sees nothing : lies down again. He keeps doing that all night.

Starts up : jerks : cries out : grits teeth : laughs in sleep.

Hyoscyamus is jealous and suspicious (*Lach.*) and has much delirium.

Opium .. .. Sleepy but cannot sleep. (*Bell.*, *Cham.*) Sleepless, *with acuteness of hearing*. Distant clocks striking and cocks crowing keep him awake.

Bed so hot she cannot lie on it: moves to find a cool place (*Sulph.*). (Bed too hard, moves to relieve soreness of parts lain on, *Arn.*)

Sleepless, full of unwelcome fancies and imaginations . . . as in delirium.

Capsicum .. Sleepless from emotions, *homesickness*, cough. Great drowsiness after eating.

Characteristic:—" Homesickness: with red cheeks and sleeplessness."

Bryonia .. Restless: could hardly sleep for half an hour; and when slumbering was continually busy with what he had read the previous evening.

Sleeplessness before midnight, with thirst, heat, ebullitions: with frequent shivering sensation of one arm and foot: then sweat.

Delusion, " away from home and wants to go home"

Cactus .. .. Sleeplessness from suffocative constriction (*Lach.*) and palpitation.

Ignatia .. Sleepless from grief, care, sadness.

Baptisia .. Restless from 3 a.m. Tosses about. Head and body feel scattered about the bed.

Abies nigra .. Sleepy by day: sleepless at night.

Indigestion with sensation of undigested hard boiled egg in stomach.

Allium sat. .. Sleep prevented by *thirst*.

Selenium .. Sleeps in cat-naps: (*Sulph.*) Wakes often: roused by slight disturbance.

Hungry in the night.

Plumbum .. Sleepiness by day: sleepless at night: from colic.

Inclined to take strangest attitudes and positions in bed.

Phosphorus .. Sleepy all day, all night restless : awakened by vivid dreams.
Sleeplessness before midnight.
Sleeplessness with drowsiness.
Phos. has fears alone, in the dark, of something creeping out of the corners.

Sepia .. .. A great remedy for sleeplessness in the *Sepia* patient : dull and indifferent : chilly, yet craves air. Hates sympathy and fuss. Often, with weariness and sagging of internal organs.

Mercurius .. Sleepless at night ; on account of anxiety, ebullitions and congestions ; from itching : from seeing frightful faces. Frequent waking.
Falls asleep late : wakeful till 3 a.m.
As soon as he went to bed, pains recommenced and banished sleep.
Night sweats.

Lueticum .. Sleepless nights : dreadful nights. All the sufferings are *worse at night.*

Always remember the nosodes of previous acute diseases, if severe or repeated : also family histories.

INDICATIONS FOR THE CHIEF REMEDIES IN COLLAPSE

Carbo veg. .. *An almost "corpse-reviver"* (as one has seen).

Lack of reaction after some violent shock, some violent attack, some violent suffering.

After surgical shock, collapse ; and danger of dying of shock.

Air-hunger : desire to be fanned : must have more air.

Cold :—Knees cold : breath cold : tongue cold : cold sweat : cold nose.

Nose and face pinched ; cadaveric.

Face : very pale : greyish-yellow ; greenish ; corpse-like.

May be distension of stomach and abdomen (*Colch.*).

Veratrum alb. .. Wonderful coldness : coldness of discharges : coldness of body.

Profuse cold sweat : cold sweat on forehead.

Fluids run out of body ; produces watery discharges.

Lies in bed, relaxed and prostrated, cold to finger-tips : blue, or purplish: lips cold and blue : face pinched and shrunken : sensation as if the blood were ice-water (*Ars.*).

Head packed in ice : ice on vertex.

One of Hahnemann's great cholera medicines.

Opium .. From fright. Shock from injury (*Arn.*), severe cases. Rapid breathing : every breath a loud moan : face livid or pale ; lips livid. Cool clammy skin : eyes fixed unequally :—or,

Long, slow expirations ; cheeks blown out : or mouth wide open.

Coldness, extremities ; or burning heat of perspiring body.

Characteristics : "painlessness, inactivity and torpor".

Increased excitability of voluntary muscles with decreased excitability of involuntary muscles.

Arnica .. From mechanical injuries (*Opium*). Concussion, with unconsciousness, pallor, drowsiness.

Cold surface; depressed vitality from shock.

Stupor with involuntary discharges.

Characteristic :—While answering falls into a deep stupor before finishing.

Camphor .. Coldness, blueness, *scanty sweat*. Scanty discharges (rev. of *Verat.*).

" *Camph.* is cold and dry. Cold, with profuse discharges, *Verat.*"

" *Camphor* in heat, wants to be covered up: his coldness is relieved by cold: wants more cold.

" A troublesome patient to nurse: the more violent the suffering, the sooner he is cold, and when cold must uncover and be in a cold room: then a flash of heat, and he wants covers on, wants hot bottles: and while this is being done, is cold again, and wants windows open, and everything cool.

" Here the camphor bottle has established a reputation*: but potentized camphor will do far more, and will put him into a refreshing sleep." KENT.

Arsenicum .. The collapse of *Ars.* is marked by restlessness, and fear. *Prostration with awful anxiety.*

" The prominent characteristics of *Ars.* are *anxiety, restlessness, prostration, burning*, and *cadaveric odours*.

" In bed, first moves whole body; as prostration becomes marked, can only move limbs. At last so weak, he lies quiet, like a corpse.

" Every symptom is *Arsenic*: he looks like it, acts like it, smells like it, and *is* it.

" Mouth black, parched and dry.

" Ceaseless thirst for small quantities often.

" With his violent chills and rigors, says the blood flowing through his veins is like ice-water (*Verat.*) then fever comes, and he feels that boiling water is going through his blood-vessels." KENT.

* N.B.—*Camphor* may need to be repeated every five minutes in desperate cases, till reaction is established. A couple of drops on a lump of sugar is the best way to administer it—or in potency.

Aconite .. Agonized tossing about. Excessively restless.
Extreme anxiety (*Ars.*). Expression of fear and anxiety ; especially *fear of death.*
Condition *sudden and violent.*
After exposure to cold, dry, wind.
Sits straight up and can hardly breathe : grasps throat : wants everything thrown off.
Anguish with dyspnœa.
As if boiling water poured into chest : warm blood rushing into the parts. (Comp. *Ars.*)
Compare *Ars.* all through : but *Ars.* comes far on in the condition, with *terrific exhaustion,* instead of *terrific violence.*

Antimonium tart. Asphyxia: from mechanical causes, as apparent death from drowning, from pneumonia, capillary bronchitis, etc., from accumulation of mucus which cannot be expectorated.
Impending paralysis of lungs.
Drowsiness or coma, pale or dark-red face ; blue lips : delirium ; twitchings.
Thread-like pulse.

Ammonium carb. Skin mottled, with great pallor. Face dusky, puffy.
Lack of reaction : livid, weak and drowsy.
Increasing shortness of breath : better cool air. Rattling in chest, but gets up little.
Weak heart, causing stasis, dyspnœa, etc.
Cold sweat : tendency to syncopy.
" One of the best remedies in emphysema."
Œdema of lungs with somnolence from poison of blood with CO_2.
Sputa thin, foamy : a dynamic state : with rattling of large bubbles in chest.
Vehement palpitation with great precordial distress, followed by syncope.
Audible palpitation : great anxiety as if dying, cold sweat : invol. flow of tears : loud, difficult breathing, with trembling hands.
Angina pectoris (*Latrodect. mact.*, etc.).
Exhaustion with defective reaction.
Hysteria ; symptoms simulate organic disease.

Carboneum sulph. Kent gives *Carb. sulph.* in black type for collapse.

Frequent attacks of fainting : asphyxia.

Violent headache till mind is affected.

Sunken, staring eyes.

Expression bewildered, as if demented.

Pushed lower jaw forward, and gnashed with it against the upper.

Great thirst : great desire for beer.

Colic about umbilicus, drawing navel in (*Plumb.*).

Asphyxia from alcohol, or coal gas.

Feeling of heavy load hanging on back between scapulæ.

Sensation of vibration and trembling of whole body.

Heard voices and believed he had committed a robbery. Sensation of a hole close by, into which he was in danger of falling.

Colchicum .. Sinking of strength, as if life will flow out from motion or exertion.

If he attempts to raise head, it falls back, mouth wide open.

Tongue heavy, stiff (? bluish, especially at base).

Bruised, sore, sensitive : *nauseated by smell or thought of food.*

Vomiting. Profuse diarrhœa and passage of blood. Stools involuntary.

Great distension of abdomen :—tympanitic.

Restlessness : cramps in legs.

Great prostration, skin cold, bedewed with sweat : cold sweat forehead (*Verat.*).

Respiration slow.

But, " without the fearfulness and dread of death of some such remedies ".

Crotalus hor. .. Rapidly becomes besotted, benumbed, putrid, semi-conscious.

Prostration almost paralytic in character.

Skin yellow, pale, bloodless with blue spots.

Rapid breaking down of bloodvessels.

SOME REMEDIES FOUND USEFUL IN SUNSTROKE WITH INDICATIONS

Glonoinum .. *Glonoine* (*Nitro-glycerine*)

Bad effects from being exposed inordinately to sun's rays:

" For over-heating in the sun, or sunstroke."

" Sudden local congestions, especially to head and chest.

" Bursting headache, rising up from the neck.

" Great throbbing: sense of expansion, as if head would burst.

" Cannot bear the least jar." NASH.

Undulating sensation in head:

Waves of heat, upwards.

Head feels larger.

Congestions; blood tends upwards.

Vessels (jugular, temporal,) pulsate.

Temporal arteries raised, felt like whipcord.

Throbbing: constriction neck, as if blood could not return from head.

Sensation of strangulation in throat (*Lach.*).

Whole head felt crowded with blood.

All arteries in head felt as distinct as though they had been dissected out.

Skull too small: brain attempting to burst it.

Even nausea, followed by unconsciousness.

" *Bell.* and *Glon.* both have the fullness, pain and throbbing, but that of *Glon.* is more intense and sudden in onset; and subsides more rapidly when relieved.

Bell. is better bending head back: *Glon.* worse." NASH.

Glon. has waves of pain, of blood, upwards.

Glon. has more disturbance of heart's action: *Bell.* more intense burning of skin.

Both have very red faces (*Mel.*).

Melilotus .. *Sweet Clover*

Fearful headaches.

Confusion of thought.

Violent congestion to head.

Violent *throbbing* headache, relieved by nose-bleed.

Most intense redness of face with throbbing carotids.

Belladonna .. Also (with *Glon.*), sudden onset.

Red, flushed face: throbbing carotids: perhaps delirium, spasms, jerks and twitchings.

Eyes staring, red, bloodshot: pupils first contracted, then greatly dilated.

Skin very red and hot: "When you put your hand on a *Bell.* subject, you want to suddenly withdraw it; the heat is so intense." KENT.

Rush of blood to head: pulsation of cerebral arteries; throbbing in head.

Inflammation of base of brain and medulla from exposure to sun.

Bell. absolutely covers the text-book description of sunstroke—even at its worst: i.e. restlessness; vertigo: breathlessness; nausea and vomiting; with frequent micturition (" even if only a few drops have accumulated "). Temperature high.

Incontinence of urine and fæces.

Stertor. Pulse rapid.

Face congested: cyanosed: and (of course) convulsions.

Early cases are best remembered! Ages ago a cottage boy who had been reading in a broiling sun had, at 5.30 p.m. a burning head, a severe frontal headache and a Temp. of 103·8. In a funny little first Case Book one finds it recorded that he got *Bell. cm.* and (in those days of inexperience) *Acon. cm.*; frequent sips. At 10.30 next morning, Temp. was 98; skin moist and cool; no headache.

Aconite .. Where there is much FEAR, restlessness, and anxiety.

" Sunstroke, especially from sleeping in the sun's rays."

Head excessively hot (*Bell.*): with burning, as though brain were moved by boiling water.

Boiling and seething sensations.

High fever. Vertigo.

Face very red (*Bell.*, *Stram.*, *Melilotus*): feels as if it has grown much larger (*Nat. carb.*).

Tingling sensations exceedingly characteristic.

One of the remedies of apoplexy: of heat apoplexy.

Acon. is one of the remedies of sudden, violently acute, painful conditions.

Amyl nitrate .. Heat and throbbing in head. Intense fullness in head.

Intense surging of blood to face and head (*Glon.*) as if blood would start through the skin.

Can't endure warmth: must throw off coverings and open doors and windows.

Difficulty of breathing is a very prominent symptom.

(One will never forget a personal experience with *Amyl nitrate*, bought for an epileptic patient. When the little glass was broken, and the contents sniffed at, the instant sensation was as if the brain would burst: there was a rush to open the window, and to take deep breaths. Soon over—luckily!) *Glonoine*, potentized, is useful to avert cerebral hæmorrhage: in crude form it might be disastrous.

Camphor .. Sunstroke, with restlessness and depression of spirits.

Contraction, tightness in head, *with coldness all over*.

Throbbing (head) with beats like a hammer; head hot, face red, limbs cool. (Comp. *Arn.*)

Rush of blood to head.

"The more violently the patient suffers the sooner he is cold, and when he is cold he must uncover, even in a cold room."

"Then, with a flash of heat, wants the covers on, and hot bottles." KENT.

Veratrum viride .. Sudden cerebral congestion: sunstroke.

Prostration: accelerated pulse.

Head full and heavy.

Intense cerebral congestion: as if head would burst open.

Congestive apoplexy: intense headache; stupid: ringing in ears; bloodshot eyes; thick speech: *slow*, full pulse, hard as iron.

? nausea and vomiting. ? convulsions.

Worse warm drinks.

Face, cold, bluish; covered with cold sweat. Or, face flushed.

Characteristic; tongue (? white or yellow) ***with a red streak down the centre.***

Cactus .. " Constrictions, contractions, congestions : the blood is always in the wrong place."

Vertigo from congestion : face red, bloated.

Irregularities of respiration : if he holds his breath, it seems as if his heart would fly to pieces. Increased pulsations also over body when holding breath.

Violent headaches ; intense heat of head ;

As if top of head would be pressed in, relieved by pressing hard on the pain.

Sounds go through the head.

Threatened apoplexy when congestion is so violent ; face flushed and purple, or very red ; pulsation felt in brain and all over. Choking as from a tight collar. (Comp. *Lach.*)

The great characteristic, constriction about heart, as if held in a vice, a wire cage ; screwed tighter and tighter.

Gelsemium .. From heat of sun in summer.

Weakness and *trembling*, of any part, or the whole body.

Headache, begins in cervical spine : with bursting sensation in forehead and eyeballs. Worse from heat of sun.

Sensation of a band around head above eyes.

Great heaviness of eyelids.

Lachesis .. *Lachesis* has also a reputation for sunstroke, or effects of sunstroke.

"Paralysis depending on an apoplectic condition of brain, after extremes of heat or cold."

Face : dark red, *bluish* ; bloated ; as in apoplexy.

Great characteristic : worse from SLEEP.

Sleeps into an aggravation.

Dreads to go to sleep, because she wakes with such a headache.

Rush of blood to head : weight and pressure on vertex.

Great sensitiveness to touch, especially throat and abdomen.

Stramonium .. Face very red: blood rushes to face.
Congestion to head: beating of carotids.
Rushes of blood to head, with furious, loquatious delirium.
After sunstroke tormenting heat in head: pain nape of neck: very sensitive to noise, to contradiction.

NASH gives a *Stramonium* mental case, in a **woman of 30**, who had been over-heated in the sun, during an excursion. She was "lost, lost, lost, eternally lost," and begged minister, doctor, everybody to pray with and for her. Talked day and night about it. She would not sleep a wink, or let anybody else sleep. Said her head was as big as a bushel . . . *Glonoine*, *Lachesis*, *Natrum carb.*, etc., prescribed on the CAUSE as the basis of the prescription, were useless. But *Stramonium* covered her symptoms, and in 24 hours every vestige of that mania was gone. She had narrowly escaped the "Utica Asylum"

Arnica .. *Arnica* may be needed. Apoplexy; loss of consciousness.
Here the great characteristic, in any sickness, is, intense soreness and bruised feeling of body.
EVERYTHING ON WHICH HE LIES FEELS TOO HARD.
Must move, to get a new place, not yet sore.
Heat of upper part of body; coldness of lower.
Face and head alone hot: body cool (*Camph.*).

Carbo veg. .. Ailments from getting over heated.
Obtuseness: vertigo: heaviness of head.
Pale greenish face, cold, with cold sweat.
Vital force nearly exhausted. Complete collapse.
Blood stagnates in capillaries: surface cold and blue. Air hunger.

Natrum carb. .. Chronic effects of sunstroke.
Headache from slightest mental exertion: *from the sun*, even working under gas light.
Inability to think. Feels stupid: comprehension slow, difficult.
Head feels too large, as if it would burst (*Acon.*).
Great debility from heat of summer.
Aversion to, and worse from milk.

Natrum mur. .. Sunstroke. Heat in head, with red face nausea and vomiting.
Rush of blood to head: headache as if head would burst (*Glon.* etc.).
Heaviness occiput; draws eyes together.
Blinding of eyes: fiery zig-zags characteristic
Worse sun: worse seaside: worse summer.

Pulsatilla .. Ailments from heat of sun.
Excessive vertigo. Headache with throbbing in brain.
Even apoplexy; unconscious: face purplish, bloated: violent beating of heart. Pulse collapsed.
Puls. is worse sitting; lying: better walking in open air. *Puls.* is apt to be tearful.

* * *

N.B. A red, or orange lining to hat, and coat along spine, is said to protect from sunstroke. One remembers well the case of an officer who, in India, had had many attacks of sunstroke, but was free from these, when he got his red linings. But his brother officers, thinking it imaginative, secretly removed them, whereupon, believing himself safe in the intense sunshine, he got his worst "stroke".

SOME REMEDIES OF HEPATITIS

WITH INDICATIONS

Aconite .. " *Sudden* inflammation of liver, first attack.
Violent, rending, tearing pains : burning.
Restlessness : tortures of anxiety : moving constantly : fear of death : great thirst." KENT.

Belladonna .. " More sensitive to jar and more sensitive to motion (*Bry.*) than almost any other remedy." KENT.
Severe pain right hypochondrium on a small spot near and above umbilicus. Worse motion : very sensitive to touch.
Acute pain, liver, worse lying right side (*Merc.*, *Mag. mur.*) ; pains go to shoulder (*Chel.*, *Crot. h.*) and neck : or spread to back (*Chel.*) and kidneys. Get rapidly worse.
Cause retching and vomiting of bile : has to bend double (*Kali c.*).
Can tolerate no pressure OR JAR.
Thirst for cold water : or thirst for water changed into thirst for beer (*Nat. m.*, *Merc.*).
Desire for lemons and lemonade which help.
Belladonna is red, and hot.

Bryonia .. " Inflammation and many liver symptoms.
Liver, especially right lobe, lies like a load in hypochondrium.
Every breath, every motion, every touch causes pain. Stitches and burning, with nausea and retching. Spits up bile.
When he coughs, feels liver will burst " (*Nat. sulph.*). KENT.

Chamomilla .. " Excessive sensibility of nerves ; so excessive that few remedies can equal it " (*Hep.*, *Nux*).
Intense irritability : and its consequences.
Hepatitis after vexation, or taking cold.
Stitching pains in liver with vomiting and chilliness : after vexation.
Jaundice after a fit of anger (*Nux*).
Vomiting of bile and food.

Chelidonium .. *One of our greatest liver medicines.*

Congestion ; inflammation ; fullness ; enlargement ; in semi-chronic and acute cases this remedy proves suitable.

Stitching ; shooting ; tearing pains from liver region through to back. (See *Bell.*, *Kali carb.*)

Characteristic pain *below right shoulder angle ;* cord-like constriction round hypochondria (*Lyc.*). JAUNDICE.

An old reputation with homœopaths for early pneumonias. " Liver and Lungs."

Better hot drinks (*Ars.*) : HOT MILK : eating.

Podophyllum .. Congestion, and enlargement of liver : acute and chronic hepatitis.

Great irritability of liver : excessive secretion of bile.

Pain, liver : inclined to rub it with hand.

Stuffed feeling : distension, liver (*Ars.*).

Worse thought or smell of food (*Ars.*, *Sep.*).

Slimy tongue : as if spread with mustard : tooth-notched.

Everything goes wrong : all dark : no light.

Cannot sit still for fidgets, body (feet, *Zinc.*).

Mercurius .. Pressing pain or stitches, liver. Cannot lie on right side (*Bell.*, *Mag. mur.*). Liver tender to touch.

Bitter taste, thirst, little appetite.

Liver swollen, hard. Distension. Jaundice.

" The liver furnishes much trouble. Our forefathers took blue mass every Spring to regulate the liver, and tapped their livers with it ! i.e. they had worse livers than if the doctors had stayed at home." KENT.

Worse Spring, night, warmth of bed.

Desire for beer (*Bell.*, *Nat. m.*); iced water ; milk ; for sweets, which disagree ; bread and butter.

Aversion to meat, wine, brandy, coffee.

Cornus cer. .. Chronic hepatitis and bilious derangements. Jaundice.

Constant working of bowels, as if they were all in motion.

Sensation as if she would break in two at waist.

Magnesia mur. Pressing pain, liver, when walking (*Hep.*, *Ptel.*), or touching it : worse lying right side (*Bell.*, *Merc.*) ; liver hard and enlarged.
Can only lie on left side for sensation of something dragging over to that side.
Chronic induration and pressive pain, extending to stomach and back.
Recurring attacks indigestion, biliousness, constipation ; large hard stools like balls.
Eats frequently to ease gnawing in stomach. (Comp. *Chel.*, *Graph.*)
Marked enlargement liver, with ascites.

Nux vom. .. Constrictive pain hypochondriac region.
Liver swollen, indurated, sensitive, with pressure and stinging : must loosen clothing.
Soreness, with pain right shoulder (*Bell.*, *Chel.*, *Crot. h.*). Acute congestion, liver.
Jaundice from anger (*Cham.*), high living.
Sufferings from much worry ; from too much mental and too little bodily exertion.
Longs for brandy, beer, fats which disagree.
Aversion to meat, tobacco, coffee, water, ale.
Chilly : irritable (*Cham.*, *Hep.*) to verge of insanity : hyper-sensitive to air, light, noise.

China .. Swollen, hard liver : sensitive to least pressure or touch.
Sensation of subcutaneous ulceration.
Obstruction of gall-bladder with colic : periodic recurrence : jaundice. Biliary calculi.
" Nerves in a fret ", feeble, sensitive, anæmic, chilly.
Periodicity in regard to pains, and complaints.

Camphora .. Constrictive pain below short ribs, extending to lumbar vertebrae.
Aching in anterior part of liver.
" With ' acute ' *Camphor* there is prostration, blueness, coldness, yet he wants to be uncovered. In *Camphor*, during heat and when pains are on, he wants to be covered up: but the cold stage is relieved by cold : he wants more cold." KENT.

Hepar .. .. Hepatitis with jaundice; with white or greenish stools.
Sticking pain in liver when walking (*Mag. mur.*).
Liver enlarged two or three inches beyond ribs.
Chronic engorgement of liver.
Useful during inflammatory process in cirrhosis of liver. Hepatic abscesses (*Phos.*, *Lach.*, *Sil.*, etc.).
Typical *Hepar* is quarrelsome: nothing pleases, everything disturbs. Becomes intensely angry; abusive; impulsive: even to violent impulses to destroy. (Comp. *Nux.*)
Oversensitive physically also, to cold, to draughts. Desire for vinegar.

Hippozæninum Hepatitis with gangrenous and ulcerative inflammation of gall ducts.
Liver greatly enlarged, often showing signs of fatty degeneration.
Useful in low forms of suppuration and catarrh, malignant ulcerations and swellings.
Abscesses.

Lachesis .. Acute pain liver; extends to stomach (*Ars.*).
Inflammation and chronic obstruction.
Cannot bear any pressure about hypochondria. (*Calc.*, *Lyc.*, *Nat. sul.*, *Nux*, *Crot. h.*, *Ptel.*)
Pain ulcerative: as from suppuration: under ribs.
Liver swollen and painful in anterior, superior aspect.
Abscess of liver (*Phos.*, *Hep.*, *Crot. h.*, *Hipp.*, *Sil.*).
Typical *Lachesis* is hot, bluish, *loquacious*, jealous, suspicious.

Crotalus hor. .. Intolerance of clothing about hypochondria and epigastric region (*Lach.*).
Pain, stitches, aching in liver and on the top of shoulder (*Bell.*, *Chel.*, *Nux*). Urine jelly-like and red like blood.
Passive hepatic congestion: acute atrophy of liver.
Jaundice; malignant jaundice: dark hæmorrhages from nose, mouth, etc., black vomit.
In malignant or malarial fevers. Specific for black water fever.

Sulphur .. (KENT says), " The liver is a very troublesome organ, with enlargement, engorgement, induration, pain, pressure and distress.

If stomach symptoms, they are exaggerated.

He becomes jaundiced, is subject to gall-stones. A victim to chronic sallowness, which increases and decreases.

Every cold settles in the liver: every 'cold', every bath, every change of weather aggravates his liver symptoms, and when these are worse he has less of other troubles.

It localizes itself in bilious vomiting and bilious headaches.

Stools black, then green, then white; alternate and change with engorgement of liver."

But in the *Sulphur* patient. Warm: hungry: loves fat, etc., will clinch diagnosis.

Phosphorus .. Diffuse hepatitis.

Hyperæmia and enlargement of liver.

Liver hard, large, with subsequent atrophy.

Hepatitis when suppuration ensues, hectic fever, night sweats, marked soreness over liver (*Hepar, Hipp. Lach., Crot. h., Sil.*).

Jaundice. Pale stools. Abdomen tympanitic.

Hepatic congestion, quantities of bright, or dark blood discharged with stool.

Craves cold food and drink: ice cream: wine.

" Bad effects from excessive use of salt."

A characteristic symptom: as soon as water becomes warm in stomach it is vomited.

Arsenicum .. Hepatitis. Tension, pressing pain in liver which is enlarged.

Painful bloating right hypochondrium with stitches which extend to stomach (*Lach.*).

Violent burning, like red-hot coals in epigastrium. Burning thirst with no desire to drink: or thirst for small quantities.

The burnings of *Ars.* are relieved by heat: by hot drinks.

Always with the *Ars.* restlessness; anxiety; prostration.

Nitric acid .. Liver enormously enlarged. Jaundice.
Urine scanty and strong smelling.
Chronic hepatitis : " ague cake ".
Stitches in liver region.

Natrum mur. .. Fullness liver, with stitching, tearing, rending pains.
Liver inflamed, swollen : skin yellow, earthy. Pain liver, after eating, better as digestion advances.
Jaundice with drowsiness.
Aversion to meat, bread, coffee.
Better on an empty stomach.
Longs for bitter things, beer (*Bell.*, *Merc.*), farinaceous things, sour things, salt, oysters, fish, milk.
Ravenous hunger towards noon.
Especially useful after malaria, and much quinine.

Lycopodium .. Tension like a cord or hoop, liver region (*Chel.*) : cannot stretch or stand upright (*Sil.*).
Sore pain, as from a blow, right hypochondriac region : worse touch.
Hepatitis, especially of children (? with pneumonia). Jaundice with flatulence.
Characteristics : worse afternoon : 4-8 p.m.
Intense flatulence : everything turns to wind.
Bloating : must loosen clothes. A mouthful fills him up to throat.
Better warm drinks (*Ars.*). Desire for sweets (*Arg. nit.*).

Ptelia .. Dragging weight in both hypochondria when walking (*Hep.*, *Mag. mur.*).
Liver swollen, sore : clothes too tight.
Congestion of liver : chronic hepatitis.
Voracious (or poor) appetite.
Repugnance to animal food and rich puddings of which he is fond ; to butter ; fats, which aggravate epigastric pain.
Hepatic and gastric symptoms worse from cheese, meat, puddings.

Natrum sulph. Cannot bear tight clothing about waist.
Liver enlarged, swollen and sore to touch.
With deep breath, violent stitch as if in liver; as if it would burst open there (*Bry.*).
Worse lying on left side (*Card. m.*, *Kali carb.*).
Nausea: vomit sour: then bile.
Worse wet weather: damp houses: sea air.
Suicidal. After head-injuries.

Carduus marianus Liver engorged: swelled laterally.
Pressure, drawing pain, stitches in liver.
Worse lying left side.
Sensitiveness and induration left lobe liver, causing difficult breathing and a cough.
Diseased liver has implicated lungs, with hæmoptysis: simple congestion, or inflammation of liver and lungs. **Vomiting of blood.**
A proving showed nausea, uneasiness, pain, vomiting, with inflation of abdomen.

Kali carb. .. Heat, burning, pinching in liver: wrenching pain on stooping.
Painful stitches right lumbar and liver: worse motion: sits stooped forward, elbows on knees and face in hands.
Must walk stooped forward, hands on knees, to steady body against motion. (See *Bell.*)
Sprained pain, liver; can only lie on right side (*Nat. sul.*, etc.)

Calcarea .. "A peculiar feature: the greater the internal congestion, the colder the surface." KENT.
Sore pain, liver and spleen.
Pressure hepatic region with every step.
Enlargement of liver.
Tight clothes about hypochondria are unbearable (*Lach.*, etc.)
Characteristics: longing for eggs: ice-cream: lemonade (*Bell.*).
Coldness: general: of single parts.
Sweat: general, of single parts. Of head during sleep.
Disposed to grow fat.

SOME REMEDIES OF JAUNDICE WITH INDICATIONS.

Aconite .. "*Acon.* alone will often remove the whole disease, or *Merc.*, provided the patient had not abused it previously, in which case *China* should be given." LILIENTHAL.

Agonized tossings. Anxiety. Urine dark and hot.

Attack sudden and with violence.

Unquenchable thirst for large quantities, but drinking increases the thirst.

Everything but water tastes bitter.

Tenderness pit of stomach.

*Mercurius sol.** Skin yellow: great itching, worse at night, worse warm in bed.

Intense thirst with moist tongue and much saliva. Taste bitter: sweet: saltish: putrid.

Tongue large, flabby, shows imprint of teeth (*Chel.*).

Profuse sweat, which does not relieve: may stain yellow.

" Rarely give *Merc.* if tongue is dry."

Characteristic, *Worse lying on right side.*

Characteristic, offensive sweat and saliva.

Chelidonium .. " Pressive pain liver region. Bitter taste in mouth.

Tongue thickly coated yellow, with red margins showing imprint of teeth.

Yellow whites of eyes, face, hands, skin.

Stools gray, or yellow as gold.

Urine yellow, or dark brown, leaves a yellow colour on vessel.

Loss of appetite, disgust and nausea, or vomiting of bile.

Patient can retain nothing but hot drinks.

A usual characteristic symptom, right infra-scapular pain.

In acute or chronic cases." NASH.

* *The liver furnishes much trouble. Our forefathers for years took blue mass every spring to regulate the liver. They physicked themselves with it and tapped their liver every spring with it, and as a result they had worse livers than they would have had if the doctors had stayed at home.*—KENT.

Digitalis .. Excessive jaundice, with slow weak heart and ashy-white stools.*

Nux vom. .. Sullen : surly : scolds and abuses if talked to.
Chilly if he moves or uncovers : can't turn in bed because if air gets clothes it makes him chilly.
Bitter taste : bread tastes
Face yellow.
Liver may be swollen, indurated, sensitive, sore.
Hyperæsthesia, mental and physical.
Jaundice after anger (*Cham.*).

Chamomilla .. JAUNDICE caused by a fit of anger (*Nux*).
" *Cham.* has a bad temper, *Nux* is malicious."
Inflamed liver from vexation or pain.
Nearly wild : " Cannot bear it ! " from pain or irritability.
Oversensitive mentally and physically (*Nux*).

Natrum sulph. Dirty greenish coating on tongue : bitter coating on tongue.
Constant taste of bile.
Jaundice after anger (*Cham., Nux*) with hepatitis.
Cannot digest starchy foods.
Food wells up—regurgitation.
Distension and weight p.c. : almost constant nausea (*Ipec.*).
Vomits slime, sour, bitter.
Liver engorged, worse lying left side.
Cutting pains in engorged liver : soreness, acute cases.

* NASH *gives an interesting case of* Digitalis *jaundice. A young man of good habits was taken with nausea and vomiting. He was drowsy, and after a couple of days he began to grow very jaundiced all over. The sclerotica were yellow as gold, as was, indeed, the skin all over the body, even to the nails. The stools were natural as to consistence,* but perfectly colourless, *while the urine was as* brown as lager beer, *or even more so. Where you could see through it, on the edge of the receptacle, it was as yellow as fresh bile. The pulse was only* thirty beats per minute, *and often dropped a beat.*

This was a perfect Digitalis *case of jaundice, and this remedy cured him perfectly in a few days, improvement in his feelings taking place very shortly after beginning it; the stools and urine gradually taking on their natural colour. The characteristic slow pulse was the leading symptom to the prescription, for all the rest of the symptoms may be found in almost any well-developed case of severe jaundice.*

Myrica cerifera	Proving shows " an accurate picture of severe catarrhal jaundice." Dull : drowsy : despondent : giddy. Eyes congested and yellow. Thick, yellow, dark, dry coating on tongue : renders it almost immovable ; also on palate. Sensation as if pharynx would crack. Taste bad, foul, bitter, nauseous. Stools daily paler, till destitute of bile. *Jaundice of infants.*
Bryonia ..	Jaundice, with liver symptoms. Liver, especially right lobe, lies like a load. Soreness to pressure : cannot move. Worse motion, touch, respiration. A deep breath causes pain through liver : it burns and stitches. When he coughs, it feels as if liver would burst.
Chionanthus vir.	Enormous liver : constipation : stools clay-coloured : Skin and urine as in severe cases of jaundice : great emaciation. Hypertrophy of liver. Obstruction of liver in malarious districts. Sore liver : stools undigested showing absence of bile : urine almost black. Chronic jaundice. Jaundice of years standing, recurring every summer. Sensation of something alive and moving in stomach (*Croc.*, *Thuja*). " Jaundice with arrest of menses." CLARKE.
Aurum muriaticum natronum	" Obstinate cases of jaundice, with alternating white and black stools." NASH.
Leptandra ..	Has a reputation for jaundice : its typical stools are " black, tarry, bilious, with a jaundiced skin ". Burnings, hepatic region. Sore bursting ache over gall-bladder or liver, extending to navel, or left scapula. < cold drinks—motion. > lying on stomach or side.

Dolichos prur. ..	Jaundice ; white stools. Violent itching over the body, without visible eruption.
Sepia	Inflammation of liver: enlargement with jaundice, pain, fullness, distension. Distress in region of liver. Typical *Sepia* has loss of affection: indifference. All-gone, empty, hungry feeling, not relieved, or not long relieved by food. "When these symptoms group themselves, gnawing hunger, constipation, dragging down sensations with the mental condition, it is *Sepia* and *Sepia* only." KENT. Bitter eructations: bitter vomiting. Nausea especially in the morning. Relief from sleep, from a short sleep (*Phos.*).
China (*Cinchona off.*)	Swollen, hard liver: with pain, worse touch. Obstruction gall bladder with colic and jaundice. Taste bitter. Aversion to bread, beer, butter, meat, fats: to warm food, to coffee. Canine hunger at night: or loss of appetite, especially in foggy weather. Abdomen distended, tympanitic: must loosen garters and waistbands. Worse fish, fruit, wine. Flatulence almost to bursting: loud eructations with no relief. Weakness and debility: worse draught of cold air.
Nitric acid ..	Jaundice: pain in region of liver: urine scanty and strong-smelling: very restless after midnight. Chronic affection of liver: jaundice. Liver enormously enlarged: clay-coloured stools. "Liver-cake" of ague. Stitches in liver region. Typical *Nitric a.* craves salt and fats. Its pains are stitching, "splinter-like" pains: sharp on touch. Depressed, irritable: anxiety about his disease.

Berberis .. Bilious colic followed by jaundice.
Sticking, stabbing pains in liver: has to bend over.

Years ago a villager used to come from time to time to beg a few twigs from our Barberry tree. He used the yellow fibres just below the bark, steeping them in beer, and drinking a wine-glassful every day, to cure his " yaller jaunders ".

Carduus mar. .. Bitter taste.
Tongue white, with tip and edges red.
Nausea: vomits acid, green fluid.
Fullness liver: tension and pressure, worse lying left side.
" Liver complaints with jaundice."
The usual clay-coloured stools and dark urine.

Plumbum .. " H. N. Guernsey claimed great powers for it in jaundice; whites of eyes, skin, stool and urine all very yellow, and I have prescribed it with success." NASH.
NASH's great indication for *Plumb.* is, *Great hyperæsthesia with loss of power.*

Iodum .. " Chronic: not due to obstruction." CLARKE.
Typical *Iodum*: emaciates while eating well.
" The same restlessness and anxiety of body and mind as *Ars.* but if the patient is hot-blooded we would never think of *Ars.*, if a cold-blooded and shivering patient, we would never think of Iodine." KENT.

Arsenicum .. Jaundice: after intermittent fevers; especially after abuse of quinine: after *Mercury.*
Induration of liver.
Painful bloatedness right hypochondrium.
Typical *Ars.* has extreme restlessness and anxiety (see *Iodum*). Chilly, with burnings relieved by heat. Prostration out of proportion, as it seems.

Arsenic causes jaundice. One remembers a case of acute arsenical poisoning. Face deepest yellow, almost black: bringing up mouthfuls of dark bloody material: unconscious: convulsed from time to time. It was a question of *Phos.*, or *Ars.* But turned out to be *Arsenic.*

Conium .. Jaundice with intense vertigo: when lying: on turning or moving head, or eyes.
Must keep head perfectly still.
Liver may be hard, swollen, tender.
Objects may look red, rainbow-coloured.
Weakness and dazzling of eyes, with vertigo.

Phosphorus .. Jaundice with liver symptoms. *Phos.* causes and may cure, congestion, fullness, pain, tenderness, induration of liver.
Phos. craves cold food and drink: ices.
Is worse lying on the left side.
Is better after sleep, even a short sleep (*Sep.*).
Usually loves salt: fears thunder—the dark—being alone.

Crotalus hor. .. "Jaundice, (?) more of hæmatic than hepatic origin.
Gained its greatest laurels in liver troubles of hot climates."
Yellow eyes, yellow face, whole body yellow.
A low typhoid state: hæmorrhagic diathesis.
Yellow fever: black-water fever.
Malignant jaundice (*Ars.*, *Phos.*, *Lach.*, etc.)
In septic or puerperal fevers.
(May have illusions of blue colours, see *Conium.*)

Lachesis .. "Has a series of liver troubles with jaundice.
Congestion: inflammation: enlarged liver and the nutmeg liver.
Cutting like a knife in liver region.
Vomiting of bile: of everything taken into stomach.
Extreme nausea: continuous nausea with jaundice. White stool.
Sensitiveness of abdomen: can scarcely allow her clothes to touch her." KENT.
Lies flat on her back, with clothing lifted from abdomen.
Excessively sensitive to touch, esp. throat and abdomen.
Aggravation from sleep: worse on waking.
Lach. is typically loquacious: jealous: suspicious. Makes mistakes in time of day.

SOME REMEDIES OF GALL-STONE COLIC

WITH INDICATIONS

KENT writes under *Belladonna* : " Spasms—general spasms and local spasms. Spasms of little canals, of the circular fibres, of tubular organs. In the ductus communis choledochus there is a clutching—or it may be in the cystic duct that the circular fibres clutch that little bit of stone and will not let it through. The passage is large enough to admit it and it has started to go through—but the irritation of the part causes a spasm and it clutches that little stone. You put a dose of *Belladonna* on his tongue, the spasm lets up, the stone passes on, and there is no more trouble ; in fifteen minutes the gall-stone colic is gone. There is never a failure in homœopathic prescribing in gall-stone colic. The symptoms are not always *Bell.*, but in this instance, where that horrible sensitiveness is present, it is *Bell.*"

Belladonna .. Extreme sensitiveness : especially to jarring.
Face red : hot.
Hyperæsthesia : extreme irritability of whole economy or nerve centres.
Extreme excitability.

Chelidonium .. Pains from region of liver, shooting towards back and shoulder. (*Hydras.*)
Pain in region of liver, extending quickly down across navel into intestines.
" Biliary calculi : chill : intense pain in gall-bladder region ; vomiting ; clay-coloured stools."
Cutting pains and stitches : constriction like a cord.
Pain inner angle of right shoulder blade, running into chest.
Yellow tongue with indented edges.
Liver region tense and tender.

One has recently seen several patients who came up many years ago for gall-stone colic, and who got Chel. 6 t.d.s. for several days, then Chel. cm. at long intervals, and who have been free for years. They used to pass gall-stones after terrific pain.

KENT says: "*Chelidonium* has cured gall-stone colic. Practitioners who know how to direct a remedy, relieve gall-stone colic in a few minutes. We have remedies that act on the circular fibres of these little tubes, causing them to relax, and allow the stone to pass painlessly. In a perfect state of health, of course, there are no stones in the bile that is held in the gall-bladder, but this little cystic duct opens its mouth and a little gall-stone engages in it, and the instant it does it creates an irritation by scratching along the mucus membrane of that little tube. *When this pain is a shooting, stabbing, tearing, lancinating pain, extending through to the back, Chelidonium will cure it.* The instant it relieves the patient says, "Why, what a relief: that pain has gone." The remedy has relieved that spasm, the little duct opens up and the stone passes through. Every remedy that is indicated by the symptoms will cure gall-stones."

China .. FARRINGTON says: "*Bell.* is useful in cholelithiasis, but the remedy to cure the condition permanently is *Cinchona.* Unless some symptom or symptoms call specifically for another drug, put your patient on a course of *Cinchona.*"

Pain in hepatic region, worse from touch.

Shooting in region of liver, tenderness and pain on touching the part. Liver region sensitive to least pressure.

Obstruction in gall bladder with colic; periodic recurrence; yellow skin and conjunctivæ; constipation with dark greenish scybala.

Biliary calculi.

Intensely sensitive to touch, to motion, to cold air.

Periodicity: pains come on regularly at a given time each day: or every night at 12 o'clock. Drenching night sweats.

Aconite .. RUDDOCK gives *Aconite* as a chief remedy for gall-stone colic. It has—

Hot, tense swelling under right short ribs.

Agony, must sit straight up; can hardly breathe; sweats with anxiety; abdomen swollen, particularly under short ribs.

Agonized tossing about. Fear of death.

Nux vom. .. Gall-stone colic with sudden severe pains right side; spasms of abdominal muscles with stitching pains in liver.

Jaundice, aversion to food, fainting turns; gall-stones. Constipation nearly always.

Liver swollen, indurated, sensitive, with pressure and stinging. Cannot bear tight clothing. (*Lyc.*, *Nat. sulph.*)

Oversensitive, irritable, touchy.

Ineffectual urging to stool, irregular peristalsis.

Chilly, if he uncovers or moves.

KENT says: " The proper medicine relaxes the circular fibres in the canal, and lets the stone pass. The remedy that ameliorates, or some of its cognates, will overcome the tendency to form stones. Healthy bile dissolves gall-stones in the sac: healthy urine does the same to a stone in pelvis or kidney."

Berberis .. " An excellent remedy for renal calculi; also for gall-stones associated with renal disease."

Pains shooting. The patient cannot make the slightest motion, sits bent over to painful side for relief.

Symptom peculiar to *Berb.* is a *bubbling* feeling, as if water were coming up through the skin.

Sticking pains under border of false ribs on right side, shoot from hepatic region down through abdomen." FARRINGTON.

" *Radiating pain* from a particular point puts *Berb.* almost alone for radiating pains. . .

Has cured renal colic many times, because of its well-known ability to shoot out in every direction. It cures gall-stone colic when these little twinges go in every direction from that locality. (*Dios.*)

The liver is full of suffering.

Sudden stabbing like a knife puncturing the liver. Dreadful suffering.

Berberis, when it is indicated, will let the little gall-stone loose, and it will pass through (*Bell.*), and the patient will take a long breath. . . . *Anything that is spasmodic can be relieved instantly*." KENT.

Dioscorea .. Hard, dull pain, gall bladder, at 7 p.m.

Neuralgia and spasmodic affections of liver and gall-ducts. Cutting, squeezing, twisting pain.

Colic begins at umbilicus and radiates to all parts of body, even extremities (see *Berb.*).

A constant pain, aggravated at regular intervals by paroxysms ot intense suffering. Unbearably sharp, cutting, twisting, griping or grinding pains; *dart about and radiate to* distant parts. (*Berb.*)

Worse doubling up (reverse of *Coloc.*, *Mag. phos.*).

Better stretching out, or bending back.

Better hard pressure.

Also, writhing, twitching and crampy pains with passage of renal calculi.

Magnesia phos. Sharp twinges, border of right lower ribs.

Severs griping colic pains, $>$ hot applications.

Spasms or cramp in stomach: clean tongue: as if a band were tightly drawn round body.

Cramping pains round navel and above it towards stomach, radiating to both sides towards back. Violent cutting pains; has to scream out: then shooting and violently contracting.

Better bending double and pressure of hand (*Coloc.*). *Better external warmth* (reverse of *Apis*).

Worse slightest movement.

Worse cold air: cold water: draughts: uncovering.

Sudden paroxysms of pain.

Better warmth: hot bathing: pressure: doubling up.

Podophyllum .. *Pod.* indicated in bilious colic.

Stools constipated and clay-coloured.

Tongue yellow or white, takes imprint of teeth.

Pain liver, inclined to rub part with hand.

(Curious), "sweat profuse, dropped off the prover's fingers."

Colic at daylight every morning.

Better bending forward: external warmth.

Lithium .. Gall-stones. Violent pain in hepatic region between ilium and ribs.

Violent pain across upper part of abdomen.

Soreness and pain in bladder ; sharp, sticking.

Red nose is characteristic.

Kali bich. .. Pain in a small spot in right hypochondrium : a sharp stitch on sudden movement after sitting.

Spasmodic attacks resembling those accompanying gall-stones.

Pains in small spots, can be covered with point of finger.

In evening is seized with violent aching pain, dragging her down, right hypochondrium, stretching round to shoulder : must undress, though not perceptibly swelled. Great oppression of breathing. Lasts several hours and subsides gradually, without passage of wind.

Carduus marianus Liver engorged. Gall-stones.

Tongue, white centre with red indented edges (reverse of *Iris*).

Crawling sensation, like the passage of a small body like a pea through a narrow canal on posterior side of liver extending to pit of stomach. (*Nat. sulph.*)

Iris .. .. Also set down for gall-stone colic.

Cutting pain, region of liver : < motion.

Tongue dry, coated on each side : red streak in centre (reverse of *Carduus*).

Great burning distress in epigastrium.

Baptisia .. Pain over gall bladder.

Pain in liver from right lateral ligament to gall bladder ; can scarcely walk, it so increases the pain in gall bladder.

Must stir about, yet motion is painful to gall bladder. May extend to spine.

Face dark red, purple : besotted.

Drowsiness. Prostration.

Rapid onset and rapid prostration.

Leptandra ..

Burnings, liver : near gall bladder.
Dull aching, liver, < near gall bladder.
Yellow coated tongue. Jaundice.
Better lying on stomach or side.

Chionanthus vir.

A great liver and gall-stone-colic medicine.
Better lying on abdomen.
Heat with aversion to uncover. (*Nux.*)
Very bitter eructations. Hot, bitter, sour, set teeth on edge. (*Lyc.*)
Hypertrophy of liver : obstruction : jaundice.
Soreness.
Nausea and retching with desire for stool.
Sensation of double action in stomach, while vomiting, one trying to force something up, the other sucked it back. (? *Nux.*)
Colic and cold sweat on forehead (*Verat.*).

Lycopodium ..

" Pain in liver ; recurrent bilious attacks with vomiting of bile.
Subject to gall-stone colic.
After *Lyc.* the attacks come on less frequently, the bilious secretion becomes normal and the gall-stones have a spongy appearance, as though being dissolved.
Lyc. patients are always belching : sour eructations like strong acid burning in pharynx." (*Chion.*)
Bloating : obliged to loosen clothes. (*Nat. sulph.*)
Worse cold drinks, often > warm drinks.
Worse afternoons : 4-8 p.m. aggravation.
Generally, craving for sweets.

Natrum sulph.

In black type for gall-stone colic.
Sore, heavy liver : stitches.
Sensation of lump below liver.
Crawling in gall bladder. (*Card. mar.*)
Cannot bear tight clothing about waist. (*Lyc.*)
Liver swollen : sore to touch : < lying left side. Colic, < rubbing.
When taking deep breath, sharp violent stitch in liver ; as if it would burst open. (Compare *Apis.*)
Worse damp weather : touch : pressure.
Many symptoms worse at 4 a.m.

Apis .. .. *Apis* is set down for gall-stone colic.

Severe burning pain under short ribs (but especially the left).

Great soreness and sensitiveness to touch.

Tension, as if something would break. (*Nat. sulph.*

The pains are stinging : exorting cries.

Apis is intolerant of heat.

Thirstless.

Cocculus .. Pressive pain hepatic region : worse bending and coughing.

Pain right hypochondriac region extends towards stomach : < bending, coughing, breathing, least touch.

Nausea from smell or thought of food.

Ipecacuanha .. Epigastric pain—colic—goes from left to right (reverse of *Calc.*). Holds him transfixed. Stabs like a knife. Cannot stir or breath. With nausea.

"Has cured cases of gall-stone colic : relief prompt and lasting."

Persistent, constant, anxious NAUSEA, *with clean tongue, not relieved by vomiting.*

Cold sweat forehead : no thirst.

Nausea with itching of skin.

Hydrastis .. Skin yellow : stools white and frequent : fullness and tenderness over hepatic region.

Catarrhal inflammation of mucous lining of gall bladder and biliary ducts.

Cutting from liver to right scapula (*Chel.*) : < lying on back or right side.

BURNETT : "I have found myself best in the painful attacks with *Hydrastis*. I have used as much as ten-drop doses of the strong tincture, given every half-hour in very warm water, and known it succeed in a few hours after everything had failed. After the attack of pain is over, it is best to set about curing the liver itself . . . gall-stones are a secondary affection, due to a previous condition of the liver, or the gall, or the gall bladder, or the lining of the ducts."

Bryonia .. *Bryonia* is also in the lists for gall-stone colic. KENT says: "It has inflammation of the liver, and many other liver symptoms.

Liver lies like a load with soreness and tenderness, and he cannot move.

Every motion, every touch, every deep breath causes pain. Breathing short, sharp, quick: burns and stitches. Stitching pains.

When he coughs it feels as if the liver or right hypochondrium would burst." (*Nat. sulph.*)

Thirsty for big, cold drinks. White tongue: constipation. *Irritable.*

Kali carb. .. Pains stitching, darting, worse during rest and lying on affected side (reverse of *Bry.*).

Cutting in abdomen, as if torn to pieces.

Violent cutting: must sit bent over, pressing with both hands (*Coloc.*) or lean far back (*Dios.*). Cannot sit upright.

Cannot bear to be touched.

Painful stitches right lumbar and region of liver. Stitches < on motion: must sit stooped forward, elbows on knees and head in palms of hands. Walks stooped forward with hands on knees.

Everything—noise, etc. felt in stomach.

Worse 2-4 a.m.

Easily startled with noise or touch.

Hepar .. .. LILIENTHAL gives *Hepar* as one of the remedies of gall-stone colic.

It has stitches in region of liver.

Hepatitis, stools white or green.

Is extremely sensitive mentally and physically

Cannot bear the slightest touch: or pain.

Cannot stand draughts: craves vinegar.

Chamomilla .. Another of the greatly sensitive remedies, mentally and physically. "*Cannot bear it!*"

Liver troubles and jaundice after anger or vexation. (One has seen this.) (*Cocc.*).

Cham. tosses in agony: bends double (*Coloc.*).

Stitches in liver region, and severe colic.

Veratrum alb. .. Is in KENT's Repertory for gall-stone colic.

It has, Hyperæmia of liver, gastric catarrh, putrid taste, disgust for warm food, great pressure on hepatic region with vomiting and diarrhœa.

In *Verat.* cases, there will be profuse sweating : *cold sweat on forehead* : hippocratic face.

Pains maddening, driving patient to delirium.

Typically ; cold skin ; cold face ; cold back ; cold hands, feet and legs, cold sweat.

Calcarea .. Cramp at navel.

Biliary colic. Calculi.

Darting pains, right to left (reverse of *Ipecac.*) with profuse sweat : has to bend double and clench hands, writhing in agony.

Tight clothes about hypochondria are unbearable.

Sweat, especially about head, feet and hands ; cold sweat, when rest of body is warm.

Sensation of damp, cold stockings.

Sensitive to cold : to wet weather.

Desire for eggs : boiled eggs.

Mercurius sol. Pressing pains ; stitching ; in liver. *Cannot lie on right side* (reverse of *Phos.*).

Jaundice : violent rush of blood to head ; bad taste : tongue moist and furred : soreness hepatic region ; from gall-stones.

Violent stitches in hepatic region, could not breathe or eructate.

Worse night : worse warm in bed : worse for the profuse sweat.

Foulness of mouth and sweat.

Merc. loves bread and butter.

Phosphorus .. Probably more important for the treatment of liver, leading to gall-stones, than for the actual attack ?

Great tenderness liver region.

Craving for ice-cold drinks, vomited when warm, vomiting followed by violent thirst.

Worse lying on left side (reverse of *Merc.*).

Anxious and restless in the dark.

Nitri spiritus dulcis	HERING says: "incarcerated gall-stones (with yolk of egg beaten up and applied inwardly and outwardly) . . . . Has the same action upon disturbed innervation as the so-called anti-spasmodics." HAHNEMANN said it should be given (in certain fevers) a few drops dissolved in an ounce of water, a teaspoonful every three hours. Desire for salt: or ailments from eating too much salt, and salt foods. < from cheese.
Ether	FARRINGTON: "In the passage of gall-stones, when remedies fail to relieve, I find that ether, externally and internally, is very good, acting better than chloroform."
Chloroformum	"Cholestric gall-stones and biliary colic." CLARKE says: "Choloform will dissolve gall-stones, and cases have been treated by injection of chloroform into gall bladder."
Hot Wet Flannels ..	Squeeze a flannel out in hot water, and apply. Have a hot bottle over this, to keep up the supply of moist relaxing heat.
Carlsbad Waters ..	Almost specific, RUDDOCK says, for gall-stone colic.

SOME REMEDIES OF THE PANCREAS

WITH INDICATIONS

Phosphorus .. *Phos.* is one of the few remedies known to act on the pancreas. Especially useful for fatty degeneration of that organ, liver, etc.

Oily stool : sometimes like frog's spawn, or like cooked sago. In diabetes and Bright's disease when preceded or accompanied by disease of the pancreas (FARRINGTON).

Phos. is also a hæmorrhage remedy : often small hæmorrhages of bright blood.

Characteristics are : thirst, for cold drinks, desire for ices. Suits tall, slender fine-haired persons; sensitive; with fears of dark, thunder, etc. One of the great remedies of diabetes.

Iodum .. Rather singular diarrhœa.

" Spleen enlarged and very sensitive. Liver affected, with white stools, sometimes whey-like : these you will find in obscure disease of pancreas. *Iodine* has such affinity for glands that it attacks pancreas also " (FARRINGTON).

Stools whitish, whey-like, fatty.

Pain, pit of stomach to navel and back.

Pancreas enlarged : abdominal pulsations.

Chronic disease of pancreas.

Iodum cannot stand warmth.

Eats often and eats much, and emaciates.

Profound debility and great emaciation.

Hypertrophy and induration of all glands, except mammae.

Spongia .. *Spongia* figures in black type for diseases of pancreas, especially for chronic pancreatitis. All glands affected ; gradually enlarge and become increasingly hard.

" Goitre heart."

A great goitre remedy.

Worse *cold, dry wind.*

Wakes, like *Lach.*, in great alarm, anxiety and difficult respiration (i.e. a great croup remedy).

Iris versicolor .. Acute affections of pancreas, inflammation or salivation.

Affects especially the digestive tract, liver, and pancreas.

Characterized by acrid, burning secretions.

" Oily nose, greasy tastes and fatty stool."

Or sweet taste.

Profuse, ropy saliva is characteristic.

Bilious, acrid watery stools burn like fire.

Curious symptom : tongue feels cold.

One of the diabetic remedies.

Conium .. Acute inflammation of pancreas. " Sudden vomiting of white substance, saliva, without any stomach contents."

Pain in liver, with enlargement.

Pressing, burning, squeezing pain from pit of stomach into back and shoulders.

Conium is one of our greatest vertigo remedies.

Affects glands, with stony hardness. A characteristic : sweats at once on falling asleep.

Parotidinum .. " Pancreatitis may start in infectious diseases —enteric, pyæmia, septicæmia, *also in mumps* : which is of interest from the structural resemblance of the pancreas to the salivary glands. . . .

" Mumps affects the pancreas, and diabetes has followed mumps, indicating that the Islets of Langerhans are affected."

Dr. X, impressed by his results with the nosodes of previous acute diseases in difficult chronic conditions, tells of two cases of diabetes which had not been progressing favourably in spite of careful prescribing.

" No. 1 suffered from neuritis and rheumatism of thighs, of several years' duration. After 3 6-hourly doses of *Parotidinum* 30, the rheumatism vanished and has not returned during the past 5 months. The blood sugar has not been tested owing to war conditions.

No. 2 had a severe aggravation, and then clinical improvement. These cases are merely suggestive."

Let us carry the matter further, on the same lines. If pancreatitis may start in infectious diseases, as enteric, pyæmia, septicæmia, and may entail diabetes, goitre, etc., we have also to consider

Typhinum, etc. TYPHINUM, PYROGEN (with which one remembers curing a case of diabetes), STAPHYLOCOCCIN, STREPTOCOCCIN, *or any other nosode responsible for or associated with previous acute illness.* In this way, triumph may lie. Very many of our hospital out-patients come for chronic conditions: and the difference in one's results, and in the improved healthy appearance of the patients since the frequent use of *Morbillinum, Diphtherinum, Streptococcin,* and all the rest, is amazing. It has to be seen to be believed.

Mercurius iod. rub. Heavy, painful sensation in liver, pancreas and spleen.

SOME SPLEEN MEDICINES

WITH INDICATIONS

Ceanothus americanus — "Where the spleen is affected from any cause, with enlargement, deep sticking pains, worse by motion, but unable to lie on left side, case will yield generally quickly to *Ceano.*"
"Pernicious anæmia, with spleen pains."
Quoted by Burnett, *Diseases of Spleen.*

China .. .. Enlarged spleen.
Aching, stitching pains in spleen when walking slowly. Pains extend in long axis of spleen.
Swelling and hardness of spleen: region of spleen hard and tender. (Intermittent.)
China is worse from slightest touch: better from hard pressure. Worse draught of air: worse every other day.
Has excessive flatulence and distension.
China has painless, very debilitating diarrhœa, with undigested food.
One remembers a striking case, when a student. A woman with an enormous spleen, etc., greatly benefited by a prescription of *Quinine* and *Arsenic*. One looked up the drugs and there was no question as to which was the curative agent, since quinine is well known as a spleen poison and a contributing cause of *ague-cake*.

Urtica urens .. With the tincture of *Urtica* Burnett cured brilliantly a case of ague-cake in a young officer invalided from Burma with malarial fever and enlarged spleen. He says: "The stinging nettle is a splenic of very high order." He gave it in ϕ, ten drops in water night and morning.

Ignatia .. Swelling and induration of spleen.
Painful pressure, spleen and pit of stomach.
Pain, left hypochrondrium: worse pressure.
Ign. is emotional: worse grief, worry.
Lies better on painful side.
"Remedy for contradictions": worse for what should relieve: better for what should aggravate. "The sighing remedy."

Diadem aranea	Swelling of spleen after checked intermittent with quinine. (Compare *Nat. mur.*) Worse wet weather. Worse damp walls. Enlarged spleen, in man subject to ague: constantly chilly, worse when it rained. Langour and lassitude. Worse every other day at same hour (*China*).
Natrum muriaticum	Stitches and pressure, region of spleen: spleen swollen. Much pain and soreness in left hypochondrium, going through to lower border of right scapula; worse lying left side. Liver and spleen swollen (Intermittent). Worse 10 or 11 a.m.: at seaside: heat of sun and stove: mental exertion: lying down. Better: air; cold bathing; "*going without regular meals*". (Allen's Keynotes.) A great remedy after much malaria and quinine. (Intermittents.) Irritable: gets into a passion about trifles: especially if consoled with.
Arnica	Pressing in region of left ribs below heart, day and night. Splenitis in intermittents (*Apis*, etc.). Stitches, splenic region: sore on pressure. Stitches under left false ribs, interrupting breathing when standing. Keynote of *Arn.* As if bruised or beaten. Bed too hard: moves for new position, which is no better; restless. Another Keynote says, "There is nothing the matter," when desperately ill.
Bryonia ..	Frequent stitches in liver, and spleen. Stitching pains in spleen during chill (intermittents). Hard swelling of spleen. Keynote of *Bry.* Worse from the slightest motion, or emotion; better, rest, mind and body. Usually better lying on painful side, to keep

Aconite .. Splenitis with inflammatory fever.
Acon. is restless : *great fear and anxiety.*
Face expresses fear : "disease will prove fatal."
"Anguish of mind and body : restlessness : disquiet not to be allayed."
Worse from dry, cold winds. Generally, sudden onset.

Citrus .. .. Affections of spleen ; painful enlargement.
Stiffness in joints, especially fingers ; as if bruised, feet.
Dyspnœa, gasping, in splenitis.

Apis .. .. Inflammation of spleen.
Considerable swelling of spleen.
Pain left abdomen, under short ribs.
Soreness and bruised feeling, most about last ribs left side.
Severe burning pain under short ribs, both sides, most severe on left ; deprives her of sleep.
Obliged to bend forward from contractive feeling in hypochondria : ? with ascites.
Apis is intolerant of heat : usually thirstless.
Worse : from sleep ; warm and heated rooms ; from getting wet ; but better washing or moistening part in cold water.
Better open air ; cold water and cold bathing.
Worse jealousy, fright, vexation.
Its pains burn and *sting*.

Asafœtida .. *Heat in spleen and abdomen.*
Asaf. is *oversensitive.* Has much flatulence and noisy, rancid or explosive belching.
Everything presses towards throat.
Better motion : open air. Worse night : sitting ; warm wraps.
Fits of violent, hard throbbing (*Ranunc. bulb.*).
One of the remedies of hysteria.

Helianthus .. Spleen enlarged and painful.
Burnett regards *Helian.* as a great spleen remedy. (Used in Russia as a remedy for malaria.)

Arsenicum .. Tensive, pressive pain in spleen. (Intermittent.)

Drawing, stitching pain under left hypochondrium.

Burning in stomach, followed by vomiting blood.

Stitches in spleen precede vomiting of blood; dark, partly coagulated. (Hæmatemesis.)

Induration and enlargement of spleen.

Liver and spleen swollen: dropsy. Soreness to touch spleen-region: worse during heat. (Intermittent.)

Spleen is expanded, tumefied.

Ars. is worse: after midnight: 2 a.m. and 2 p.m.; from cold; cold drinks and food; lying on affected side; better from heat; *burning pains relieved by heat.*

Great characteristics: great prostration: restless: anxious.

"The greater the suffering, the greater the anguish, restlessness and fear of death."

Anthracinum .. Enlargement of spleen: especially a spleen remedy.

"Epidemic spleen disease, the main seat of anthrax."

Pains of *Anthrac.* are "horrible, burning pains".

Sudden prostration with great abdominal soreness, worse epigastrium, with vomiting, and cold limbs.

Great restlessness: trembling: spasms.

Cyanosis: ecchymoses.

Headache is described "as if a smoke with a heating pain was passing through head."

A great remedy for septic conditions—very like *Arsenicum*, but more so!

Iodum .. .. Left hypochondrium hard and acutely painful to pressure: enlarged spleen after intermittent.

Characteristics: Profound debility with great emaciation: ravenous hunger, eats well: better when eating: yet *loses flesh all the time.*

Excessive nervousness.

Nitric acid .. Spleen large after yellow fever.
Liver enormously enlarged : liver-cake of ague.
Kent gives it as one of the notable spleen remedies.
Longs for fats, herring, chalk, lime, earth. But fat food causes acidity and nausea.
Aversion to meat ; bread. Worse milk.
Curious symptom : Urine strong-smelling, like horses' urine ; cold when it passes.
" Splinter-sensation " in suffering part.

Nux .. .. Pain region of spleen : very perceptible enlargement of spleen.
(But a great liver medicine, with bilious attacks : jaundice.)
Nux is worse, at 4 a.m. : from mental exertion ; over-eating ; touch ; noise ; anger ; alcohol ; dry, cold.
Better damp, wet weather.
Nux is particular, careful, irascible.
Oversensitive physically and mentally.
Quarrelsome : every harmless word offends.

Nux moschata .. Stitches in spleen : must bend double.
Enlarged spleen, loose bowels.
Colic after eating and drinking, with *dry mouth and thirstlessness*.
Diaphragmitis.
Drowsy : sleepy : inclined to faint. *Great indifference to everything*.
Worse cold : wet : wind : changes of weather. Cold food : driving in carriage.
Better : warm, dry weather, room. Wrapping up.

Secale .. .. Burning in spleen : thrombosis of abdominal vessels.
" Similar to *Ars*. But cold and heat are opposite."
Skin feels cold to touch, yet cannot tolerate coverings.
In all diseases, worse from heat.
Better cold air : getting cold ; uncovering.
Swelling of spleen after checked intermittent fever with quinine. Worse damp weather.

SOME SPECIAL REMEDIES OF APPENDIX AND CÆCUM

WITH INDICATIONS

" Acute Appendix " is one of the pitfalls of the unwary. While it may be slight and subside without treatment, or may be easily curable by the appropriate homœopathic remedy, before it has gone on to suppuration, yet danger may lie in what appears to be a favourable termination—the sudden cessation of pain. Where this occurs training and experience suggest the possibility of the onset of mortification, when doctor and patient are faced with a dangerous peritonitis. We feel bound to preface our remedial suggestions with this serious warning. Appendicitis is one of the danger spots for carelessness and ignorance.

Belladonna — Years ago, when making diagrams to show the action of remedies on parts of the body, one grasped the fact that two drugs seemed to share the honours in this area—*Belladonna* and *Mercurius corrosivus*. And one knows that *Bell.* has earned a great reputation for early, simple inflammation of appendix. Among its symptoms are :

Great pain in right ileo-cæcal region. Cannot bear the slightest touch, not even of bed covers. Tenderness aggravated by *least jar*. (Kent says, " The jar of the bed will often reveal to you the remedy.")

Bell. has much swelling. Its inflammations throb : feel bursting.

Kent also says, " There are instances where *Bell.* is the remedy of all remedies in appendicitis."

Mercurius .. Painful, hard, hot swelling, movable, near right ilium ; prevents extension of thigh.

Hard, hot, red swelling between umbilicus and inferior spine of ilium. Must lie on back, leg flexed. Fever, thirst, red dry tongue.

Constipation ; red urine. (Typhlitis.)

Merc. characteristics : Offensive breath, mouth, sweat. Worse heat of bed, but sensitive to draughts and damp cold. Thirst with salivation. Typically : large, dirty, tooth-notched tongue.

Mercurius corr. Kent has this drug down in black type for appendicitis.

Merc. corr. is violent and active.

Has far more activity, excitement and burning.

Cæcal region and transverse colon painful.

Bloated abdomen.

Characteristic : Great tenesmus of rectum, the " never-get-done " remedy.

Abdomen bruised, bloated, tender to least touch. Tenesmus of bladder, also. Hot urine passed drop by drop.

Opium .. .. Opium, morphia, aspirin and such pain-killers in old school dosage are absolutely contra-indicated in acute intestinal affections. They mask symptoms, whose urgent gravity is not recognized. They also prevent the possibility of discovering the homœopathic remedy.

But *Opium*, in homœopathic potency and dose is one of our most useful remedies here. Typically the face is red, bluish, bloated. " For continuous stertorous breathing, gives *Opium*."

Opium is painless, inactive, torpid : or, develops extreme nervous excitability, especially to noise, " hears flies walking on the wall ".

Paralytic conditions of bowels and bladder : inability to strain.

A curious determining symptom, if present : Says *he is not sick when desperately ill* (*Arn.*).

Pupils contracted : in fatal cases, they dilate.

Plumbum .. Large, hard swelling in ileo-cæcal region. Sensitive to touch and motion (*Bell.*, *Lach.*).

Plumb. has terrible colic : relief from bending double and hard pressure. Typically, *has retraction of abdomen* (*Plat.*).

Navel and anus are violently retracted, as if abdomen were drawn to back.

Sudden constipation.

Anæsthesia, or excessive hyperæsthesia.

Cold sweat, or absolute absence of sweat.

Lachesis .. Lies on back with knees drawn up: tenderness, pain, and swelling neighbourhood of cæcum.

Great sensitiveness to contact, especially of clothes (*Bell.*, *Hepar*, *Lyc.*). (Typically, also, of neck.) Worse after sleep; from warm bath (*Opium*). Hot flushes; hot sweat.

Purple puffiness of face is characteristic.

"Acute *Lachesis* has nausea and increased choking from warm drinks: chronic *Lach.* has nausea from a cold drink."

Lycopodium .. Is given as one of the remedies of inflammation of colon and cæcum.

Colicky pains right side abdomen, extending into bladder, with frequent urging to urinate.

Balloon-like distension of abdomen (rev. of *Plumb.*)

Abdomen sensitive to pressure and weight of clothes (*Lach.*).

Desire for sweet things and warm drinks.

Worse afternoon.

Bryonia .. Appendicitis: peritonitis.

Must keep very still; stools hard, dry, as if burnt.

Pain in a limited spot: dull, throbbing or *sticking*. *Bry.* is better lying on painful side, for pressure and to limit movement. Lies knees drawn up. Better for heat to inflamed part.

Phosphorus .. Weak empty feeling in abdomen with burning between the shoulder blades.

Loud rumblings in abdomen; distension, though much flatus is passed.

Tympanites, especially about cæcum and transverse colon.

Nausea and vomiting; better cold drinks till they get warm in stomach; then are vomited.

Regurgitation of food by mouthfuls.

Worse thunderstorms, dark, cold.

Hepar	Deep, circumscribed swelling in ileo-cæcal region; lies on back with right knee drawn up. Decreased peristalsis. Worse cold, dry air, wind; uncovering, touch. Better damp weather; warm wraps. Chilly; oversensitive, mind and body. Sweats easily; dare not uncover. Hasty, irritable, dissatisfied.
Crotalus horridus	Typhlitis and perityphilitis. Low type. Red-tipped tongue. Prostration: no stool; or discharges very offensive. Prostration of vital force. Sudden purpura hæmorrhagica. *Lach.* is cold and clammy. *Crot.* cold and dry. *Lach.* is bluish. *Crot.* yellowish (or bluish); jaundiced appearance, skin, whites of eyes. Deep-acting remedy of *sepsis*. Characteristic: swelled tongue.
Crotalus cascavella	Has a reputation here; but its mental symptoms are very strange and pronounced.
Apis	Abdomen bloated: feels inflated. Sensitiveness of ileo-cæcal region. Pains burning, *stinging*, sore. Extreme sensitiveness to touch. Worse: after sleep (*Lach.*); hot rooms; better open air, cold water and bathing.
Arsenicum ..	*Burning like fire, only relieved by heat*, calls for *Ars.*, with restlessness, anxiety, anguish. *Ars.* has coldness externally, with internal, burning heat. Tongue bluish, brown, blackish: dry.
Colchicum ..	Distension with gas: cannot stretch out legs. Cæcum and ascending colon much affected. Characteristic: *Smell painfully acute; nausea and faintness from odour of cooking food.* Loathing of food, still more of its smell. Abdomen immensely distended; feels it will burst.

Rhus .. .. Inflammation of cæcum and appendix.
Pains like a knife right abdomen ; walks bent from pain and contraction in abdomen.
Ailments from getting wet, especially after being over-heated.
Tongue dry, sore, red, cracked ; with great thirst.
Great restlessness, anxiety, apprehension.
Can't lie in bed ; must change position.
Fear at night. Fear of poison.
Cravings are for oysters, beer, sweets, cold milk. Or aversion to beer, spirits, meat.

Caladium .. Burning in abdomen (in typhlitis).
Abdomen swollen and tender to touch.
Dreads to move (*Bry.*).
Red, dry stripe centre of tongue, widens at tip.
Sensation of a long worm writhing in transverse colon or duodenum.
Characteristics : Sweet sweat attracts flies.

Iris .. .. Has been found useful (Clarke).
Characteristic : acrid, burning excretions.
Acrid vomiting : bilious, acrid watery stools burn like fire.

Cocculus .. Constant pain right iliac region near cæcum worse least touch ; pain remits, returns much aggravated : during pain, drawings through whole abdomen, causing her to work the limbs constantly : can find relief in no position.

Echinacea .. (In Repertory for Appendicitis.) Boericke says : " It acts on appendix and has been used for appendicitis. But remember, it promotes suppuration, and a neglected appendix with pus formation would probably rupture sooner under its use."

China .. .. *China* is also given as useful here.
Abdomen distended (Comp. *Lyc.*, *Colch.*, etc.), wants to belch ; eructations afford no relief.
Periodicity : colic at a certain hour each day.
Better hard pressure, and loose clothes.

SOME KIDNEY AND BLADDER REMEDIES

WITH INDICATIONS

Apis .. .. Pain in region of both kidneys.

Swelling of left kidney : acute Bright's disease.

Hyperæmic state of kidneys (organic disease of heart).

Albuminuria during desquamation of scarlet fever.

Vesical tenesmus with frequent discharge of red urine ; morbid irritability of urinary organs.

Agony in voiding urine.

Frequent, painful, scanty, bloody urination.

Retention of urine : bladder but slightly distended.

Cystitis, in hydrocephalus, typhoid, typhus, etc.

Scanty, high-coloured, often scalding, urine : or

Scanty, milky, albuminous, dark, with sediment like coffee grounds : contains uriniferous tubules and epithelium.

Urine has the odour of violets. (*Strophanthus.*)

Half the bulk of urine is albumen.

Urine scanty and fœtid : or frothy.

Apis is worse at night ; from cold, yet worse warm room.

Its pains are of a stinging character. Has swelling and puffing up of whole body.

Cantharis .. Paroxysmal cutting and burning pains in both kidneys, the region sensitive to slightest touch ; alternating with pain in tip of penis. Urging to urinate ; painful evacuation, by drops, of bloody urine ; at times, of pure blood.

Dull, heavy, distensive pain in region of kidneys, either side ; no relief in any position : rolling and twisting of body with groans and cries ; resulting in nausea, retching and vomiting. . . .

Painful urging to urinate but was not able to

Violent tenesmus vesicae and stranguary.

Cantharis (*continued*) .. Painful discharge of a few drops of bloody urine, causing very severe sharp pain, as if a red-hot iron were passed along urethra. . . .

Violent pains in bladder; frequent urging: intolerable tenesmus. Urging to urinate from smallest quantity of urine in bladder.

Violent cutting and burning pains in bladder, before, during and after micturition.

Paralysis, neck of bladder. Nephritis.

Cantharis is worse from coffee; from drinking cold water.

Terebinthina .. Nephritis. Violent burning and drawing pains in kidneys; hæmaturia.

Pain, renal region, extending down ureters: in right kidney, extending into hip.

Dropsy dependent on congestion of kidneys. Smoky urine.

Early stages of albuminuria when blood and albumen abound more than casts and epithelium.

Affections of kidneys, worse from living in damp places.

Violent burning and cutting in bladder alternate with similar pain in umbilicus.

Helonias dioica Burning, kidneys: can trace their outlines by burning.

Pain and congestion in kidneys, with albuminuria.

Burning, scalding when urinating; frequent desire and urging.

Involuntary discharge after bladder seemed to be emptied.

Diabetes. Dropsy.

Burning, stomach and spine.

Berberis .. Sticking, or tearing digging pain in either kidney, as if suppurating. Worse deep pressure.

Bubbling, left kidney region, extends across into bladder. Burning pain in bladder, sometimes when full, sometimes empty.

Drawing sticking in one or other side of bladder extending down into urethra; or arises in lumbar region and extends along ureters.

Berberis (*continued*) .. Painful cuttings left side bladder into urethra, comes from left kidney along course of ureter.

Violent sticking pain in bladder extends from kidneys.

Blood-red urine, speedily becomes turbid, deposits thick, mealy, bright red sediment, slowly becoming clear, but always retaining its blood.

Or pale yellow urine with gelatinous sediment which does not deposit.

Berb. affects kidneys, liver, bladder, back (lumbar region).

Bubbling sensations, kidneys (*Med.*).

Berb. is worse for movement ; JAR (*Bell.*).

Benzoic acid .. Nephritic colic, with very offensive urine.

Urinous odour exceedingly strong.

Brownish, very repulsive-smelling urine.

Cannabis sativa Ulcerative pain, kidney region.

Pain in neck of bladder and in both kidneys.

Frequent urging to pass urine, or retention.

Patient walks very slowly with legs stretched apart : cannot walk with legs close together : it hurts urethra.

Painful jerks, abdomen, as if something alive there. (*Crocus. Thuja.*)

Cannabis ind. .. Pain in kidneys when laughing. Sharp stitches in both kidneys.

Loses himself : forgets his last words and ideas : speaks as if tired.

Constantly theorizing.

Hallucinations and imaginations innumerable.

Time and space exaggerated.

Laughs immoderately. Horror of darkness.

Mercurius cor. One of the violent medicines. It has violent burnings.

Tenesmus vesecae with intense burning in urethra.

Discharge of blood and mucus with, or after, urine.

Micturition frequent, urine in drops with much pain.

Mercurius cor. (*continued*) Urine scanty, or increased; hot, burning, bloody.
Albuminuria.
Pinched and shrivelled face.
Vertigo with coldness: cold perspiration.
Ptyalism, with salty taste.

Arsenicum .. Difficult urination.
No desire, and no power, to urinate.
Suppression of urine. Retention of urine.
Or great desire, but passes no urine.
Scanty urine, passed with difficulty. Burning during discharge.
Urine like thick beer: rotten smell. Turbid, mixed with pus and blood.
Albuminuria. Fatty degeneration or atrophy of Bellinian tubes, tufts, and capsules of Muller.
Ars. is very restless, very anxious: jerks about till exhausted.
Worse: from cold, cold foods, fruit. Wants to be wrapped up warmly: better warmth in general: warm fire.
Worse during stool: when vomiting may occur.

Phosphorus .. Bright's Disease.
Fatty or amyloid degeneration of kidneys, especially if associated with similar condition of liver.
Nephritis. Dropsy accompanied by diarrhœa.
Bladder is full, but urine does not flow because of absence of urging.
Especially useful in a typical *Phos.* patient:—tall, slender, refined.
Desire for salt, fear of thunder, etc.

Thuja .. .. Kidneys inflamed.
Bladder feels paralysed, has no power to expel urine.
Sensation of moisture running forward in urethra. Orifice closed with slimy fluid, or serous liquid, or a lump of mucus.

Plumbum .. Granular degeneration or cirrhosis of kidneys: marked tendency to uræmic convulsions.

Morbus Brightii, contracted kidney. Hæmaturia. Diabetes.

Not able to pass urine, apparently from want of sensation to do so.

Urine scanty, high-coloured, passed in drops. Dribbles. Stranguary.

Typical pain; as though abdomen were drawn in, towards backbone: as though a string inside were drawing it in. (See *Tereb.*, *Verat.-v.*, *Zinc.*)

Lycopodium .. Aching in kidney, worse before and better after urinating.

Renal colic, especially right ureter to bladder. Red sand in urine.

Cystitis: turbid, milky urine, with offensive, purulent sediment.

Dull pressure, or bearing down over bladder.

Left kidney affected. Pain in back before urinating.

Frequent hæmaturia: large clots of blood in urine.

Retention: or, no urine secreted.

Urging: must wait long before urine will pass, with constant bearing down. Supports abdomen with hands.

Urine of strong, pungent odour. Causes eruption where it comes in contact with skin.

Nux vom. .. Nephritis from stagnation of portal circulation caused by suppression of habitual sanguineous discharge. Burning in loins and region of kidneys; after suppression of hæmorrhoidal flow, abuse of liquors, or when caused by a calculus.

Renal colic, especially in right kidney, extending to genitalia and right leg. Better lying on back.

Violent pains in small of back, as if bruised. Cannot move.

Pain culminated every little while in distressing retching and vomiting.

Nux vom. (*continued*)

Painful ineffectual urging to urinate: urine passes in drops with burning and tearing. Spasmodic stranguary.

Paralysis of bladder: urine dribbles. Paralytic incontinence of urine.

Involuntary micturition when laughing, coughing or sneezing.

Nux is irritable and sullen. Scolds.

Cannot turn over, must rise to do so.

Strong aversion to open air (rev. of *Puls.*).

Zincum .. Pressing, stinging, soreness in kidneys. Pressure, left kidney.

Retention of urine when beginning to urinate.

Sits with legs crossed, bending forward, and cannot pass water, or but very little. Feels bladder will burst.

Zincum can't keep still: keeps feet in continual motion.

Asked why she swung her feet incessently, the child said it was to prevent urine escaping.

Pulsatilla .. Pains in kidneys; also on urinating.

Tenesmus of bladder: stinging, neck of bladder.

Urine scanty, bloody, with mucus; reddish. Involuntary.

Incontinence in bed. Before making water, a sensation as if it would gush away. Can scarcely wait.

Bladder region very sensitive to pressure.

Remedy of changes. Pains change character, position: are very severe, then suddenly mild. *Puls.* is easily excited to tears.

Sulphur .. Violent pain in kidney regions, after long stooping.

Hard pressure in bladder.

Itching and burning in urethra.

Sudden, imperative desire to urinate: if not gratified, urine escapes.

Sulph. is worse on waking: after eating: from milk; from bodily exertion; from water and washing; on getting warm in bed.

Very painful passage of stool and urine.

CONCERNING THE REMEDIES

The remedies are put up as medicated granules, their most convenient form of carrying, and for keeping in condition.

A DOSE consists of half a dozen granules—less or more

It may be given dry on the tongue, to be dissolved before swallowing.

Or, when quick effect is wanted in acute conditions, dissolve half a dozen granules in half a tumbler of water, stir, administer in doses of a desertspoonful six hours apart, or in very urgent conditions, every hour, or half hour for a few doses, till reaction sets in, then stop, so long as improvement is maintained

CAMPHOR ANTIDOTES MOST OF THE MEDICINES So the camphor bottle must be kept away from the medicine chest.

POTENCIES.—The best potencies for initial experiments in Homoeopathy are the 12th and the 30th.